EDUCATING BLACK DOCTORS

EDUCATING BLACK DOCTORS

A *History of*

Meharry Medical College

JAMES SUMMERVILLE

FOREWORD BY LLOYD C. ELAM, M.D.

The University of Alabama Press

Library of Congress Cataloging in Publication Data

Summerville, James, 1947–
  Educating Black doctors.

  Bibliography: p.
  Includes index.
  1. Meharry Medical College—History. I. Title.
R747.M49S95   1983   610'.7'1176855   82-15883
ISBN 0-8173-0143-7

*This book is for
Sherman Paul.*

Contents

Foreword

For one hundred years, Meharry meant opportunity to thousands of black Americans and some others, but the history of the institution is told, not by the changes in the futures of those fortunate men and women who became graduates, but by the action of a few in each generation with the vision to attack the vestiges of slavery, poverty, and excess morbidity through the building and operation of a medical college. The college was conceived just after the Civil War when many thought the problem of the ex-slaves would soon disappear because their death rate was so great and the absence of health care was not a focus. The institution would be national, but its setting was a bankrupt city that had the fourth worst health statistics in the world. It was started by a missionary who had no money or medical experience at a time when there were more who objected to this work than applauded it. However, the desire of those students who begged that a medical school be started and the future of the many people who would be touched by its services were enough to motivate the founders to embark on this venture.

A number of documents have existed chronicling the events of the institution, but when requested by an academic society to provide one book that gave the most accurate history of the institution, I knew that no recent such book had been written. This book satisfies the need for such facts to be available. It also provides a journalistic, well-documented account of the varying approaches to providing opportunity and improving health for black Americans.

In the hundred years covered, medicine went from a craft to a specialty profession based on biological sciences and to an industry using and providing the greatest achievements of mankind. In that 100-year period blacks in America were trying to make up for years of education lost, to catch up in a rapidly moving industrial society, and to adjust to an ambiguous status assigned them.

The book is written at a time when all the ingredients are still present—higher prevalence of illness among blacks, greater shortages of black professionals, education and socioeconomic hindrances to the study of medicine and dentistry, and little money or desire by outside benefactors to provide the resources to solve the problems.

Many of the resources were original documents of oral interviews. Two deserve mention: the unpublished manuscript of Dr. Harold West that included much of the master's thesis material of Grace Harrison Ferguson, and *Meharry Medical College, A History* by Dr. Charles Victor Roman, written almost fifty years earlier. The history of Meharry by Dr. Roman (1934), now out of print, is a fascinating stylistic account of the first fifty years of the institution by one of Meharry's most poetic faculty members. After Dr. West retired from the presidency he began the work for this book, which was to be completed by the centennial year. His sickness and untimely death prevented his completion of the work, and Dr. Leslie A. Falk, Chairman of Occupational Health, picked up the project. The interest of James Summerville was independent, but fortunately he not only made use of the earlier documents but also cooperated with Dr. Falk, which added an insider's flavor to his work.

Mr. Summerville's painstaking and insightful account makes the point in the title that the history of Meharry is a history of the education of the black doctor during the century covered, and it is a point well made since this one institution educated over half of the practicing black doctors during much of the period. In some ways this is the end of a period—a period when most blacks were educated in predominantly black institutions and non-blacks could largely ignore the question of the education of minorities. Although it is the end of a century of isolation, it is not an end to the contribution of Meharry and other institutions of which it is an example. The faculty and friends of Meharry will applaud the account of the input that was necessary to make the education of black doctors possible. What is not covered is the contribution of the alumni, which would be the subject for another volume. The achievements of Meharry, in the face of overwhelming odds, speak to a future that will require the continued work of this institution, and others like it, which provide opportunity for those with restricted opportunity and seek solutions to the health problems that preferentially affect black people.

Meharry Medical College

Lloyd C. Elam, M.D.
Chancellor

Preface

One hundred years of any medical school is a significant story. This story of one is unique: Meharry Medical College, since its founding in 1876, has graduated approximately half the black doctors in the United States. Having achieved international recognition as a leader in medical education for service to the community, especially to poor and minority people, Meharry has a history that must be told.

Meharry is one of two comprehensive, predominantly black colleges of medicine, dentistry, and health sciences in the United States. (The other is Howard University School of Medicine.) Meharry began as the medical department of Central Tennessee College. It survived the demise of that institution and its successor, Walden University, and continues today, albeit with serious problems.

From its founding until now, the goals of Meharry Medical College have included liberating people through education and preparing them for service to others. Its early students were former slaves or descendents of slaves. After their graduation they practiced in the disease-ridden cities and impoverished countryside of the post–Civil War South. Some of these alumni pushed forward the frontiers of prevention, diagnosis, and therapeutics.

As the decades passed, students and faculty members of all races and many nations came to learn and teach at Meharry. Its communities widened to include all of America, the Caribbean, Africa, the world. Administered primarily by black physicians, dentists, and research scientists, Meharry has had a racially integrated student body since 1957.

Meharry drew its first sustenance from the Methodist Church and the benevolent societies of the time. Conceived and created by a minister, the Reverend John Braden, and two physicians, George Whipple Hubbard and William Joseph Sneed, the college became an endeavor of scientists steeped in both compassion and corporeal reality. In 1915 it was chartered as a

secular institution, but it has maintained ties of friendship and cooperation with churches and other community organizations.

The beginning of Meharry's second century was an impetus for the
writing of this book. No survey of the institution's history existed, although there had been several notable contributions. A commemorative
centennial volume was originally to have been the work of Meharry's fifth
president, Harold Dadford West, Ph.D., the first black chief executive of
any medical school in the United States. Following his retirement in 1966,
he was commissioned by the college to write such a book, but illness and
then death stilled his hand. He left some 120 typed pages of manuscript,
which dealt with the years from 1876 to 1944. Dr. West's work drew
heavily on a thesis by Mrs. Grace Harrison Ferguson, "Hubbard Hospital
and Meharry Medical College for Negroes," written in 1945 for a University of Chicago master's degree in social work. Her offering followed in
time a memoir by Dr. Charles Victor Roman, *Meharry Medical College, A
History,* published at Nashville in 1934. *Educating Black Doctors* uses each of
these sources, fully crediting the extent of such use in the footnotes, but it
is entirely the product of original research on Meharry's first century.

No part of this manuscript has been submitted to Meharry officials for
editing, review, or approval, nor is it endorsed by the college or any of its
trustees, officers, faculty members, or alumni. An independent inquiry, it
emphasizes Meharry's social and educational significance. Scholars interested in technological and scientific contributions made by the faculty and
alumni have further fertile ground to till.

Dr. Leslie Falk suggested the leading theme and certain sources through
which to pursue it, supplied a number of research items, and offered a draft
of this preface as well as comments on earlier versions of the manuscript.
Other faculty members, alumni, and community friends of Meharry gave
interviews, and these indispensable contributions are recognized in the
works cited.

Further acknowledgment is made to the Kresge Learning Resources
Center and Library at Meharry, particularly the archives. The latter is the
repository for many of the college records used in the writing and is hereby
credited for all of the photographs that appear in the book. Cheryl Ham-
berg, Connie McKissack, and Joe Pass of the Kresge Center deserve mention for their special help.

Some of the sources used in writing the first three chapters were
gathered by Mr. Samuel Cameron and Ms. Gloria Leath, formerly research
assistants in the Department of Family and Community Health at Meharry. Mrs. Patricia Augustine of the United Methodist Publishing House
supplied important materials relating to Meharry and the Methodist
Church. At The University of Alabama Press, Malcolm M. MacDonald and
the staff, together with the Press's peer reviewers, provided the cogent

criticism, editorial judgment, and marketing skill that helped transform a manuscript into this book.

A civil servant and teacher of sociology, whose special interest was human resources, James Mapheus Smith (1901–68) lived a life committed to racial tolerance and social justice. The estate of Professor Smith, a Tennessean, provided a grant to The University of Alabama Press in support of publication. Proceeds from the sale of *Educating Black Doctors* repay the principal that honors his memory.

EDUCATING BLACK DOCTORS

1

An Oft-Told Tale

LATE ONE DAY in 1826, sixteen-year-old Samuel Meharry was hauling a load of salt along a wilderness road in Kentucky toward the ferry that would carry him to his home on the other side of the Ohio River. It was a lonely passage, leading through a swamp and lying some distance from the nearest town. As the way darkened, young Meharry's wagon slipped over the edge of the road and became mired. Night was falling, and Samuel looked desperately around him for some source of help. Deep in the woods, there was a dim light. Making his way toward it, he came upon a rude slave cabin. When he explained his plight, the black family gave him supper, a place to sleep, and breakfast. The next morning the man of the house helped him raise the wagon out of the mud, and Samuel was able to go on his way. The kindness of the black family touched Samuel Meharry deeply, and he resolved to repay it. "I have no money," he told the man upon parting, "but when I can, I shall do something for your race."[1]

No one knows the name of this black family whose charity would result in the founding of a medical college. Perhaps it even receded in the mind of Samuel Meharry as he grew to manhood and prosperity through the years of sectional conflict and Civil War that followed the encounter in the swamp. But he did not forget his promise. More than two score years later, as the war was ending and black people were beginning the long struggle up from slavery, the opportunity came for him to redeem it.

The first Christmas of the peace was a joyful time for many of Nashville's people who had fought in the Union or Confederate armies. Blazing coal fires kept the icy winds without the eaves and gables; the tinkle of bells brought the season's delicacies from kitchen or cellar; the company of spouse and children mellowed the bitter memories of war.

Outside such comfortable parlors, however, the capital of Tennessee was teeming with human misery. As slaves, black men and women had been tied to their masters, forbidden to go anywhere. When they learned the previous spring that they were free, their response in the main had been to leave their homeplaces for somewhere else. Throughout the summer and fall of 1865, thousands of them wandered aimlessly about the South. Some crowded around military posts where they were given rations. Many congregated in the cities, where large numbers of Federal soldiers were stationed, in the hope that military power could protect their newly acquired rights.[2] Nashville, having been in Federal hands since February 1862, had been a haven for freed men and women throughout the war.[3]

Most who settled there found no means to earn a living. The few who did worked for meager wages. Some believed the rumors that the lands of their former masters would be distributed among them and therefore saw no reason to take work in the city. Others, having never been taught better, thought that freedom meant unrestraint and indiscipline, regardless of contracts or the criminal laws, and that it released them from any and all forms of labor. As the winter of 1865–66 drew on, Nashville's muddy streets were crowded with these impoverished former slaves, begging pennies from any well-dressed passersby. At night robbers worked the same thoroughfares, but with blade or club rather than hat in hand.

To accommodate the hundreds who had no means, several small cities, bearing the local names of "By-Town," "Hell's Half-Acre," and "Black Center," sprang up within the larger one.[4] Wending along the Cumberland River and also circling the inner city, they consisted of sheds and hovels built of refuse lumber. Rough, unpainted, without dooryards, outbuildings, or sometimes even a roof, a single dwelling might be home to a dozen people. The Negro newcomers could also be found living under railroad bridges and in trenches remaining from the Battle of Nashville. "The amount of want, present and prospective, in this city is beyond the telling of tongue or pen," declared the *Republican Banner* two weeks before Christmas.[5] Its editorial columns daily carried stories of assaults, of people freezing to death, of starvation in the open streets, of widespread illness.

Throughout the war, the government at Washington and private benevolent organizations had been trying to assist the destitute former slaves in the areas of the South embraced by the operations of the Union armies. Nearly 400 secular benevolent societies and auxiliaries sent volunteers among the freed people of the South during and after the Civil War. The most active in Tennessee were the American Freedmen's Union Commission, the Western Freedmen's Union Commission, and the Western Sanitary Commission. The interdenominational American Missionary Association, which founded Fisk University, and the Freedmen's Aid Society of the Methodist Episcopal Church, which founded many black colleges, were the leading church-sponsored relief agencies.[6]

To coordinate this work, Congress, in March 1865, created the Bureau of Refugees, Freedmen, and Abandoned Lands. The Freedmen's Bureau, as it came to be known, was placed in the War Department and given authority over all subjects relating to refugees and freedmen in the former rebel states. The secretary of war was directed to issue provisions, clothing, fuel, and shelter to the destitute, both black and white, on a temporary basis. The bureau was also given the power to set apart tracts of abandoned lands for the use of the freedmen and "loyal refugees."[7]

On May 12, 1865, President Andrew Johnson organized the bureau. Major General Oliver Otis Howard was appointed its head, with the title of commissioner. Brigadier General Clinton B. Fisk was named assistant commissioner for the district comprising Kentucky and Tennessee, with Nashville as his headquarters. Entering upon the formidable job at once, General Fisk sought to place the former slaves in a position to help themselves. "Do not expect us to do all, nor half, but put your shoulders to the wheel and do for yourself," he told a group of freedmen soon after his arrival in Nashville.[8]

Through persistent canvassing, he persuaded many black people who had crowded into Nashville to return to the country and resume farming. By autumn he had disbanded some of the refugee camps and homes in the city and had drastically reduced the government's outlay for the aged, infirmed, orphaned, and sick.[9] At the same time, physicians and surgeons of the bureau's medical department supplied treatment, including hospitalization, to the poor. They also inaugurated stringent sanitary measures to combat the smallpox and cholera prevalent in the city, representing perhaps the first public health program ever undertaken there.[10]

In General Howard's view, the most urgent want of the freed people was education.[11] From the beginning, the bureau made the strongest commitment to providing instruction to them and their children. At first this schooling was at the reading and writing level. But as students advanced in knowledge and as their intellectual hunger grew keener, the schools began to offer advanced courses. The bureau's educational work was carried on in close cooperation with benevolent societies from the North. Teachers recruited by these associations had moved South throughout the war, a few steps behind the Union soldiers. They intended to provide for the general welfare of the freedmen and in particular for their spiritual and educational needs.

In 1863 the United Presbyterian Mission had founded the first school for the Negro children of Nashville. By the time the Freedmen's Bureau entered the city, six such schools were in operation there, meeting in barracks, barns, basements, and in the open air.[12] They supplied instruction of the most basic sort in reading, writing, arithmetic, and geography. Sometimes, classical studies like Greek, Latin, and philosophy ("dialectic") were given.[13] Nearly always, classes were conducted with a strongly Christian emphasis, since the school's parent associations were strongly evangelical and many teachers had been selected as much for their religious zeal as for their intellectual abilities. Serious conflicts among the schools, turning on disputed points of dogma or polity, were not uncommon. Upon its arrival in Nashville, the Freedmen's Bureau set about cooling this heated sectarian atmosphere and coordinating the work of the benevolent society schools. Using funds derived from the rental of abandoned property, it fitted up former military buildings as classrooms, supplied desks, books, and rations, and contributed to salaries for teachers.

The freed people responded enthusiastically to the educational opportunities. Their desire for learning, however stimulated by the bureau and missionary societies, had deeper roots. In bondage, Negroes had exhibited an avid interest in the master's books and in the Bible, which they were taught to revere, but laws had forbidden the instruction of slaves. Nonetheless, some had been taught to read and write, especially those who lived among the Scotch-Irish people of Tennessee and Kentucky. For others the first meaning attached to the word "freedom" was the chance it offered to become literate.[14]

During 1866 and 1867 children began to attend the schools in larger numbers than before, while adult leaders among the black people began to assume roles in the financing and operation of the schools. The bureau, desirous of fostering self-sufficiency among the freedmen, and eager to turn over the schools under its administration to civil authority, encouraged this trend. Opposition to the presence of Northern teachers was growing among Southerners, and it was hoped that schools conducted by the freedmen themselves would be left alone. Missionary teachers had already been driven from many rural areas, where the reaction was especially virulent. Even though this increased the number of teachers in the cities, there was still a shortage of them. In Nashville the freedmen's schools labored under teacher-pupil ratios of 1 to 40 up to 1 to 400.[15]

The growing hostility toward outsiders, the lack of teachers, and the policy of retrenchment imposed by Congress on the Freedmen's Bureau led General Howard to conclude that if Negro education was to survive in the South, it must depend upon the Negroes themselves. Accordingly, he directed bureau funds in significant amounts to help establish normal schools and schools of higher learning to prepare black teachers and other black leaders.[16]

The first of these in Tennessee was Fisk University, founded in Nashville on January 1, 1866, by the American Missionary Association with assistance from the Freedmen's Bureau and others.[17] Housed in a one-story barracks that had been an army hospital during the war, Fisk promptly began to furnish Tennessee and other states with a steady supply of teachers.

In July a second college began offering advanced studies to Negroes in Nashville. Incorporated by the Tennessee legislature under the name of

Central Tennessee Methodist Episcopal College, it was the latest benevolent work of that denomination, which had begun missionary activities among the slaves of Tennessee as early as 1829.[18]

Central Tennessee College's immediate forebear was Clark Chapel, a freedmen school organized in Nashville in 1865 by the Missionary Society of the Methodist Episcopal Church and the Reverends John Seys and O. O. Knight. Opening at first in Andrew Church on Franklin Street in south Nashville, Clark Chapel soon felt the pressure of expanding enrollment and moved to a former Confederate gun factory. This building, located nearby on College Street, was donated by the Freedmen's Bureau.[19] Several decades later, the Reverend John M. Walden, Methodist bishop of Cincinnati at the end of the war, recalled how Clark Chapel acquired its home:

> In 1866, as corresponding secretary of the Freedmen's Aid Society of the Methodist Episcopal Church, I called at General Fisk's headquarters in Nashville to consult about housing our opening school work in that city; and he turned over to us a large building known as the "Gun Factory." Early in the war the Confederate authorities had seized it for the purpose of establishing a manufactory of arms, but they were not given time to consummate the purpose. That this building should be first used as a school house for the freedmen instead of a Confederate gun factory, as had been proposed, is still an interesting fact. . . . Here was the early and rude seat of the school which . . . has grown into Central Tennessee College. The use of the Gun Factory, through General Fisk's agency, not only gave an impulse to the school, but determined its location in the southern section of the city, which has been a great advantage.[20]

Like most of the other missionary schools for freed people, Clark Chapel attempted to encompass the entire educational gamut, offering the most basic studies through advanced subjects. It was on this latter basis—and in particular "for the general and theological education of colored people"—that the Methodists obtained the charter for their college from the Tennessee legislature.[21]

The Methodist Episcopal Church had begun to aid the emancipated black people more than two years before Appomattox, through workers, missionaries, and schools. For a time it united its humanitarian efforts with those of other denominations in the Freedmen's Union Commission. But even before the war ended, this coalition began to split over the question of whether educational and religious needs of black people should be served by the same organization.[22] Determined that religious beliefs and values should be taught to black children in conjunction with school subjects, a convention of leading Methodist clergymen and laymen met at Cincinnati in August 1866 and organized the Freedmen's Aid Society with the object of elevating the former slaves intellectually and morally.[23]

These two purposes were inseparable, the convention declared. Exhorting those going forth to take up the cause of the impoverished Negro, Bishop Davis W. Clark wrote: "The emancipation of four millions of slaves has opened at our very door a wide field of calling alike for mission and educational work. It has devolved upon the church a fearful responsibility. Religion and education alone can make freedom a blessing to them. The school must be planted by the side of the Church; the teacher must go along with the missionary. . . ."[24]

Bishop Clark's clarion call was heard in Nashville at the first Tennessee annual conference of the Methodist Episcopal Church, held in the fall of 1866. Leaders of the meeting organized a freedmen's aid society to foster locally the work of the parent group.[25] Several ministers were transferred from Ohio conferences to assist in this endeavor. Two of them, the Reverends G. H. Hartupee and John Braden, became important figures in the early days of Central Tennessee College. Reverend Hartupee served as principal (or president) of the embryonic school the first year, 1866–67, being relieved by Reverend Braden for the following year. In 1868–69 Hartupee again took the helm, until Braden was installed, in 1869, as the first permanent president of the college.

John Braden was born in New York City in 1826 and, after an early life unsettled as to vocation, graduated from Ohio Wesleyan University in 1853. Soon thereafter he was licensed to preach by the Cincinnati conference of the Methodist Church. In his early appointments he taught in church-related schools and served as minister to several congregations. At the request of Bishop Clark, he went to Nashville in 1867, where he would devote the rest of his life to Central Tennessee College.[26]

Braden, Hartupee, and the first trustees of Central Tennessee College received a total of $21,500 from the Methodists' Freedmen's Aid Society and the Freedmen's Bureau to purchase a site and to erect buildings for the new institution. With this money they bought a lot in south Nashville near the University of Nashville medical department. A distinguished faculty of physicians, surgeons, and scientists had earned for the university an international reputation in medicine. Black students were not admitted, however, and the residents in the neighborhood vehemently opposed the erection of a college for Negroes there. They succeeded in procuring a decree from Chancery Court annulling the sale.[27]

Eventually, Central Tennessee College was able to buy frontage on Maple Street (later renamed First Avenue, South) in the southeastern part of Nashville not far from Clark Chapel and the Gun Factory. Standing on this lot was a two-story building of fifteen rooms. The school year of 1868 opened in these quarters, and during the winter, construction proceeded on two new buildings.[28] One contained a large chapel with dormitories above it, and the other held classrooms and more living quarters. Al-

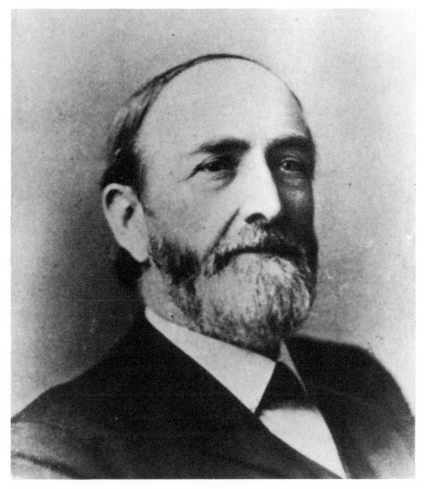

John Braden

together these facilities could accommodate 200 students. Central Tennessee College's first catalog, published in 1869, showed an enrollment of 192. All of these students had mastered the Second Reader, and many had entered upon higher courses of study.

At first, Central Tennessee College held its primary purpose to be the preparation of teachers and preachers. As the pupils advanced in their studies and thus were prepared to teach, the Normal Department was

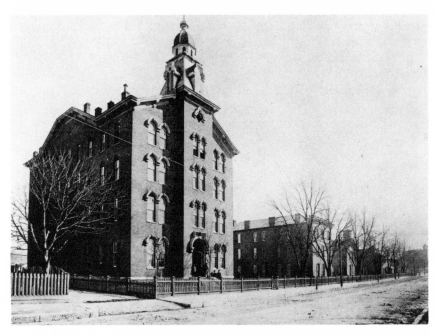

Central Tennessee College in 1894

organized. Then followed the Theological, Preparatory, and Collegiate courses of study.[29]

The opening of advanced classes at Central Tennessee College was delayed because many students left to teach or preach as soon as they were at all competent to do so. As late as 1872 John Braden told the Board of Trustees: "The demand is so great for teachers that it hardly seems just or right to keep young men and women plodding through Greek and Latin while thousands are perishing for lack of a little learning."[30] All did not feel that their life's work was preaching or teaching, however. "The halls are crowded with students preparing to teach school, *practice law or medicine,* or teach the glorious Gospel," declared the annual report of the Freedmen's Aid Society in 1869. (Emphasis added)[31]

During the 1870s the institution's leaders made an effort to fashion Central Tennessee College into a university by setting admissions standards, offering algebra, geometry, and natural sciences, and requiring rigorous examinations.[32] Young black people who had been born slaves were thus showing themselves fully competent to study medicine. The gnarled finger of death pointed toward the need for them, as epidemic and endemic illnesses ravaged the freed people of the South. The plight of this black population, the devotion of two white former soldiers—one Union, one Confederate—and the generosity of Samuel Meharry and his family provided the impetus and the means.

2

"A Most Dangerous Inheritance"

T HUS DID DR. JOSEPH JONES, appointed Nashville's first health officer in 1867, describe the houses and shanties huddled together in the environs of the city after the war.[1] Mrs. Thomas Henry Huxley, who accompanied her husband, the English physician-biologist on his triumphal visit to Tennessee's capital in 1876, would long remember the miasmas of the city. "I am not surprised at anyone getting any illness in Nashville . . . ," she recalled more than a decade later. "It always struck me as about the most unhealthy place we ever were in."[2] Nashville had the highest death rate of any city in the United States in that centennial year and, of those reporting, the fifth highest in the world.[3] Five times in the previous fifty years, cholera had ravaged the city (numbering former President Polk among its victims in 1849), and sometimes diphtheria vied with it in severity.

In the years immediately after the Civil War, the medical officers of the Freedmen's Bureau had treated a million former slaves and refugees throughout the South,[4] and in Nashville they undertook sanitary measures to combat epidemics.[5] But, as in education, the bureau sought to turn over responsibility in these matters to civil authority. Faced with the closing of the bureau hospital and with the danger of new outbreaks of cholera and smallpox, Nashville's mayor and aldermen were forced to take a few steps in the direction of a public health program. With aid from the Freedmen's Bureau, the city government opened a small charity hospital,[6] and the city council in July 1866 created a Board of Health. But before Dr. Joseph Jones could be installed the following spring, the cholera claimed 800 lives.

Even then, had a program of sanitary reform been allowed to proceed under Jones's direction, more tragedy might have been averted. But the government of Nashville, under the carpetbagger mayor, Augustus E. Alden, was sliding into bankruptcy. The board collapsed, and when the city went into receivership in 1869, a program of vaccination for smallpox was stopped in order to save money. Not until 1874, in the wake of another wave of cholera that drove 10,000 people from the city, was another Board of Health created.[7] Unfortunately, it was exceedingly cautious in urging expensive sanitary measures. Its members spent their time collecting mortality statistics and reminding the public that cleanliness was important.[8]

These pious proclamations went largely unheeded, and, in 1876, Nashville remained extremely dirty, with poorly drained streets, open sewers, and foul garbage heaps. Privies and kitchen pipes at the State Penitentiary, located a mile west of the public square, seeped into open streams flowing through the town. Several slaughterhouses discharged their offal in the same manner. Garbage and human wastes were commonly pitched from windows to the already saturated ground. Wells, even in the best parts of the city, were often contaminated, and the purity of the water in the reservoir was questioned when it was noted that four cemeteries, a public dump, a tannery, and innumerable privies drained into the Cumberland River a short distance above the intake pipes. The number and variety of ill odors arising from alleys, backyards, and outhouses to pervade the air of Nashville reminded one visitor of Cologne as depicted in Coleridge's poem by that name.[9]

Most of Nashville's black people still lived where they had come to rest in the turbulent summer and fall of 1865: in the innermost city, in old stables situated upon alleys, in the midst of privy vaults, in wooden shanties remaining from the war, or in huts on the outskirts of town.[10] In the summer of 1876, the *Daily American,* Nashville's principal newspaper, recorded the almost incredible density of the black population occupying these blighted quarters and took note of the consequences: "From three to ten live crowded up together until diseases seize them and they die."[11]

The causal connection between living conditions and disease was just beginning to be recognized in the highest scientific, intellectual, and religious circles. Most black people were uneducated in even the simplest laws of personal and community hygiene, and, like white Nashvillians, did not ordinarily perceive any relation between their exposure to filth and the onset of sickness. When illness did befall them, most could not afford the services of those few courageous white physicians who accepted black patients. And by 1876 there was no more public money for even the gravest hardship cases. Strapped under its terrifying debt and beset by the national depression, Nashville closed its hospital.

Even when medicine or clinical care was available, black people often ignored or actively resisted them. Negro folklore was rife with signs of coming death, and many believed that "a man never dies before his time." Widespread faith in voodoo and sorcery, flourishing in the city as it had on the plantation, reinforced these fatalistic attitudes. It also allowed "trick doctors" and "witch doctors"—who made their fellow men believe they could produce and heal sickness—to ply their trade in the streets.[12] "Voodoo doctors, conjurers, and quacks here find a most inviting field," wrote

Dr. George Hubbard. "This superstition is apparently of African origin, modified and changed, with large additions derived from the white man and the Indian. In some of its phases it closely resembles the old New England witchcraft, with other names which signify the same thing. When a person is said to be 'tricked' it means the same thing as good old Dr. Mather would have called bewitched. . . ."[13]

There were various other types of black healers—bleeders, midwives, herb doctors—and they may have met a small part of the medical needs of the impoverished freed people. Nonetheless, many black Nashvillians, even in times of severest illness and epidemics, received no bona fide medical attention whatsoever,[14] in part because there were so few black physicians. Only two black practitioners are known to have worked in Nashville before 1877. Dr. A. T. Wood's advertisements, in the year after the Civil War, urged blacks to "patronize [their] own physician" and identified Wood as "a graduate of Cambridge University, late missionary to Africa, and a member of the Indiana Conference." Wood's name does not appear in Venn's *Alumni Cantebrigienses* or on supplementary lists in the University archives. A tantalizingly brief note in a local newspaper is the only known record of Dr. Aaron Jennings, "body servant and assistant surgeon" to another Dr. Jennings, presumably his master, in antebellum Nashville.[15]

Forced by poverty to live in the filthiest places in an unclean city, uneducated in health matters, and without doctors to treat them, blacks died in numbers far in excess of their proportion in the population.[16] The mortality of black infants was also markedly greater than that of white infants.[17]

The idea for a medical college to prepare the physicians for black people was attributed by John Braden to a student, who asked him early in the life of the school, "Will there be facilities for a medical education furnished at Central Tennessee College?"[18] As the death rate among blacks soared—leading some observers to believe that they would die out altogether—the necessity of such instruction became every year more apparent to Braden, the Board of Trustees, and the leaders of the Freedmen's Aid Society.

While the college was struggling in the early 1870s to prepare pupils for advanced studies, two friends were developing independent plans for a school in Nashville to train young Negroes in nursing and auxiliary health work. It is not known just when and where Dr. William J. Sneed and George W. Hubbard became acquainted. Probably they met in the last days of the Civil War; certainly, they remained close companions and colleagues for the rest of their lives. The friendship must have seemed improbable at the start. Sneed, a Tennessean, was a Confederate surgeon, while Hubbard, a native of New Hampshire, had served in the Union Army as a member of the Christian Commission. From the first, however, they held each other in high esteem, and Hubbard promised to come to Nashville after the war and study medicine under his old friend's tutelage and sponsorship. In an undated manuscript headed "Half a Century Among the Freedmen," Hubbard recounted, many years later, his wartime service and the beginning of his "providential call":

> In February, 1864, I had a six weeks' term of service in the Christian Commission with the Army of the Potomac, then preparing for an advance on Richmond. The headquarters of the Commission at that time was at Brandy Station, Virginia, some 60 miles south of Washington. . . . Its business was to furnish the army with religious literature, hold religious services, and aid the chaplains in their work, and its efforts were successful to a considerable degree.

In August 1864 Hubbard was commissioned for the same work in the Army of the Cumberland, which, under General Sherman, was besieging Atlanta. On reaching Nashville, he learned that General Nathan Bedford Forrest had severed the railroad line south. "While waiting for it to be repaired," he continued, "I was assigned to teach a colored school in the basement of the Nelson Merry Baptist Church, where I remained until the close of the school year." At the end of the term, in July 1865, Hubbard was employed as an instructor by a regiment of black troops, whom he taught "the elementary English branches." When mustered out at Huntsville, Alabama, in February 1866, Hubbard wrote, "a large proportion of the men were at least able to read and write."

In the company of his former student-soldiers, Hubbard spent some months on an Alabama plantation. In August 1866 he contracted "malarial fever" and left the South for Kansas, where he taught in a rural school and acquired a parcel of farmland. By the following winter, he was again able to take up his vocation among the former slaves: "In February I returned to Nashville, where under the supervision of William Mitchell, a brother of the celebrated astronomer, Maria Mitchell, I opened a school in a government barracks on Summer Street. This school was supported by the Pittsburgh, Pennsylvania Freedmen's Aid Commission." A year later, George Hubbard's school was merged with another one to form the Belle View Public School. He was made principal of the new institution, in which post he remained for several years.[19]

At some time during this first decade of their friendship, W. J. Sneed and George W. Hubbard decided to start a school that would train young black men and women in nursing and other health subjects. The genesis of the project, according to one account, came about when the two men received charge of a friend who became seriously ill. No information about this man survives—not even his name—except that he came from Illinois to Nashville and that his condition was desperate.

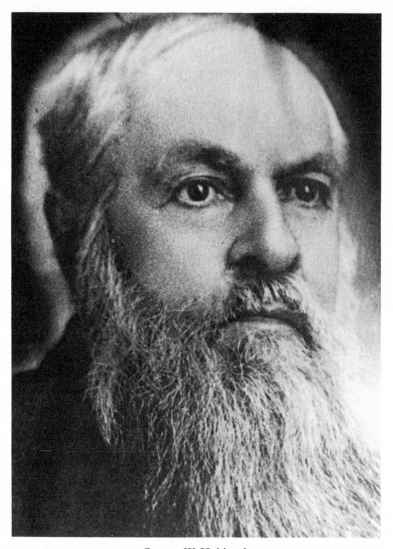

George W. Hubbard

Dr. Sneed examined the patient and issued a guarded prognosis. At the very least, he said, their friend would require constant attention. To provide it, the account continues, he and George Hubbard hired a young Negro woman of Nashville who had once cared for an invalid in the home of her former master. So grateful were they to her when their friend began to recover that they decided to found a school where other black men and women could learn skills like hers. It was said that they often discussed their proposed program with John Braden.[20]

The plans for this venture may have revived George Hubbard's dormant ambition to become a physician, or perhaps the orderly days of a professor's life left him restless. In any case he was at last prompted to carry out his long-standing promise to himself and W. J. Sneed. "In 1875," his memoir continued, "I attended the Medical Department of Vanderbilt University and of the University of Nashville, graduating from Vanderbilt University in 1876. I spent that summer on my farm in Kansas."[21] Deliberately, Hubbard chose these months of leisure, his last for fifty years. Events at Central Tennessee College that would show him the chief work of his life were moving rapidly toward culmination. John Braden and his students were on the eve of realizing their long-postponed design, a course of studies in medicine.

Braden had failed in efforts to interest other schools of higher learning in Nashville in a joint program of health education. As his advanced students were refused admission to every medical school in the South and most of those in the North, he and the trustees began to consider their repeated requests for training in medicine. By 1874 or 1875 Braden was posed to begin a medical department. His daughter, Mary, chronicled his dinnertime musings and his hopes of bringing Drs. Hubbard and Sneed to Central Tennessee College:

> The development of a training program for physicians was repeatedly discussed by my father at mealtime around the family table at which two or more members of the faculty or friends of friends of Central Tennessee College were usually to be found. Whenever the study of medicine or the opening of a medical department . . . was mentioned, Father always suggested that we would have to wait until young George Hubbard graduated, then he would convince him and Dr. Sneed to train physicians instead of Practical Health Workers. . . .[22]

In the fall of 1875 Dr. Sneed began to teach classes in anatomy and physiology for a few undergraduates at the college, preparing them in the basic studies. The following spring George Hubbard received his M.D. degree, and John Braden began the campaign to recruit him. Mary Braden continues the story: "On a hot summer afternoon, soon after his graduation, in the coolest place in the house south of the Chapel, Dr. Hubbard and Father talked over the matter together and the decision was made to open a Medical Department at the College for the training of physicians."[23]

Besides selecting Sneed and Hubbard to commence the teaching of medicine, Braden and the trustees secured the initial finances. To buy the necessary apparatus, chemicals, and drugs, and to pay faculty salaries, they placed at Hubbard's disposal an endowment provided by the Meharry brothers—Samuel, Hugh, David, Jesse, and Alexander. These five were the sons of Alexander and Jane Meharry, both of whom had been born in Scotland. In 1774, when Alexander and Jane were still small children, both their families had been forced by religious persecution to flee Northern Ireland.

Alexander and Jane were married in County Craven in the spring of 1794 and sailed for America in May of the following year. From New York they went on to Philadelphia, then to Lancaster County, Pennsylvania. In 1798 they fitted out a flatboat and embarked westward on the Ohio River. Although they considered making a new home in Kentucky, their abhorrence of slavery led them to settle instead at Manchester, Adams County, Ohio, in the spring of 1799. At a site about eight miles northwest of the town, they cleared out a dense forest. Illness, destruction of the first year's crop by frost, and suspicion and distrust on the part of their neighbors made life hard for the Meharrys the first year. But they ultimately succeeded in making the farm prosperous.

Soon after arriving in America, both Alexander and Jane had joined the Methodist Episcopal Church. Their religious convictions were deeply felt and openly expressed, and they raised their children in an atmosphere of fervent piety. It was while traveling home from a camp meeting on a summer night in 1813 that Alexander Meharry met a sudden, violent death. Riding with a friend and deeply engaged in conversation, he was felled in the road by a limb from a falling tree.

The management of the farm devolved on Jane and her eight children (the five sons mentioned and Thomas, James, and Mary). As they grew in age and strength, they took up work their father had left unfinished, cleared more acres, and kept profitable those already in production. In early manhood the boys went to Indiana and Illinois, where they bought land at low cost and established homes of their own.[24]

The Meharry family first proposed to create an endowment for Central Tennessee College in 1874. That spring the Reverend Alexander Meharry of the Cincinnati conference, a friend of John Braden, visited the campus, where Braden told him of the need for secure, permanent income to assure the institution's growth and usefulness. The Reverend Meharry appealed to his brother, Hugh, of Shawnee Mound, Indiana, who conveyed a tract of farm land valued at $10,000 to the trustees.[25]

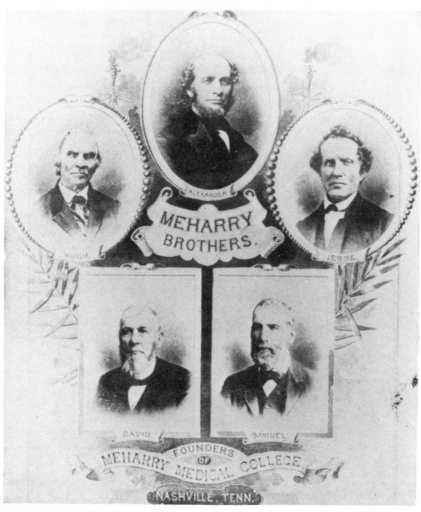

The Meharry brothers. Clockwise from top, left: Hugh, Alexander, Jesse, Samuel, David

When John Braden sought funds for a medical department, George Hubbard's friend from Illinois—the boy whom he had nursed back to health after the war—recalled the story about Samuel Meharry and the black man on the wilderness road. It was a tale often told throughout southern Illinois and Indiana.[26] Braden appealed to Samuel Meharry directly, and Meharry saw the chance to keep the promise he had made in the swamp. To his 1875 donation of $500, evidently the first gift specifically designated for medical studies, his brothers added more. Ultimately the five men gave over $30,000 in cash and real property to Central Tennessee College.[27]

The Freedmen's Aid Society and the John F. Slater Fund also gave money to start medical classes. These gifts, other smaller private donations, and student fees enabled John Braden and George W. Hubbard to open the Medical Department of Central Tennessee College, as it was first called, in October 1876. The following spring the trustees changed the name to the Meharry Medical Department at the suggestion of its faculty.[28]

To study medicine at Central Tennessee College, an applicant had to be of good moral character and pass an examination in the "common English branches." The medical course consisted of two terms of five months each. Anatomy, physiology, chemistry, materia medica (pharmacology), and dissecting were taught the first year. The second year consisted of surgery, obstetrics, diseases of women and children, theory and practice of medicine, and surgical anatomy. Textbooks included Gray's *Anatomy*; Steele on chemistry; Biddle on materia medica; Ashhurst on surgery; Hartshorne on the theory and practice of medicine; and Leishman on obstetrics. (The medical writings of John Wesley, the founder of Methodism, are not mentioned in early catalogs.) Tuition was ten dollars a term, payable in advance; board and other expenses were about eight dollars a month; the graduation fee was ten dollars. To graduate the student was required to be twenty-one years old, to have studied medicine two full terms and attended two full lecture courses, the last one at Central Tennessee College. The prospective doctor was also required to pass an examination in the course work and to present an original thesis on some medical subject.[29]

During the department's first years, students faced a well-prepared faculty whose members often did multiple duty. George W. Hubbard, in addition to being dean, was professor of chemistry, materia medica, and therapeutics. Hubbard was born on October 11, 1841, in Charleston, New Hampshire, whose citizens honored his grandfather as one of the town's first settlers. Hubbard studied at the New Hampshire Conference Seminary and the New London Literary and Scientific Institute. In February 1864 he began service with the Christian Commission, which, as previously recounted, led him to Nashville, to medicine, and Meharry.[30]

The professor of surgery and surgical anatomy was William Joseph Sneed. Although he is considered one of the founders of Meharry Medical

College, little is known about Dr. Sneed. He was born in Brentwood, Tennessee, in 1835 and received his early education in the western part of the state. He took his medical degree from the University of Nashville with high honors and thereafter practiced for a time in Logan County, Kentucky, where he was remembered for interposing himself between a mob and a young Negro boy whom it was about to lynch.

At age twenty-six Sneed entered the Confederate army as a surgeon. Upon returning to Nashville after the war, he served as professor of anatomy and surgery at his alma mater before teaching the first preparatory classes in medicine at Central Tennessee College. He was a master Mason, and although many of his forebears had been Methodists, he was an energetic Presbyterian. After thirty years service to Meharry, he died in Nashville on March 17, 1907.[31]

John F. McKinley was a member of the class of 1879 of the Meharry Medical Department and was thus evidently the first alumnus to join the faculty. Following his graduation he attended the medical department of Michigan University and then returned to Meharry as demonstrator of anatomy and professor of physiology and histology. He held that post through the 1883–84 school year, then relocated in Texas. Between 1900 and 1902, McKinley was again teaching at Meharry as lecturer on diseases of the eye, ear, and throat.[32]

Professor of obstetrics and diseases of women, James Balaam Stephens was born on October 18, 1834, at Chapel Hill, Marshall County, Tennessee, and educated at the University of Nashville. In 1875 he began practicing in Nashville where he became one of the best known physicians in the city. He was a Mason, a member of the Primitive Baptist Church, and an officer of the Nashville Gynecological Society, organized in 1889. Returning from a visit to a patient, Stephens was killed on the evening of December 10, 1910, when his buggy collided with a taxicab.[33]

Newton Guilford Tucker was the first professor of the theory and practice of medicine. Born in Williamson County, Tennessee, on March 28, 1839, he graduated from the medical department of the University of Nashville in 1861. For the next thirteen years he practiced at Lewisburg, Tennessee, and was elected its mayor in 1870. Three years later he returned to Nashville. Subsequently he was elected to the Common Council and, in 1877, made its president. In the summer of that year he joined the faculty of the Meharry Medical Department. An officer in local and state medical societies, Tucker was a Mason and a Presbyterian. He died in Nashville on January 8, 1899.[34]

Completing the first faculty was Joseph Whitney, professor of medical jurisprudence. Born in Warrenton, Massachusetts, on November 21, 1834, Whitney was first trained as a lawyer. When war broke out, he enlisted at President Lincoln's first call for volunteers and remained in the army until the South's defeat. Taking a theological degree and holding a pastorate in

Wisconsin, he then taught at Central Tennessee College, serving on the medical faculty during the first year of Meharry's existence. In 1879 he returned to the ministry in Wisconsin, where he lived until his death in 1916.[35]

These teachers, black and white, were beginning a momentous work on the campus of Central Tennessee College in south Nashville. The first commencements of the Meharry Medical Department gave John Braden and George Hubbard cause for rejoicing and prayers to God for continued success. But two challenges during the last years of the century would draw upon every spiritual and intellectual resource of Meharry's faculty, leaders, and graduates. The first was the new standards being wrought in medical education as a result of discoveries in the laboratories, perfection of new techniques in the surgical theater, and reforms in licensing and practice. The other was the long night of "Jim Crow," whose shadows were beginning to deepen as the Meharry Medical Department's first graduates received their diplomas and entered upon their work.

3

Trumpet Voices

CENTRAL TENNESSEE COLLEGE was ten years old when its first medical students met for recitation and laboratory work in a small room in Tennessee Hall, the college's main building, in October 1876. They were allotted additional space in the basement for practical demonstrations in anatomy.[1] Poverty, illness, and distractions from study caused some of this first class, eleven in number, to leave the college altogether and others to fall behind. The result was that James Monroe Jamison of Nashville was the only student to receive the degree of M.D. with the Class of 1877, Central Tennessee College. Jamison may have completed some of the requirements under Dr. Sneed during the 1875–76 school year, since he won his diploma in a single session.

Little is known about this pioneer, who was Meharry's first graduate and the first black physician to be formally trained in the South. He was born in either 1851 or 1853 and thus was about twenty-five when he became a doctor. Following his graduation, Jamison resided in Nashville, apparently practicing medicine. In 1880 he was elected the first president of the State Colored Medical Association, formed by Meharry's early graduates and comprising some of the score of black doctors then residing in Tennessee.[2] Jamison moved to Topeka, Kansas, in 1884, where he had a prosperous practice among both black and white citizens. He died there on December 30, 1921.[3]

Three more new physicians—John Silas Bass, John C. Halfacre, and Lorenzo Dow Key—graduated on February 22, 1878, at the first separate commencement of the Medical Department. The Reverend John Braden conducted the proceedings, during which, in fulfillment of the requirement for an original thesis, Lorenzo Dow Key presented a paper on malaria. It was an interesting mixture of the miasmatic and bacterial theories of disease. The word "malaria," Dr. Key told his audience,

was derived from two Latin words which mean "bad air." It is supposed that air in certain portions of this and other countries is filled with germs that

21

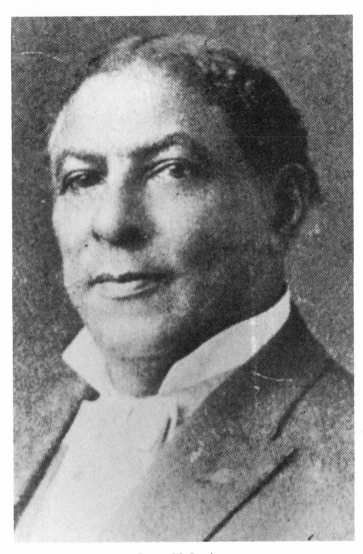

James M. Jamison

are formed by the decomposition of animal and vegetable matter, and it is thought by a large number of writers on the subject that persons who inhabit these districts take into their systems during respiration these germs, which enter the circulation. . . .

From the etiology of the disease, Key proceeded to the principal remedies, several of them still experimental.

Dr. John C. Halfacre followed his classmate at the podium, speaking on "Physician's Qualifications and Responsibilities." Then Dr. John S. Bass delivered an address on "Our Aim as Physicians," noting:

> The question is often asked: "Why do more colored people die in a given period than whites?" Simply because they more frequently violate the laws of health. Why are they more liable to violate these laws? Because they have been deprived of men of their race capable of teaching these laws and urging the necessity of observing them. I know that there is a class who say that we will gradually die out, but the Medical Department of Central Tennessee College is engaged in preparing physicians who, in a few years, will prove that assertion to be false, by decreasing the mortality which is now so great among our people. . . .

Dr. George Hubbard addressed the audience on some of the causes that produced the high mortality rate in Nashville and proposed measures to reduce this toll among the city's black citizens. He advocated the creation of a pure public water supply open to the poor without charge; penalties on property owners who rented houses unfit for human habitation; and the acquisition by Negroes of their own homes, or, if they could not afford them, relocation to the West, where demand for labor exceeded the supply and land was cheap. Finally, he called for dissemination in the public schools of information about the laws of health.

Dr. John Braden then delivered the commencement address, whose power has not since been diminished:

> Gentlemen of the Class of 1878:
> I congratulate you tonight, first, because you are recognized as men. You were born slaves, the recognized property of others. . . . Tonight you are on your own; no fetters bind your limbs, no human law manacles your intellect, no earthly master has the keeping of your conscience. . . . I hail you as *men*.
> Your position here tonight is the trumpet voice of encouragement to the poor young men who have the desire to secure a thorough education. Your example tells them that they need not wait for others if they will use the powers God has given. . . .
> Your school days are about to end, but not your student life. . . . Know what is in your books; as soon as possible, get the best and dated works on

medicine; read the best medical journals you can find. Be married to your books and dare allow to think for yourselves. Study your patients, notice carefully the various forms of disease, the effects of every prescription, the surroundings of the sick. . . . Remember that internal remedies will not remove dirt on the skin, or tonics overcome the destructive influences of bad ventilation, dampness, and filthiness. Get your mind filled with the idea of healthy surroundings for your patients, and labor to secure everywhere observance of the laws that will prevent disease as well as heal the sick. . . .

You cannot go to Africa as a people and it is doubtful if that would be best. Your home is here, and you are no carpetbagger. Generations in the future will find your people here. Cultivate for these generations the friendliest relations with your professional brethren and others of the Anglo-Saxon race, and by your diligence in study, modesty in deportment, fidelity, and kindness to your patients, and your earnest efforts to promote the highest welfare of your people, demand the respect of the entire community. . . .[4]

Dr. Bass is remembered for his work among victims of the yellow fever epidemic that struck Chattanooga in 1878. He treated patients there through the full wrath of the plague, and upon his return home to Murfreesboro, he was given a public reception by the white citizens of the town.[5] The yellow fever also swept through Memphis and western Tennessee. Dr. Key, namesake of the evangelist, spiritualist, and healer Lorenzo Dow, continued to practice at his home in Mason, Tennessee, while many fled inland from the disease-infested city and the lands along the Mississippi River.[6] He relocated to Greenville, Texas, about 1890. Their classmate, Dr. John C. Halfacre, successfully practiced at Columbia, Tennessee, where he owned property. He also taught "Theory of Medicine" at Meharry from 1892 through 1893.[7]

In his address to the 1878 graduates, George Hubbard declared it to be the Medical Department's intention to send out an increasing number of carefully trained physicians who "like our common Master, spend their lives going about doing good." As classes increased in size, he and other leaders recruited new faculty members, constructed and equipped new facilities, offered additional courses, and added departments of dentistry and pharmacy. With continuing assistance from the Meharry brothers and the Freedmen's Aid Society, the Central Tennessee College trustees were able to erect for the Medical Department a new building of its own. During the summer of 1878, the Reverend Alexander Meharry visited Nashville in the company of his brother, Samuel. They selected a pleasant elevation at the corner of Maple and South Franklin Streets. This lot adjoined, and thus enlarged, the campus of Central Tennessee College.

The cornerstone of the department's new building was laid on May 14, 1879, by Dr. J. W. Freeman of New York City.[8] The completed facility was

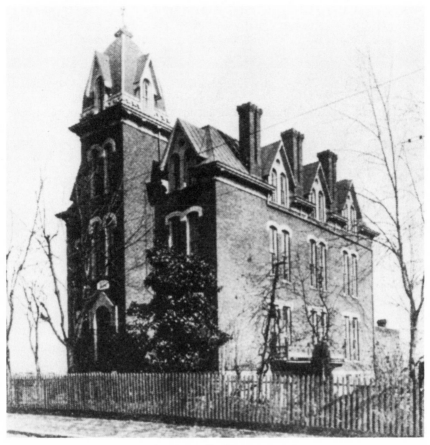

Meharry Medical Department

dedicated on October 13, 1880, just as Nashville was celebrating its centenary. The new department stood four stories tall. The ground floor was the chemistry laboratory, and the second floor had offices, a museum, and dwelling apartments. The third floor was a lecture hall seating 100 persons and a storage area for materia medica. The top floor served as a dormitory.[9]

Meharry students were, in the words of Dr. Freeman, "taught to practice until they knew." The earliest catalogs for the department, published about 1880, showed that anatomy, physiology, chemistry, botany, dissecting, and chemical analysis were required of first-year students. In the second year they studied surgery, gynecology, obstetrics, surgical anatomy, theory and practice of medicine, histology, microscopy, and medical chemistry. Medical jurisprudence and Bible history and doctrine were also required.[10]

Thoroughness and practicality were the announced aims of Meharry's early faculty members, such as Drs. Henry T. Noel and Charles O. Hadley. Both were alumni, both taught fundamental courses in anatomy, and both served as charter officers of the association of black physicians that Dr. James M. Jamison founded at Nashville in 1880.[11] They and their colleagues sought to teach students to apply lessons from the classroom to the particular conditions that awaited them upon graduation. An early statement of purpose declared:

> There is no reason why the colored physician should not be as thoroughly educated as any other. There are special reasons why he should be thoroughly equipped. . . . The ignorance, the irregular habits of life, and the great mortality among colored people in many parts of the South renders it absolutely necessary that those whose work is especially among this class should be thoroughly prepared to grapple with the difficult problems which present themselves. . . .[12]

Lectures, recitations, and frequent quizzes were the chief teaching tools during the first decade of Meharry's life. But from an early date, the didactic approach was supplemented by practical exercises. By the mid-1880s students were doing laboratory work in chemistry that included qualitative analysis, urinalysis, and toxicology. In obstetrics and gynecology, they learned the use of instruments by means of a manikin. Surgical classes gave particular attention to venereal diseases, bandaging, and minor operations. The Medical Department's microscopy collection contained hundreds of slides, and there were demonstrations in "the therapeutical application of electricity in medicine and surgery."[13] Students also dissected cadavers, at least some of which were obtained through grave robbing or secret purchases. An aura of horror still clung to dissection at Meharry as late as 1890. It was done in a separate building, and students were required to sign pledges not to reveal what occurred there.[14]

By 1900 medicine was becoming increasingly specialized. Anatomy, chemistry, and physiology remained the core of medical education, but they deepened in complexity. In 1906, the year of his graduation from Meharry with honors, Dr. Thomas Henry Elliott became head of the chemistry department. His curricular reforms, including the addition of courses in physiological processes to Meharry's basic offerings in organic and inorganic chemistry, reflected the depths that contemporary students of medicine were expected to plumb.[15]

Fundamental work behind them, upperclassmen proceeded to obstetrics, gynecology, and surgery. They also recited in histology, bacteriology, diseases of the genitourninary organs, dermatology, medical ethics, mental diseases, opthalmology, otology, and laryngology.[16] These requirements meant days and nights bent over one's books and instruments. "We had little time for anything except hard, grinding, and difficult work," a student from this period wrote. "In materia medica, we were required to know the origin, physical properties, incompatibilities, physiological effects, toxicity, medicinal uses, and doses of any drug." The final examination in qualitative analysis, requiring at least a week to complete, consisted of identifying an unknown solution. In anatomy, all portions of the brain had to be committed to memory.[17]

The comprehension needed to pass one's courses required facilities that could illustrate textual material. When Dr. John Henry Holman, Class of 1897, began teaching histology and bacteriology that year, Meharry's laboratories were without even such basic equipment as lamps. Work tables and benches had to be arranged around the walls to take advantage of light from the windows. Although the medical department owned microscopes and slides, it lacked other proper equipment for the study of bacteriological and pathological preparations. Dr. Holman is remembered for his efforts to bring Meharry's laboratories into line with evolving national standards for such facilities. He regularly visited other campuses in the East, examining their stores of scientific supplies and viewing the teaching techniques employed.[18]

As long as medicine remained a matter of dogma and rote learning, its fundamental elements could be mastered in a short time. But as experiments began replacing authorities and as diagnosis became more sophisticated, longer periods of study were required. Almost immediately after the department's founding, Meharry leaders began to stiffen entrance requirements and to prolong the time necessary to complete the course of study. These reforms paralleled ones being undertaken throughout the nation in response to the proprietary schools of medicine, which admitted everyone able to pay tuition and which graduated thousands of pseudo-physicians each year. By the end of the century, Meharry had adopted the admissions rules of the Association of American Medical Colleges, another of the reforms coming from within the profession. These rules required each student to pass a difficult examination in English, arithmetic, algebra, physics, and Latin before admission.

Meharry strongly urged prospective students to complete college before enrolling there to study medicine. Applicants who presented college diplomas or certain other credentials could be excused from the entrance examination. Those who failed it might still be admitted to the first-year class but not to subsequent study until the deficiencies were satisfied. Meharry also continued to impose an age requirement of eighteen and to insist that entering students be of "good moral character."[19] This last remained very important. Older applicants of known good character could sometimes gain admission even though they did not meet all the other criteria.[20]

Graduation from Meharry was also made more difficult through the lengthening of the course of study. Beginning in 1879 a third year was added to the course in medicine. The department encouraged students to be in residence for all three sessions, but it permitted some preliminary studies to be pursued at home under the direction of faculty members or some regular physician. The fourth year was added in 1893, and students were required to pass examinations for each year's work before being admitted to the next higher class. By the end of the century, the candidate for a degree had to have attended medical school for four sessions of at least six months each, with the last session at Meharry.

In recognition of the labor required to excel in these rigorous requirements, the most outstanding students from each class were asked to present addresses at commencement. Certain members of the faculty also awarded medals or other prizes to the new doctors deemed most knowledgeable in each discipline. Competition for these awards was keen. Prior to the commencement of 1897, for example, a faculty committee of judges debated for three days before proclaiming a tie for the prize in surgery.[21]

Evidence that the State of Tennessee recognized Meharry alumni as fully qualified is found in the records of the board of medical examiners from its establishment in 1889. Upon presentation of their diplomas to the board, Meharry graduates were issued certificates permitting them to practice within the state. These certificates were registered on the public lists of practitioners kept in each county courthouse.

In 1884, at the urging of some of the first medical alumni, the trustees directed Central Tennessee College officials to investigate the practicality of dental studies. Two years later, the new course was begun within the Meharry Medical Department "to provide the Colored people of the South with an opportunity for thoroughly preparing themselves for the practice of dentistry."[22] Dr. William Henry Morgan, the first dean of Vanderbilt University's dental school and an acknowledged leader of the profession in the South,[23] helped to establish the new department. He also lectured and gave demonstrations in clinical dentistry. Dr. John P. Bailey, a Vanderbilt graduate, was placed in nominal charge of the program, reporting to Dr. Hubbard. He taught operative and mechanical dentistry and recruited several white Nashville dentists to offer other courses.

Like prospective medical students, applicants to the dental school were required to be of reputable character and to pass an entrance examination or to present evidence of having completed a course in some normal school, academy, or college. At first, two years were required to earn the degree of D.D.S., but by 1893 the course was lengthened to four years. First-year students recited daily in anatomy, chemistry, and physiology, then worked

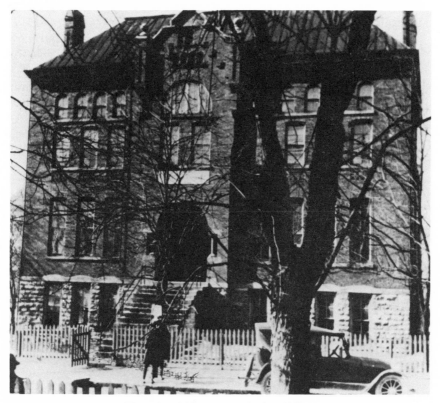

Dental and Pharmaceutical Building

two hours in the chemical laboratory and one hour in the dental infirmary. In the second year, the curriculum continued with anatomy, materia medica, hygiene, and practical work in the laboratory or dissecting room. Before a candidate could graduate he was required to treat a patient in "all the usual dental operations" while being observed by the professor of operative dentistry. He was also required to prepare a specimen case for deposit in the museum and to pass an examination before the dental faculty. Upon graduation the new dentist received a diploma that was recognized everywhere.

At the American Association for the Advancement of Science convention at Philadelphia in 1884, Dr. Hubbard obtained contributions in money, laboratory equipment, and books from dental supply houses.[24] Early students were asked to bring their own tools if they owned any. The first textbooks, in addition to some of those utilized by the Medical Department, included Harris's *Principles and Practice* and *Dictionary of Dental Surgery*. Reference works were Tomes's *Dental Surgery,* Taft's *Operative Dentistry,* Richardson's *Mechanical Dentistry,* and Wildman's *Instruction in Vulcanite Work.* Tuition was thirty dollars per year, and the graduation fee was ten dollars. Dental and study materials were furnished at cost. Room, board, fuel, lights, and laundry amounted to nine or ten dollars a month for those residing on campus.

The first dental students, nine in number, included three Meharry medical graduates, Dr. Henry T. Noel (Class of 1879), Robert Fulton Boyd (Class of 1882), and John W. Anderson (Class of 1885). Dr. Noel devoted the rest of his life to Meharry as a member of the faculty. Dr. Anderson also taught at Meharry for a time. Later, he became an enormously successful practitioner and businessman in Dallas and donated to his alma mater the funds to build an anatomical hall, which was named in his honor. The work of Dr. Boyd is the subject of a subsequent discussion.

When Dr. John Bailey returned to private practice in 1890, the leadership of the dental department devolved upon the shoulders of young James B. Singleton. For more than a quarter of a century, Dr. Singleton, who received the degree of D.D.S. in 1892, served as head of dentistry at Meharry. Upon his retirement in 1921, Dr. Donley H. Turpin, his colleague and successor, credited the success of the dental school during its early years—when it labored under shortages of money, equipment, and teachers and yet graduated well-prepared practitioners—solely to Dr. Singleton. Besides his administrative duties, Dr. Singleton taught operative dentistry, orthodontics, dental metallurgy, and engaged in the practice of dental surgery. He was also an officer of the Peoples Savings Bank and Trust Company of Nashville and president of the Economical Steam Laundry Company, where, he said, Negroes might call with their bundles to avoid "the public insults flaunted in their faces daily."[25]

In October 1889 the School of Pharmacy of the Meharry Medical Department opened in specially prepared rooms in the new dental building. The first announcement promised to confer the degree of Graduate of Pharmacy (Ph.G.) upon those who completed two twenty-week sessions, passed their examinations, and possessed four years' practical experience in compounding drugs and medicines in an established pharmacy.

Entrance requirements were much like those for medicine and dentistry, although more emphasis was laid upon knowledge of physics and Latin. The first pharmacy students were required to study botany, medical chemistry, toxicology, materia medica, microscopy, pharmacy, and urinalysis. During the first session, in addition to daily recitations, students performed experiments in weighing and measuring various substances and finding their specific gravity. During the second session, they were given a thorough course in qualitative analysis, urinalysis, and toxicology.

At first the faculty was small, but it grew as more students enrolled. West Patterson, professor of chemistry, was the most distinguished early teacher of pharmacy. He kept the keys to the cabinet of drugs, which held most kinds and compounds then employed in pharmacy. Professor Patterson also supervised Meharry's herbarium of 2,500 specimens, which yielded vegetable material for manufacture into drugs.

The first class in pharmacy was graduated at the Meharry commencement of 1890. Its one member, John T. Hobbs of Nashville, presented a dissertation on opium. The first pharmacy graduate recruited to teach was Dr. William Sevier, a member of the Class of 1892. Subsequently he earned the M.D. degree (Class of 1898) and a diploma from the Northwestern College of Pharmacy in Chicago.

Upon the death of West Patterson in 1904, Dr. Sevier became head of pharmacy and served in that capacity for twenty-seven years. Administrative duties did not distract him from his vocation as a teacher. Throughout his career he taught a wide range of courses, including urinalysis, qualitative analysis, toxicology, medical chemistry, and materia medica. The wide ties, brilliant stickpins, and fashionable suits that Sevier wore contributed to his reputation as one of the most colorful figures on the faculty. There were those who considered him eccentric for declining a lucrative career in private practice, but his devotion to pharmaceutical studies at Meharry made that subject increasingly important. Under his leadership, students and teachers of pharmacy were able to give crucial support to the clinical and hospital services that Meharry began soon after the turn of the century.

The pharmacy school attained its highest enrollment in 1929, with 159 students. As the Depression settled over the nation, the number fell sharply, and the school was forced to close in 1938. During the half century of its existence, more than 600 pharmacists were trained at Meharry. While a majority evidently were employed in drugstores, a considerable number opened their own retail establishments, strengthening the black business class in their locales.[26]

A course for nurses was established at Central Tennessee College by 1878, fulfilling George Hubbard and W. J. Sneed's original plan to offer such training to young black women. Instruction was given in anatomy, physiology, hygiene, the use of simple medicines, caring for the sick, and the preparation of suitable food for the sick.[27] The following year the first three women—Henrietta Davis, Florence Holmes, and Julia Thomas— were admitted to classes in the Meharry Medical Department. They all attained junior class status in 1881, but for unknown reasons they did not receive degrees.[28]

It was not until 1893 that the first women graduated from Meharry. Annie D. Gregg, who completed the "Special Course in Obstetrics," thereafter practiced in south Nashville and was active in alumni affairs. Her classmate, Dr. Georgia Patton Washington, is also remembered.

Georgia Esther Lee Patton was born in Grundy County, Tennessee, in 1864. After completing the normal course at Central Tennessee College in 1890, she entered the Meharry Medical Department that fall. Upon her graduation she became the first black woman to receive a license to practice medicine and surgery in Tennessee. Three months later, in May 1893, she sailed for Liberia, the first Meharrian to go to Africa. The following August, from Monrovia, she wrote a letter that gave an account of her first months' labors as a missionary:

> For the first days after my arrival, the surroundings looked very discouraging for my professional work. On examining my first case, remarks made by natives were: "Patients in his condition never get well; we always expect them to die." After careful treatment and watching for two months, he was able to leave his bed and finally went to work. The next two cases were also considered to be hopeless, yet both recovered.

Later Dr. Patton wrote: "I have treated over one hundred cases and have lost four."

Failure of her health and lack of financial support forced Dr. Patton to return to the United States in 1895. She located in Memphis, where she enjoyed a large and lucrative practice. In 1897 she married David W. Washington.

Dr. Georgia Patton Washington was called "the gold lady" by the clerks in the office of the Freedmen's Aid Society because of her cash contributions to the schools in which she had been educated. One of her characteristic letters survived her untimely death, at age thirty-six, in 1900.

> Memphis, Tenn., May 24, 1900
> Dear Brother Mason,—Some weeks ago I sent you a letter with a little money inclosed. In reply you said, "Dear Brother." I am not a brother. Do you not remember Georgia Patton? Well, it is she, with a little more attached. I send ten dollars more, and hope to be able to keep sending until I have given $100, asked by you of the alumni of the schools; and even more if possible.
> Yours, with best wishes for the Society,
> G. E. L. Patton Washington
> P.S.—Say "Sister" next time.[29]

The first woman to teach at Meharry and the first to attain a position of leadership there was Dr. Josie E. Wells, Class of 1904. Prior to studying medicine, Josie Wells received training as a nurse and had worked in that capacity. Earlier women physicians, both black and white, had practiced in Nashville, but when she received her degree, Dr. Wells was the only female doctor of either race residing there. As a clinician she devoted herself entirely to diseases of women and children. Besides dispensing medicine and treatment without charge two afternoons a week, she performed surgery in serious cases. Dr. Wells later became a close associate of Dr. George Hubbard. "Under a more favorable environment," a colleague observed, "she might have risen to fame."[30]

Home was the "best and highest field for women, but not for all women," declared Bellina A. Moore in her valedictory address to the pharmacy class of 1897. Men had "held the heights so long that they were selfish and wanted women to stay on the lower levels." Nonetheless, she concluded, women were "entering every profession and succeeding in all."[31]

Classmates of Patton, Wells, and Moore, and other early Meharrians, kept personal accounts of these pioneer days. In his autobiography, *Forty Cords of Wood,* John Edward Perry, Class of 1895, gave a vivid picture of student life at Meharry near the end of the nineteenth century. Like most of his fellow students, Perry was born a poor boy in the South just after the Civil War. To earn money to attend school, he sold wood. Forty cords brought enough for him to enter Bishop College in Wiley, Texas, a school for black students conducted by Baptist missionaries from the North. After graduating, Perry taught school for the means to attend Meharry. Many of his fellow students also worked long hours while in medical school to pay expenses. Farm labor in the countryside around Nashville supported some of them. The only recreation Perry could recall, aside from "fireside jollification," was an hour's walk after dinner.

Lister's theories concerning the relationship of bacteria to infection were much discussed. Perry and his classmates observed various bacteria under the microscope. "I shall always remember the first time I prepared a slide from the sputa of a patient and saw under the microscope the tuberculosis bacilli," he wrote. He also listened as Dr. Newton Tucker, by now an old man, drew upon his vast clinical experience in discussing diseases of the circulatory system.[32] Perry later became a member of the Board of Trustees of Meharry Medical College, enacting Dr. Charles Victor Roman's observation that to thousands of young black people the meaning of Meharry was opportunity.[33]

Roman, Class of 1890, is himself remembered as another chronicler of these early days, in his anecdotal, aphoristic memoir, *Meharry Medical College, A History.* Like George Hubbard, whose confidant he became, Roman had roots in the Northeast. Born at Williamsport, Pennsylvania, on July 4, 1864, he was raised and educated in Ontario, where his parents moved when he was eight. It was in that same year that Charles, fascinated by the prospect of adventure and of earning a few pennies, accompanied an old root doctor on an herb-gathering expedition. He soon began dispensing herbs himself to anyone nearby who complained of illness or discomfort.

His practice flourished, then ended abruptly when the relatives of a patient apparently cured by one of Charles's prescriptions became anxious nonetheless. The bona fide physician who took over the case prophesied, "You'll be a doctor someday."

Having recently graduated from Hamilton Collegiate Institute in Hamilton, Ontario, Roman came south in 1885 to Columbia, Tennessee, where he accepted a teaching post. From his salary he intended to save enough to return to medical school at McGill University in Montreal. But fate led him to board in the home of Dr. John C. Halfacre, who revived in the young man "early ambitions and prophecies" and directed him toward Meharry, where he enrolled in October 1887 as a freshman.

Roman observed that personal conduct and paying one's bills on time were just as important to graduation as the formal requirements of the day. College rules governing these matters were "interpreted with Puritanic strictness and New England penetration," he wrote. "Board bills, love affairs, and tippling were deadly evils if discovered and not remedied. Failing in one's examinations meant repetition. Having paid tuition, one could attend until he passed or got tired."[34]

One whose life and work flowered briefly, but intensely, after his preparation at Meharry was Henry Alonzo Napier (Class of 1880), who bore the name of a distinguished Nashville family. He was the son of William Carroll and Jane Napier, former slaves who purchased their freedom prior to the Civil War. William Carroll Napier kept a livery stable in Nashville and by the mid-1880s was one of the city's oldest and best-known citizens. Henry's grandfather, Elias W. Napier, was a white planter, physician, and iron foundry owner.[35] J. C. Napier, Henry's brother, became a Meharry trustee and leader in Nashville's black community. From 1911 to 1915 he was United States Treasury Registrar, and his signature appeared on all bank notes issued during that period.

Some accounts say that Henry Alonzo Napier attended West Point. According to another, he was in the same class as George Hubbard at the University of Nashville-Vanderbilt Medical Department, from which he was dismissed when it was discovered that he was black.[36] He is known to have taught in the public schools of St. Louis, Missouri, both before and after graduation from Meharry. In 1876 he served as principal of Salem School in Nashville, probably a public school for Negro children.

Henry Napier visited Kansas in 1875 to investigate whether immigration there was feasible for black Tennesseans wanting to flee local oppression. "Feeling that whatever would be to the interest of the whole people would be to the interest of each," he reported his "discreet and thorough exploration" of the plains country. Although he found that, politically, there was "no better state for colored people than Kansas," the prospective settler needed at least $1,000 "to make the first crop."[37] Napier's statement was used by anti-immigration forces to buttress their arguments.

According to early alumni records, Dr. Napier was a man of more than ordinary ability and one of the best anatomists to attend Meharry in this period. His light was extinguished abruptly in December 1882 when he was thrown from his buggy and died from the injuries within a few days.[38]

Napier's colleague, Robert Fulton Boyd, was also drawn into the tumult in which black Nashvillians found themselves during this repressive era. Among the first black doctors to earn a living with the full-time practice of medicine or dentistry in the city, Boyd was one of the most distinguished men ever educated at Meharry. Born a slave in Giles County, Tennessee, in 1858, Boyd was brought by his mother to Nashville in 1866 to live with Dr. Paul Eve, an internationally renowned surgeon. He attended night classes at Fisk and for the next fourteen years taught in various rural schools. During the months of recess he lived in Nashville, studying at Fisk and Central Tennessee College. In 1880 he entered Meharry, graduating with first honors two years later.

Throughout the spring and summer of that year, Boyd practiced medicine and taught school in New Albany, Mississippi, becoming perhaps the first licensed black physician in that state. In the fall he returned to Central Tennessee College to pursue the college course. At the same time he held an adjunct professorship in chemistry in the Meharry Medical Department and taught hygiene and physiology at Central Tennessee College. In 1886, after graduating with honors from the college department, he commenced the study of dentistry. The next year, the degree of D.D.S. in hand, Boyd opened an office on North Cherry Street to practice his professions.

"Colored physicians had not been a success here. . . . Very few good families had ever given colored doctors their practice," Boyd wrote in 1890. "I married to my office, slept there, ate all my meals there. . . . I went to see everybody that sought my services." Boyd's practice grew until he alone could not supply the demand. "It is becoming the rule for colored families to have colored doctors. There has been a great change during the past three years."[39]

Dr. Boyd made some of the earliest detailed observations about health conditions among city-dwelling black Americans in his paper, "What Are the Causes of the Great Mortality Among the Negroes in the Cities of the South, and How is that Mortality to be Lessened?" From the pulpits of Nashville churches and in other public forums, he taught the etiology and transmission of tuberculosis and showed his audiences the ways to resist this killer.[40] Following still more studies at the Chicago Post-Graduate School of Medicine, Boyd became professor of gynecology and clinical medicine at Meharry in 1893. His experience of work in a teaching hospital in Chicago proved to be highly consequential to his alma mater.

Patients who called at the Medical Department's classrooms for treatment provided the only clinical experience for Meharry students, although seniors were permitted to treat homebound sufferers under supervision of

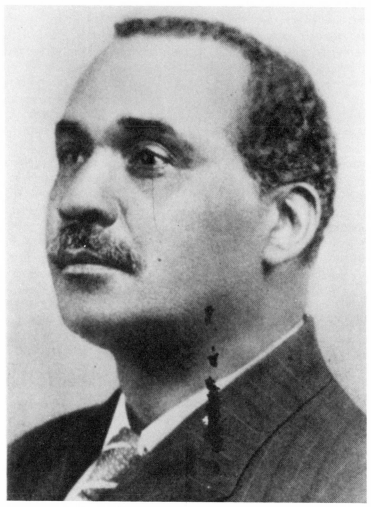

Robert Fulton Boyd

a faculty member.[41] George Hubbard and the trustees of Central Tennessee College recognized the need for a teaching hospital, but their efforts to obtain funds from the Freedmen's Aid Society to build one proved futile.[42] When Nashville opened a city hospital, about ten minutes by foot from the campus, Dr. Hubbard sought privileges for students there, pointing out that half the patients were black.[43] For a time the wards and clinics were opened to Meharrians; then, without reason, city officials abruptly revoked the permission.

That adversity ultimately proved a boon to Meharry, for it stirred the resourcefulness of Robert Fulton Boyd. In a building that he owned on Cedar Street, he founded in 1893 the first hospital for black people in Nashville. Although it was Boyd's private property, it served from the beginning as the teaching hospital for students in the Meharry Medical Department. Clinical privileges were open to all, while obstetrical cases were attended by members of the senior class.[44] Students were avid for this practical work and observation. John Edward Perry recounted how he and his classmates made a mad dash for the streetcar whenever an announcement was made that surgery was pending in the Boyd Infirmary. In his senior year, Perry sat in the front row of the surgical room while Dr. W. J. Sneed worked carefully dissecting tissues and ligating blood vessels "with poise and assurance."[45]

The year 1893 was otherwise memorable for Boyd, whose intelligence, ambition, and personality had vaulted him to prominence in Nashville. Regular biennial elections to fill the offices of city government were set for October. But it was generally acknowledged that the next mayor would effectively be chosen in the Democratic primary in September. The Democratic Executive Committee met in the summer and voted to limit the franchise to white citizens. The Republicans selected their slate at a private, segregated club.

Robert Fulton Boyd had previously sought a seat in the Tennessee legislature as a Republican. Now, with both parties closed to them, the city's black leadership selected Dr. Boyd to head an independent ticket as candidate for mayor of Nashville. As expected, Mayor George Guild, the Democratic nominee, was the winner and succeeded himself, receiving 2,843 votes to 213 for the Republican nominee and 135 for Dr. Boyd. Nevertheless, by their turnout the black voters had shown that they were determined to resist the bipartisan effort to deprive them of the right to vote.[46]

Black doctors generally shared the lot of all black people as systematic segregation, economic exploitation, and legal abridgement of Negroes' civil rights followed the end of Reconstruction. Denied hospital facilities, membership in medical societies, and a forum in their professional journals, Negro physicians and dentists nevertheless had to prove their competence. Until they could establish their own institutions, associations, and scientific periodicals, the chief criterion for success was the acquisition of money, property, and the respect of influential white people.

Meharry students studied and later practiced at the sufferance of the white leadership elite in their communities, and they were expected to do their part, as leaders of their race, to quell not only their resentment at injustice but also any appearance of aspiration to social equality. On one occasion, around 1890, it became the fashion among medical students at Central Tennessee College to sport "plug hats" and Prince Albert coats. When the fad was at its height, President John Braden summoned them all to the chapel and delivered an impassioned address on gratitude. What would be the reaction of the benefactors of the institution, he asked, if they should come to the campus and find the objects of their charity dressed better than they were? The coats and hats disappeared immediately.[47]

Braden's finest energies were necessarily spent in securing the good will—and the money—that sustained his beloved college. For the latter he continued to rely upon the Methodist Freedmen's Aid Society, private gifts, tuition, and cautious investment. But income from any and all of these was uncertain. Projections and plans based on them were, at best, chimerical. Promises and pledges came easily; hard cash had to be hard won. In a year of financial crisis—1882, for example—Braden asked Cincinnati for $2,000 and was promised $500, but delay forced the trustees of the college to seek a buyer for some of the Meharry properties. The private gifts, though given in largeness of spirit, were too small to meet the gravest need of the college—new buildings. And despite the growing number of students, tuition barely kept pace with expenses for salaries. Many students, being poor, were irregular in their payments: large amounts were perpetually due from former graduates for tuition and board.

John Braden and the Board of Trustees valiantly tried at every turn to find new sources of revenue and to cut expenses. One plan, put forth in 1884, to organize a troupe of singers to raise money in the North only incurred a deficit when an unusually hot summer and the distraction of the national political campaign kept people away from the concerts. By the 1892–93 school year, the college had to borrow money commercially to make repairs on the physical plant.

No such frustrations accompanied the fiscal affairs of the Meharry Medical Department, which had more private donors than all the other departments combined. The gifts from the Meharry family earned a considerable return upon investment. In 1884, the same year as the singing troupe fiasco, the college trustees had $1,000 in medical endowment funds to invest, compared to only $200 from the theological department. The rising enrollments and the increasingly stringent standards for medical education stretched the Medical Department's income; George Hubbard often remarked that he had to make a dollar do the work of ten. But with his scrupulous management, each year's income sufficed to improve the department's facilities, add to its store of equipment, pay its faculty on time, and widen and deepen the learning opportunities.[48]

John Braden's first love remained Christian theology, and his life's work was the training of ministers and missionaries. Mutual admiration and respect preserved a surface peace and cooperation between Dean Hubbard and President Braden. But as the support for theological studies dwindled while that for medicine grew, John Braden's affection for the Meharry Medical Department cooled.

By 1890 Hubbard held the reins of power and authority in the department, and the connection between it and Central Tennessee College had become only nominal. From his position as dean and a seat on the Board of Trustees Executive Committee, he presided over medical affairs with undiluted power. He worked to weld together the department's scattered alumni, recruited faculty members, and raised money. Even such routine matters as the corporal punishment of students, he took into his own hands, carrying out the painful ceremony in his dean's robes.

John Braden was a visionary, an orator, a sunlit personality, while George Hubbard, large of body and slow of speech, was diffident, secretive, indirect. Braden stirred his listeners' emotions, whereas Hubbard moved by persuasion that was gentle, albeit relentless. When he called upon alumni ("my boys") in their homes, he never left without soliciting a contribution. He was also certain to urge the brightest and most esteemed to accompany him back to Nashville to teach at Meharry. Despite his distinct New England drawl and his furtive look, Hubbard held fast these prospective donors and teachers until they gave in to his requests for their money or their lives.

As one of the pioneers and the first leader of Meharry, George Hubbard deserves a foremost place of honor in its history. Hubbard built the first physical plant with gifts secured by Dr. Braden and the early trustees. The idea and the plan for a medical department at Central Tennessee College had sprung from Braden, but the skill and work that made it an actuality came primarily from Dr. Hubbard and the faculty of black doctors whom he and Dr. Sneed trained and then associated with themselves.[49]

As the fortunes of Central Tennessee College continued to sink after 1900, those of Meharry rose. Over the next decade George Hubbard recorded his greatest service, and his faculty saw their students carry the name of Meharry out into the world.

4

"By the Power That Is Within You"

W HEN JOHN BRADEN DIED ON June 10, 1900, another link between
Central Tennessee College and its Meharry Medical Department
dissolved. In voting to change Central Tennessee College's name to Walden
University the following October, the trustees recognized that Meharry
had earned a separate identity. From this time it was known as The Meharry
Medical, Dental, and Pharmaceutical Colleges of Walden University. The
change of name from Central Tennessee College to Walden University was
ostensibly done to "federate the several schools" composing the college and
to honor John M. Walden, the aging bishop of Cincinnati who had devoted
his life to the education of black people in the South. As corresponding
secretary of the Freedmen's Aid Society of the Methodist Church, Walden
had, in 1867, acquired the Gun Factory, the first site of the institution that
now bore his name.[1] The change was also an effort by the Board of Trustees
to strengthen the university's ties to Cincinnati and to loosen the society's
purse strings for the school's needs.

By whatever name, Meharry was growing in size and prestige. By 1890
approximately 130 physicians had graduated, and they numbered more
than half of the black practitioners in the South. The 1890s saw a spectacular growth, with between thirty and forty diplomas presented at each commencement.[2] Meharry is the "most useful medical school in the United
States for Negroes," said a newspaper report in 1908. "Students from all
over the world are attending."[3] The quality of Meharry's faculty, most of
whom were alumni, was one of the reasons for this flowering. In addition to
teaching their skills and attending patients, they served in administrative
posts at the college and worked at the center of black leadership and enterprise in Nashville.

John Angelo Lester, for example, began teaching physiology at Meharry
in 1896, the year after his graduation. Twenty years later, in 1916, he
became dean of the medical faculty and was a tireless fund-raiser in the
college's behalf.[4] Arthur Melvin Townsend (valedictorian in medicine,
Class of 1902) joined the faculty as professor of pathology. He was also a

successful private practitioner, executive of a black Baptist publishing house, and from 1913 to 1918, president of one of Meharry's sister schools in Nashville, Roger Williams University.[5]

Another pathologist compiled a record of service surpassed in length only by Dr. Hubbard himself. Dr. Ferdinand A. Stewart was not a Meharry alumnus, although he had taken a baccalaureate degree at Fisk University in 1885. After he received an M.D. degree from Harvard Medical School in 1888, Dr. Stewart returned to Meharry as lecturer in pathology, assisting Dr. William J. Sneed. Eventually, Stewart succeeded this Meharry pioneer and remained on the faculty until 1931, when he retired after forty-two years' service as a teacher of medicine.[6]

Forces that united these and other black doctors were strong: the challenge of facts to be mastered and taught, a vision of reducing illness and death that beset their people, the political and social oppression that they and their students endured. They held in common the fact of being excluded from membership in the American Medical Association and local medical societies. Formation of professional associations of their own was thus a natural and necessary action.

In several states, including Tennessee, Texas, and North Carolina, Meharry alumni had already founded black medical societies.[7] In 1892 Dr. Miles V. Lynk (Class of 1892) called for "an Association of Medical men of color, national in character" in his *Medical and Surgical Observer,* the first Negro medical journal in America.[8] Lynk and Dr. Robert Fulton Boyd both attended the Cotton States and International Exposition in Atlanta in October 1895. With ten other black physicians present in the city for the occasion, they met and organized the national fraternity of black doctors that Lynk had editorially proposed and elected Dr. Boyd as its first president. Dr. Daniel Hale Williams of Chicago was named vice-president.[9] Meharry Medical College supplied many of the early leaders of the American Medical Society of Colored Physicians and Surgeons, as it was first called. The chartered name was later changed to the National Medical Association.

President from 1904 to 1905, Dr. Charles Victor Roman was often called the Sage of the NMA. His early statement of purpose expressed the organization's abiding goals: "Conceived in no spirit of racial exclusiveness, fostering no ethnic antagonisms, but born of the exigencies of the American environment, the National Medical Association has for its object the banding together, for mutual cooperation and helpfulness, the men and women of African descent who are legally and honorably engaged in the practice of the cognate professions of medicine, surgery, pharmacy, and dentistry."[10]

"Mutual cooperation and helpfulness" was much in evidence at the early conventions of the association. Delegates attended surgical clinics and heard medical papers from their colleagues. The lectures given by the black doctors who had managed hospitals for the care of the sick and the training of medical and nursing students were always sure to be packed. But some means for continual dialogue and proposal was needed, especially by members who practiced in the isolated small towns and countryside of the South. In 1909 the National Medical Association published the first issue of its *Journal,* under the editorship of Dr. Charles Roman. He served as editor for ten years, assisted by a managing editor, Dr. John A. Kenney of Tuskegee Institute.

More state associations of black doctors were formed following the creation of the NMA. Large cities also had affiliate societies. The Tennessee Association of Colored Physicians, Surgeons, Dentists, and Pharmacists (later called the Volunteer State Medical Association) was begun in 1903, evidently as a corporate successor to the Colored Medical Association that the first Meharry graduates organized in 1880.[11] In Nashville the Society of Colored Physicians (later named the R. F. Boyd Medical Society) comprised Meharry alumni and faculty members. Black dentists organized the Capitol City Dental Society there in 1919.

"Nashville was an exciting spot for the National Medical Association," Dr. John Edward Perry wrote. Three times in its early years—1897, 1903, and 1913—the NMA's annual convention met there with Meharry, its faculty, alumni, and friends as hosts. Only a few doctors were present at the 1897 meeting, held in conjunction with the Centennial Exposition of Tennessee, and membership rolls remained short for the next decade. However, the 1913 convention was attended by scores of registrants and observers, eager to exchange scientific information and patient care experiences and to chart a direction for the future. The session was not all work. Perry remembered it as marked by "pomp and splendor" and the consumption of a vast amount of fried chicken.[12]

Besides serving their alma mater as teachers and their community as leaders, Meharry graduates who returned to the campus provided a third important service. Indeed, the example and encouragement given the black student by the presence of a black doctor at the lectern was the culmination of their work. But the hiring of alumni to teach apparently tended to retard change at Meharry at a time when medical schools throughout the nation were being opened to new influences. The most important was the German method of organizing and conducting medical education, as it was introduced at Johns Hopkins University. Medical schools in Germany were departments of a larger university. Their faculty members devoted full time to teaching, caring for patients in modern affiliated hospitals, and working in well-equipped laboratories, one for each of the proliferating specialties. Dissection rooms and clinics were also recognized as indispensable to medical education.[13]

The idea of paying full-time wages was beyond Dr. Hubbard's ken, so the energies and talents of many of Meharry's teachers were divided between their classrooms on campus and their consulting rooms elsewhere in Nashville. And although there were laboratories for dentistry, chemistry, and histology, these did not lend themselves to—and thus discouraged—development of specialized studies. When Dr. Roman returned to Meharry from postgraduate study in Chicago and London, he was shocked to learn that his students were illiterate in the terminology required for clinical work in opthalmology and otolaryngology, and he resolved to involve himself in a fight for higher standards in the college.[14]

The most serious consequence of drawing teachers from among the graduates was the perpetuation of the lecture-quiz system of teaching. Alumni-teachers tended to impart what they had learned years before as students and by the same methods. John Edward Perry noted that even by the second year of medical studies no member of his class had viewed a surgical procedure. In reviewing the causes, symptoms, and treatment of diseases of the circulatory system, for example, Perry and his classmates read the available literature and then underwent examinations. There was little bed-side teaching. The study of medicine at Meharry was, in the 1890s, still "more didactic than practical," Perry wrote in his memoirs.[15]

Increasingly, medical schools would be measured by the new ideas in medical education being brought from Europe. A teaching hospital, attached to the medical school, was chief among these. In opening his infirmary to Meharry students, Dr. Robert Fulton Boyd had recognized the importance of clinical teaching. But the Boyd Infirmary was small and ill-equipped. Opportunities for students to treat patients were limited, and surgery was a rare event. Meharry's continued existence as a proper medical school demanded bedside instruction and practice facilities. It required a hospital where students could learn about diseases and their treatment through observation and experience that brought to life the printed page of their textbooks.

Dr. Hubbard's express desire for a hospital at Meharry arose in part from his compassion for the sick among black people of Nashville. But he was not insensible of the tremors that were shaking the foundations of medical education. In 1899 he traveled to Chicago to attend a conference on standards and curricula and to see what teaching talent he might find. On this particular journey, he would unwittingly set in motion events culminating in the building of a teaching hospital at Meharry.

Hubbard's principal quarry on his journey was Dr. Daniel Hale Williams, whom one fervent admirer called the "bright and morning star in the firmament of Negro surgery."[16] Williams earned that sobriquet in 1893 when he performed the first successful heart surgery in history, a suture of the pericardium to repair the wound made by the thrust of a knife.[17] Although it brought him international acclaim, the operation was only the most spectacular among the many challenging ones done by Williams before he was forty years old. By the end of the century, his profound anatomical knowledge and uncanny surgical judgment had placed him in the front ranks of American surgery.

Born on January 18, 1856, at Hollidaysburg, Pennsylvania, Williams graduated from the Chicago Medical College (later Northwestern University School of Medicine) in 1883, after having been apprenticed to former U.S. Surgeon General Henry Palmer of Janesville, Wisconsin. The eminent pathologist and surgeon, Christian Fenger, was another of Williams's mentors.

In 1891 Williams founded Provident Hospital in Chicago. While serving the city's black population, it provided clinical training to nursing and medical interns, including some from Meharry. Between 1893 and 1898, Williams was surgeon-in-chief at Howard University's Freedmen's Hospital in Washington, D.C., bringing new organizational and scientific ideas to that pioneer institution.

On his visit to Chicago, Dr. Hubbard, at the urging of Drs. Robert Fulton Boyd and Ferdinand Stewart, called upon Williams to ask him to hold surgical clinics at Meharry. Williams was inclined to refuse. But a few moments after Hubbard left his office, Dr. Charles Roman, then a student at the Post Graduate Medical School, arrived. Williams asked the younger man's opinion. At the close of their conversation, he wrote Hubbard a letter of acceptance.[18] In the fall of 1899 Williams arrived in Nashville. By lamp and candlelight, he performed four successful operations in the cramped rooms of the Boyd Infirmary. These facilities did not impress him, despite the claim of "excellent" put forward in the Meharry catalogs.

Before returning home, Williams expressed his reservations frankly to Dr. Hubbard, in the presence of Boyd and Stewart. There was no use, he said, in Meharry's teaching black people to become doctors if it could not provide a hospital experience. A medical student who has had the advantage of the hard practical drill in a hospital, Williams insisted, is ten years ahead of one who is not given it. If Nashville's public hospital would not permit clinical privileges to black students or admit black doctors to practice, then there was only one thing to do. "We can't sit any longer idly and inanely deploring the existing conditions," he said. "We must start our own hospitals and training schools."

Hubbard was dubious. But Boyd and Stewart listened closely as Williams told how Provident Hospital was founded. When he finished, Boyd asked, "Will you come down and tell that story to our people here?" Stewart promised, "We'll gather them in, if you'll just talk to them as you've talked to us today." In January 1900 Williams came back to Nashville for that purpose. On a wintry evening he addressed a capacity audience at the Phyllis Wheatley Club. Nashville and every other city in the South with a population of 10,000 black people must have a black hospital and nurse training school, he told his listeners. The first step they must take, he said, was to believe that it was the right thing. They must examine themselves and determine to their own satisfaction that they had the qualities within them or among them for organization, industry, perseverence, and self-sacrifice. After that, they should choose a leader, someone with influence and enthusiasm, and bring to him "all the support possible."

Williams advised them not to build a hospital immediately: "Rent a house of ten or twelve rooms, preferably one with a basement, furnish it modestly, so that it can be cleaned and kept clean. Select a level-headed graduate nurse for superintendent. . . . Appoint to your staff the best physicians obtainable. . . . Then, when you have done your preparatory work, open your doors and your success will be assured!"

Williams did not leave them without a word about the obstacles they faced. "Do not be deterred," he warned, "by the thought that you may encounter antagonism. Few enterprises, even those for the betterment of mankind, have smooth sailing from the start." He then mentioned the name certain to stir them, Frederick Douglass, and he repeated Douglass's words, spoken to him years before: "The only way you can succeed is to override the obstacles in your path. Hope will be of no avail. . . . By the power *that is within you,* do what you hope to do."

By September 1900 the black people of Nashville had their hospital, a two-story brick structure located at 811 South Cherry Street. Mercy Hospital held, at first, twelve beds, later twenty-three, then thirty-five as it prospered. Its appointments were arranged and its operations managed along the lines suggested by Daniel Hale Williams. From the first, senior medical students from Meharry attended patients.

The post of leader that Williams suggested was soon filled by Robert Fulton Boyd. According to Dr. Roman, Mercy Hospital came into being primarily through the application of Boyd. It was he who bought the building on South Cherry Street—and it was he who drew the fire of the opposition that Williams had predicted. Soon after Boyd closed his purchase, word spread that he was going to establish a hospital. Some of the residents of the area, angry at the prospect, went to court and sought an injunction to prevent the facility from opening, but Boyd proved equal to the challenge. He simply put two workmen to bed and called in a prominent white physician to attend them. At the hearing he pleaded *res adjudicata*—the matter is already settled—and produced the influential doctor, who testified to attending patients at Mercy Hospital. The injunction was denied, and a sympathetic judge mollified to some degree the visceral opposition of the plaintiffs.

Not long after the opening of the 1900–01 school year at Meharry, Daniel Hale Williams began at Mercy Hospital the series of clinics that were to profoundly influence the lives of the students and faculty members who observed him at work. The Meharry catalogs listed the "rare and difficult operations" he performed, including the removal of fibroid tumors, diseased ovaries and tubes, ovarian cysts, and appendixes. Williams was meticulously attentive and methodical, yet his procedures were rapid in the absence of an adequate general anesthetic.[19] The hundreds who crowded into the operating room received a memorable demonstration of an educated touch applied to affliction requiring surgical treatment. After a time, white doctors began joining the students. "They never saw such a clean, swift operator," said Dr. J. H. Holman. "Why, Dr. Dan could sew up a man faster than any sewing machine ever made!"

The Williams clinics were the highlights of each school year at Meharry.[20] Some of the students he trained, including William A. Reed, Julius A. McMillan, and John Henry Hale, graduated with honors and joined the faculty. Reed was professor of materia medica.[21] McMillan's speciality in diseases of the genitourinary tract and his skill in abdominal operations made him one of the South's leading surgeons.[22] The career of John Henry Hale is the subject of a subsequent discussion. These three and others trained by Dr. Dan sustained a Williams tradition at Meharry.

At the same time, divisive forces were inadvertently set in motion on the campus by Daniel Hale Williams's best efforts. It would be years before the full, bitter harvest was reaped. The seeds had indeed been sown prior to Williams's appearance. Under the brilliant light of his work in Nashville, they germinated.

As described by Dr. Charles Roman, the trouble rose from two sources.[23] The first was the faculty, which was split by factions and jealousies. Most of its members had given long service to Meharry. Over the years, Roman wrote, several had developed temperamental idiosyncracies, while others claimed prerogatives, real or imagined, solely for themselves. Dr. Hubbard might have been part of the solution. Instead, Roman averred, he became a second problem. For all his administrative ability, Hubbard had difficulty managing conflicts. He avoided intemperate and unpleasant discussion whenever possible. Moreover, he had few impulses to collective action or cooperation. He arrived at his conclusions and then issued them as edicts, not subject to debate. He convened the faculty, which he regarded as *his* faculty, only to announce, never to discuss or mediate.

It was no doubt difficult to be a forceful advocate for Meharry Medical College before a suspicious, even hostile outside world and, at the same time, be a conciliator, counselor, and democratic dean of one's peers. Even if he had been temperamentally inclined, this last would have been impossible for Hubbard. As the white leader of a black institution, he was expected to preserve an attitude of paternalism and to exercise firm control.

It is possible to speculate that the younger, highly able faculty members, keenly aware of the new currents in medicine, knew also that a struggling black college within a floundering university was likely to remain limited in physical and financial resources. Roman's reference to the claiming of pre-rogatives, real or imagined, suggests that the factions among the faculty may have been caused by competition. One instance of open conflict among ambitious young faculty members is preserved in Roman's memoir. Shortly after Daniel Hale Williams's first visit to the campus, several Meharry teachers began to vie for a place next to him in the public eye. When it became apparent that this would fall to Robert Fulton Boyd, as head of surgery and proprietor of Mercy Hospital, a rival raised a challenge.

By any measure, John T. Wilson (Class of 1895 and clinical instructor),[24] a large man with an attractive personality, was a formidable opponent. He had a reputation as a surgical genius, which dated from an evening not long after he had opened his office in Nashville. An obstetrical patient, whose case was edging into complications, came under his observation, and he determined that a Caesarean delivery would be necessary. Being black, the patient could not be admitted to the public hospital. So in a cramped room by the light of a coal oil lamp, Wilson opened her abdomen and found two babies instead of one. Mother and children survived, and Wilson's name became widely known.

His surgical ambitions kept pace with his fame. Claiming that he had not been fairly dealt with at Meharry, he opened a facility, the Wilson Infirm-ary, to compete with Mercy Hospital. Then he demanded of Dr. Hubbard that the portion of Meharry's annual budget paid to Mercy be divided between his facility and Dr. Boyd's. Dr. Josie Wells widened Wilson's indict-ment. Meharry itself was not being treated equitably at Mercy, she told Dr. Hubbard. Some members of the faculty supported Boyd, some Wilson, and some remained neutral. Partisans held their views fiercely. But, accord-ing to Roman, each one gave an overriding loyalty to Dr. Hubbard.

A meeting of the entire faculty with the dean presiding might have ended the controversy. But Hubbard, preferring the intimate chat and the solitary decision, could not or would not attempt such a conference. There-fore, it fell to Dr. Boyd himself to put forward an idea that all could support, under the unifying power of the dean's name. Before an assembly of the faculty, he proposed the building of a hospital to be named in honor of Dr. Hubbard.

Boyd's motion called upon the spirit instilled in many by the Williams clinics. Mercy Hospital, the scene of those spectacular occasions, had be-come more and more crowded; Meharry, moreover, did not even own or operate it. The time had come, Boyd insisted, to build the hospital attached to Meharry that Williams envisioned at the Phyllis Wheatley Club on that cold evening in 1900. Boyd's colleagues adopted his idea, and The George W. Hubbard Hospital Association, comprising prominent Nashvillians and friends of Meharry, was created to raise money. Ten thousand dollars, they estimated, would be required to complete the first unit. Even the most optimistic thought that such a sum could not be attained for several years. Nonetheless, within a few months, the Executive Committee—Robert Fulton Boyd, chairman, Charles Victor Roman, vice-chairman, John A. Kumler, Henry T. Noel, and Arthur M. Townsend, secretary—posted more than half that amount to its credit. The effort exhausted solicitors and donors alike. As the school year 1909–10 opened, the association's effort was at a standstill.

Dr. Hubbard assembled the Executive Committee for a council of desperation and invited the venerable Bishop Walden, who had spent a lifetime turning adversity to account. After several doleful speeches, Walden's among them, Hubbard turned to Roman for a cheerful word. Roman recalled what then took place: "Maybe the thought was unconsciously generated and needed the stimulus of speech. Be that as it may, I answered at once, 'Charge, Chester, charge! On, Stanley, on!' I move that we break ground at Commencement and dedicate the building at the opening of the next session!"

"God bless you, young man!" cried Bishop Walden as the motion was greeted with an enthusiastic chorus of ayes. With a new letterhead featuring Dr. Hubbard's portrait ("Shall we honor him while he lives?") and a sketch of the hospital ("now in process of erection"), the drive to meet Roman's deadlines was mounted. Brochures, broadsheets, and articles in friendly newspapers extolled Hubbard's career and unhesitantly reminded alumni of the obligations—financial as well as spiritual—that they owed as individuals and as black people to Meharry and its dean: "These should remember that Dr. Hubbard did not hold his means selfishly. Likewise, they should not hold their means selfishly. . . . These should not forget that Dr. Hubbard at great personal sacrifice and inconvenience to himself made it possible for many of them to graduate while still owing money to the school."[25]

Work began on the site, on Second Avenue, South near Chestnut Street, in April 1910. The first operation was performed in the building in October, and by mid-December the wing surrounding the surgical theater was complete. It was three stories tall and sixty feet long. Besides the operating room, where as many as twenty-five students could observe, there were twenty-two rooms. At first Hubbard Hospital did not have outpatient clinics—Dr. Hubbard opposed them—but during the first year as many bed patients were admitted as the institution could accommodate. Although still unfinished when it was dedicated in November 1912, Hubbard Hospital had by that date beds for 80 sick people and could receive up to 100 in emergencies.

The dean, faculty, and trustees all wanted to finish construction as soon as possible. Andrew Carnegie gave $10,000, half the estimated cost of completion, and Julius Rosenwald, $1,000. When Dr. Robert Fulton Boyd

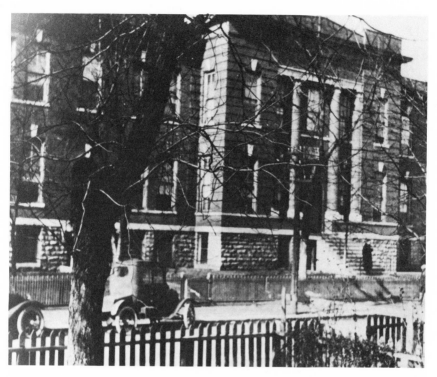

Hubbard Hospital (c. 1915)

died in July 1912, $5,000 was willed from his estate. The balance came from smaller individual, church, and corporate gifts. By 1916 construction was complete. Dr. Josie Wells, formally reporting to Dr. Hubbard as superintendent, had charge of the institution. Speaking to a local congregation in the interest of the hospital's development, she said, "One object of the hospital is to come into touch with the home life of the people."[26]

Where black people established their hospitals, Dr. Daniel Hale Williams had observed in 1900, the way was open for nursing education. Soon after its founding, Mercy Hospital began offering a training program for nursing, enlarging the work begun at Central Tennessee College two decades before. Between 1900 and 1906, twenty-five nurses graduated from Mercy Hospital. When the George W. Hubbard Hospital opened in 1910, the training school for nurses was transferred there. Two types of programs were offered: a "non-professional course," which required two years of nine months each, and a "professional course," which required

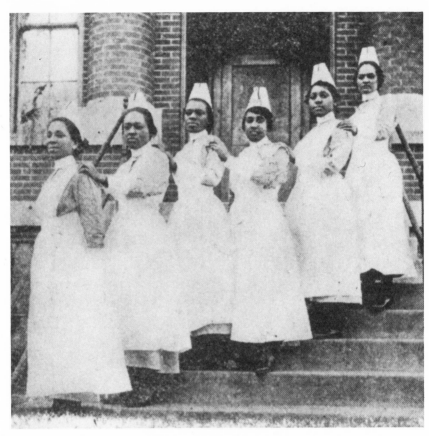

Nurse training class, 1918

three years of the same duration. The former, open to students who could not devote all their time to training, was soon discontinued.

Charmian C. Hunt, a graduate of the nursing school of the Women and Children's Hospital in Boston, was employed as the first superintendent of the George W. Hubbard Training School, as the nurse education program was called. At first, two graduate students composed the entire faculty; thus, some classes were taught by physicians from Meharry. Twelve students enrolled in the first class. Two—Lula Woolfolk and Hulda Margaret Lyttle—completed the course in 1912. They were joined by Rhoda A. Pugh, trained at the Wilson Infirmary, so there were three graduates in the first nursing class of Hubbard Hospital.

That same year, Hubbard nurses attempted to take the examination required for a license from the State of Tennessee. When they arrived at the prescribed time and place, the secretary of the licensing board refused to administer the test to them. Protests by black citizens and the Rock City Academy of Medicine led state officials to reconsider the prohibition.

In 1914 two graduates of the Hubbard Training School were permitted to take the examination under conditions of pressure and difficulty. The two, Minnie D. Woodward-Smith and Rhoda Pugh, were employed by the health department of Nashville at the time. Called from their work one afternoon, they were presented an examination over ten nursing subjects. Although allowed no time for review, they both earned passing grades. Thereafter, Meharry's nursing graduates were admitted to the state examination without opposition.

Several new courses of instruction had been added to the nursing curriculum by 1920, and two years later the entrance requirement was raised to the completion of a four-year high school course. In addition to a mastery of nursing subjects, teacher's training was required of faculty members. Hulda M. Lyttle (Class of 1912) had resigned a teaching post at the Southern University School of Nursing in 1916 to return to Meharry as director of Nurse Training. In 1921 she was named superintendent of Hubbard Hospital. Although her titles and the nomenclature of the department changed, she remained head of the nursing program for more than twenty years. By the mid-1930s, more than 200 women had graduated in nursing at Meharry's Hubbard Hospital and were established in nursing practice in nearly every state in the Union. Many held positions in hospital administration, on the faculties of nursing schools, and in public health centers.[27]

The period between the opening of Hubbard Hospital and World War II saw the construction of many great medical centers and research institutions. Large outlays of money were spent for new facilities and equipment. Innovations in diagnosis and therapeutics followed one another with bewildering rapidity. The medical literature reporting these developments became so vast that no single physician could possibly read more than a fraction of it.[28]

This revolution in medicine and medical learning was given impetus in June 1910 by the publication of a little book with the unprepossessing title, *Medical Education in the United States and Canada: A Report to The Carnegie Foundation for the Advancement of Teaching.* Popularly called the Flexner Report after its author, Abraham Flexner, the book was a climax as well as a prelude. Efforts to reform medical schools had been under way for half a century, carried on by medical educators and various associations that they formed. Although these efforts achieved some successes, grave abuses and defects remained. The majority of medical schools in America were still

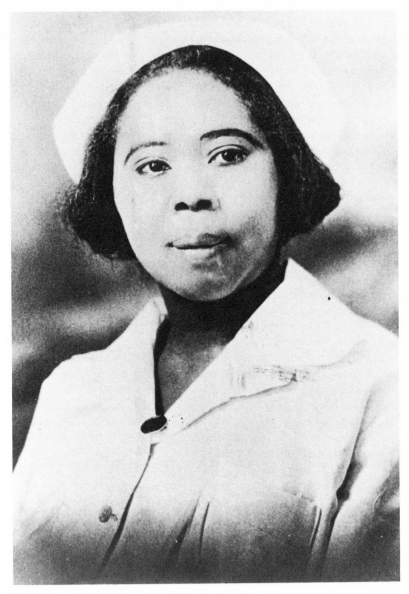

Hulda M. Lyttle

privately owned and commercially operated for profit. Academic standards were low. Curricula varied from school to school, so that the degree of M.D. was held by both frauds and bona fide practitioners, by faddists and skilled surgeons. Entrance requirements were nonexistent or unenforced. Many schools drew unprepared young men out of industrial occupations by the use of advertising. In general, anyone who was able to pay tuition could attend some medical school. The result, Abraham Flexner noted, was "an enormous over-production of uneducated and ill-trained medical practitioners." America had four or five times as many physicians in proportion to the population as did some European nations.

In the first part of his report, Flexner proposed ways to reduce the number of medical school graduates and suggested reforms in medical teaching so that those who did graduate might be physicians of high caliber. He strongly favored a scientific medical school organized around strong basic science departments and thus designed a curriculum—one with fundamental courses taught in laboratories and lecture rooms during the first two years, and clinical work in medicine, surgery, and obstetrics the last two years. Junior and senior students would be assigned to assist with the care of patients in the medical school's own hospital. Flexner recommended that a college diploma with credits in chemistry, biology, and physics be required for admission, and he suggested a fifth year of medical school, the internship.

The ideal medical school, the report continued, would encourage research and employ a full-time faculty, all of whose members were at once physicians, scientists, scholars, and teachers. There would be no room for "the scientifically dead practitioner whose knowledge had long since come to a standstill and whose lectures, composed when he first took his chair, like pebbles in a rolling brook, get smoother and smoother as the stream of time rolls over them."

As for the commercial schools, the bane of the profession, Flexner proposed to close them down rapidly and systematically. He thought that state governments had an obligation to protect the public by passing rigid licensure laws enforced by vigilant, incorruptible registration boards. Such boards would make it impossible for schools whose first interest was profits to survive. They could not afford full-time faculties, laboratories, and teaching hospitals, and without these, their students could not hope to learn enough medicine to pass state examinations.

In the second part of the report, Flexner described the facilities and methods of instruction at the medical schools he had visited in preparing his study. When he came to the fraudulent, the incompetent, the inefficient, he did not mince words. Two medical schools in Arkansas were "without a single redeeming feature." Three medical schools in Texas were "without resources, without ideals, without facilities." Establishments at

Knoxville and Chattanooga were "utterly wretched." He reserved praise only for those that approached creditable standards. Turning to black medical schools, he reported:

> Of the seven schools for Negroes in the United States (Howard University in Washington, D.C.; Flint Medical College at New Orleans; Leonard Medical School at Raleigh, N.C.; Knoxville Medical College at Knoxville, Tenn.; the Medical Department of the University of West Tennessee at Memphis; Meharry Medical College at Nashville; and National Medical College at Louisville), five are at this moment in no position to make a contribution of value. . . . Flint at New Orleans, Leonard at Raleigh, the Knoxville, Memphis, and Louisville schools are ineffective. They are wasting small sums of money annually and sending out undisciplined men whose lack of real training is covered up by the imposing M.D. degree.
>
> Meharry at Nashville and Howard at Washington are worth developing, and until considerably increased benefactions are available, effort will wisely concentrate upon them. . . . The upbuilding of Howard and Meharry will profit the nation much more than the inadequate maintenance of a larger number of schools.[29]

The Flexner Report aroused considerable ire among educators whose schools it pronounced worthless. But almost as soon as it appeared, two influential groups endorsed the reforms it recommended and urged the nation's medical schools to adopt them. The first was that segment of physicians organized as the American Medical Association. Its Council on Medical Education designed a system of accreditation based on the report. Having opened Hubbard Hospital, Meharry met one important criterion fixed by the AMA. It obtained an "A" rating when the council first awarded accreditation, with the understanding that certain other standards for teaching were to be met within a specific period of time.

The second group was the foundations headed by such wealthy men as Andrew Carnegie, John D. Rockefeller, Julius Rosenwald, George Eastman, and Edward Harkness. They thought that American medicine would be improved and the public benefited if Flexner's ideas could be implemented. They realized, however, that the medical schools themselves could never raise enough money through tuition or investment to build the laboratories and hospitals and to pay the faculty salaries that Flexner envisioned. If these things were to be done, the resources of medical schools would have to be supplemented by philanthropy.

In selecting medical schools to receive assistance, the foundations followed Flexner's advice closely. As earlier noted, Carnegie and Rosenwald funds helped complete Hubbard Hospital. These gifts together with the annual contributions from the Freedmen's Aid and Southern Education Society, student tuition, and alumni support enabled Dr. Hubbard to manage without a deficit. But he was not always certain, as each new academic year began, where the money would come from to see Meharry through to the end of the spring session.

At a meeting of the Board of Trustees in January 1919, authority was given to Bishop Thomas Nicholson and Dr. P. J. Maveety, trustees and officers of the Freedmen's Aid and Southern Education Society, to represent Meharry in an application to leading foundations for grants to begin an endowment fund. Such a fund would allow Meharry to budget and to plan for expansion.

The following March the two men reported that the Carnegie Foundation and the General Education Board of the Rockefeller Foundation had each agreed to give Meharry $150,000, provided certain conditions were met. The first was that, upon Dr. Hubbard's retirement, "a man of scientific training in medicine" be appointed to succeed him. Second, the money would be paid "provided the reorganization of said medical school is carried out along modern lines." Third, the trustees of Meharry and the Methodist Church would be required to raise an additional $200,000 so that the college might have, upon payment of the grants, a total endowment of a half million dollars.

Dr. Maveety assumed responsibility for leading the fund-raising drive. The alumni, faculty, and student body assisted him with a pledge of $10,000. The Methodist Church, embarking upon the Centenary Movement, which celebrated 100 years of Methodist missions in America, raised a million dollars for all its black schools and colleges. In 1921 the managers of the Board of Educational Institutions for Negroes, successor to the Freedmen's Aid and Southern Education Society, announced that the funding conditions set by the foundations had been met, and the money was promptly paid over.[30]

The required reorganization of Meharry began with a new legal life, a charter from the State of Tennessee granting it separate existence from the failing Walden University. Although considered by some to be the best of the Freedmen's Aid Society schools, Walden University had continued its downward course after the death of President John Braden. By 1910 it desperately needed new buildings and an endowment to command and pay a faculty of recognized worth. In cooperation with the society, the pastors and members of the Tennessee Conference of the Methodist Episcopal Church made valiant efforts to raise money for Walden. Conference leaders directed that a financial rally be held in each church during the second week in May, culminating in "Walden Sunday." Funds raised during these campaigns were sent to the university. The alumni also organized a campaign to pay for the construction of a new administration building. But these efforts did not put the school beyond the constant threat of bankruptcy and collapse.[31]

George W. Hubbard, dean of Meharry, had succeeded John Braden to serve as acting president of Walden for the year 1900–01. In 1902 Dr. J. Hamilton Benson of New York was installed as president. As seen earlier, Meharry's ties to its parent university were weakening during this period. No sooner had the medical department attained solvency than it was called upon to share its resources with the larger institution. As Walden continued to sink for lack of support, deepening its dependence upon Meharry, Dr. Hubbard began to have doubts about their affiliation. These doubts were exacerbated by personal conflicts between him and President Benson. According to Charles Victor Roman, the formal truce observed between the university and the medical college shattered upon Benson's installation.

A horrifying disaster widened the breach between the two men and their schools. Near midnight on December 18, 1903, a fire broke out in one of the two residential units on the Walden campus. Six young women burned to death, six more were killed as they leaped from windows to escape the flames, and many others were seriously injured. Lawsuits for more than $150,000 were filed in state and federal courts, naming Walden and its administrators and managers as defendants. As long as these were pending—and several years were required to settle them—the university's lawyers advised Walden not to erect new buildings or to purchase new equipment.[32]

As shrewd investors, the Carnegie and Rockefeller trustees were not prepared to see their grants to Meharry encumbered by possible judgments against Walden or attached to pay the university's debts. Separation of the two schools seemed the prudent course. Dr. Hubbard agreed.

But as evangelical Christians, determined to instruct students morally as well as intellectually, leaders of the Methodist Church were reluctant to relinquish control of Meharry. Some members of the Board of Managers of the Freedmen's Aid and Southern Education Society denounced the terms of the proposed new charter. In no wise, they said, should the Church surrender Meharry "for the sake of a thousand or a few thousand dollars." Vanderbilt University, also in Nashville, had been lost to secular hands when these same two foundations extended their philanthropy. Meharry's fate would be the same if it were to become independent.

Bishop Francis J. McConnell responded in favor of the Carnegie and Rockefeller grants and their attached conditions. He argued that a medical education was of a special technical character, involving no ethical or religious principle that would be jeopardized by a new charter. Moreover, the church simply could no longer support Meharry as it needed to be supported. McConnell concluded by saying that he saw no other way than to permit Meharry its own separate existence.[33]

His view prevailed, and the Freedmen's Aid Society came to an agreement with the trustees of Meharry and the foundations on the terms of a new charter. The Church would retain ownership of most of Meharry's property, and the society's financial and spiritual support for the college would continue as it had, unbroken, for half a century.

On September 30, 1915, a dozen leaders, both black and white, from medicine, religion, and education applied for a charter of incorporation in the name of Meharry Medical College. Two weeks later it was granted. By the charter's terms, the incorporators assumed the management of Meharry and its schools of medicine, dentistry, pharmacy, and nurse training. They were also given the power to operate "a hospital or hospitals" and "such other privileges as are usually possessed by medical colleges, including the power to confer degrees." The following January, these leaders adopted bylaws and provided for the governance of Meharry through an eighteen-member board of trustees.

While Meharry was establishing itself on an independent footing, the Freedmen's Aid Society was considering closing Walden University altogether, so that its land and buildings could be turned over to the medical college. This expansion, together with the prospective endowment from the foundations, the society reasoned, would place Meharry in the front rank of American medical schools.

The idea remained dormant until 1922. By that year the number of students declined so far as to make impractical Walden's continued existence as a four-year college. Instead, the Board of Educational Institutions for Negroes renewed support for the school as a two-year campus, purchased a new site for it, and allowed Meharry possession of the old one.[34] With independence from Walden, a part of the changes urged by the foundations was complete. But there remained the reorganization of teaching and administration at Meharry along modern lines, essentially those set out in the Flexner Report. Reforms in curricula, in the role of the faculty and the place of the hospital, and in qualifications of students and graduates required no money. They did require a willingness to surrender traditional views in the face of the new standards proposed for medical education.

To the managers and trustees of Meharry, assembled under the new charter, fell the responsibility of selecting the college's first president. Of course, no one other than Dr. Hubbard was considered for the post, since he had devoted his entire life to Meharry's development. But George Hubbard, nearing eighty years old, was withering in body and weakening in mind. The year-to-year struggle to make old buildings, old equipment, and old methods serve ever-larger classes was taxing his strength beyond the point of renewal. Bold plans such as those Flexner proposed seemed to mock his efforts. The swifter the current grew, the more he strained against it. The irresistible forces of change and the immovable object representing years of devotion and mission and labor were set against each other; the result was disaster. Beginning with Dr. Charles Roman, historians of Meharry have called these years of Hubbard's presidency "the tragic period."

At his inauguration in Meharry's auditorium on October 19, 1916, Hubbard reviewed the forty years of the college's existence. He pointed to the more than 500 students enrolled as of that date in medicine, dentistry, pharmacy, and nurse training, and to Meharry's 2,000 graduates who were practicing all over the United States and as missionaries in Africa. At the conclusion of his address, the alumni presented President Hubbard a check for $10,000, chiefly the gift of Dr. John Wesley Anderson (M.D., Class of 1883; D.D.S., Class of 1888), to be used for the construction of an anatomical sciences building. The dedication of Anderson Anatomical Hall in October 1917 was evidently Dr. Hubbard's last concession to innovation at Meharry.[35]

One night not long after his inauguration, Hubbard lapsed into a coma. Although he was roused without general alarm, he soon began to exhibit symptoms of serious physical decline and mental conflict. Two matters, especially, had weighed upon him for years. The first was his failure to interest the sons and daughters of the five founding Meharry brothers in the school that bore their name. The other was the ostracism he suffered from white people because of his work in helping to educate black men and women. His decline had also been hastened by a second brief term as acting president of Walden University, during the 1913–14 school year. The new president of Walden, Dr. George F. Durgin, sought to reassert the university's control over Meharry and to compel Dr. Hubbard to report to him. Hubbard drew heavily upon his physical and mental capacities to preserve what he considered his due authority.

The final separation of the two schools aged him perceptibly. Many of Walden's graduates blamed him for the failure of the university's other departments, rather than congratulating him on the success of his own. A more serious complication grew out of Meharry's new charter. When Dr. Hubbard assumed the title "President," several candidates offered themselves for an apparent vacancy in the deanship. Their campaigns divided the alumni and further beset Hubbard.

During 1919 and 1920 he experienced the worst mental aberrations of his long illness. His physical infirmities alternated with his mental difficulties. He sometimes went about his duties befogged; at other times, he lay helpless in body, though perfectly lucid in mind. "Matters went from bad to worse," Dr. Charles Roman recalled, "until the trustees decided to take the reins out of Dr. Hubbard's hands." In the winter of 1920 they accepted his resignation. With funds from the college treasury and alumni gifts, a new home was built on the campus for the former president and his wife.

The death of Mrs. Sarah Lyon Hubbard in 1921 deepened the shadows over Dr. Hubbard's life. But for nearly three years he was able to go auto riding and to entertain friends who came to call. He apparently bore no resentment over the trustees' action in forcing his resignation, nor did he attempt to interfere in the management of the college.[36] In August 1924 George Whipple Hubbard died in Nashville, the last of the Civil War missionaries in the South.

5

Wider Horizons, Deeper Roots

Dr. JOHN J. MULLOWNEY was installed as the second president of Meharry Medical College on February 1, 1921. Immediately he set to work to dispel the atmosphere of despair that had settled over the campus in the last months of Dr. Hubbard's faltering stewardship. There was plenty of reason for despondency. Meharry in the winter of 1921 was deep in crisis. Its buildings were in a state of disrepair, their staircases broken, their banisters loose, their windows smoke-begrimed. Its library consisted of only 2,500 books, many on religious and pseudoscientific subjects. A sink, two dozen microscopes, and a few jars of specimens were all the tools available for the teaching of pathology and bacteriology. At Hubbard Hospital patients were neglected, asepsis was entirely absent, and surgery proceeded with inadequate equipment in cramped, infectious surroundings. Students commonly absented themselves from their classes, or else whiled away the hour over a newspaper, awaiting their turn at a microscope. Members of the faculty were overworked and underpaid, and there was no money to hire more.[1]

Dr. Mullowney came to Meharry knowing its problems. They had cost the college its "A" rating when the American Medical Association made its second inspection of the nation's medical schools. Thirteen states refused to admit graduates of class "B" institutions to license examinations. Half of those states were in the South, where Meharry graduates were badly needed. At his first meeting with the faculty, Mullowney pledged to help them win back the AMA's highest evaluation. They could do it, he said, through work—work for everybody, work all the time, work everywhere.[2]

Hard work, sometimes of the hardscrabble variety, had been John James Mullowney's lot throughout his life. Born in England in 1877, Mullowney lost his father and then his mother before he was eight years old. The orphanage in which he was placed soon sent him to Canada to work on a farm. There was little opportunity for books and schooling on the frontier; nevertheless the boy's desire for an education blossomed. Still in his teens,

60

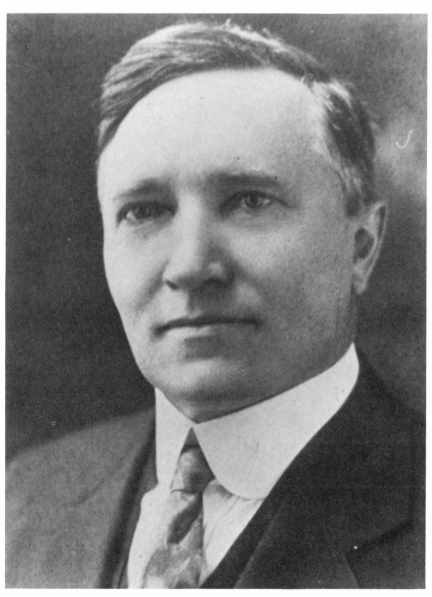

John J. Mullowney

he crossed the border and settled in a New Hampshire village, taking any odd job for the wherewithal to finish high school. His ambition and energy earned him the sympathy of the local Methodist minister and the principal of the high school, both of whom encouraged him to continue his studies. Diligent application to books became overwork, however, and it brought Mullowney to the point of collapse. He contracted tuberculosis and survived it only through the same methodical devotion to deep breathing and physical exercise that he had given to study.

The Methodist Church lent him part of the money he needed to attend the Medical Department of the University of Pennsylvania, the oldest medical school in America. When Mullowney enrolled it was throbbing with the vital influence of Dr. William Osler, one of the greatest clinicians of the nineteenth century.

While still a medical student, Mullowney became interested in working as a Christian missionary. He offered his services to the Methodist Board of Foreign Missions, and upon his graduation in 1908 he was sent to China. For three and a half years he served in the Hopkins Memorial Hospital in Peking and taught at North China Union Medical College (which later became Peking Medical College), a teaching service of Harvard University School of Medicine. For his work among victims of the bubonic plague, the Chinese government awarded him several decorations in the name of the nation.

Returning to America Dr. Mullowney began pursuing a special interest in public health and preventive medicine. He held several posts in the health departments of the City of Philadelphia and the Commonwealth of Pennsylvania before joining the faculty of Girard College. There he was chairman of the Department of Science. It was this position that he resigned to become, at age forty-two, president of Meharry Medical College.[3]

The emphasis that Mullowney laid on continuous activity "caused some creaking in the machinery," Dr. Charles Roman observed.[4] But in a short time the new president and the faculty, working together for the first time in anyone's memory, wrought more improvements at Meharry than had been seen in twenty years. Nine months into the new administration, in November 1921, Dr. N. P. Colwell of the American Medical Association made another inspection tour of Meharry. This time he found a "well-arranged, well-conducted medical school where active teaching is everywhere in evidence." Entrance requirements were being rigidly applied. Laboratories were in better order than in previous years, and the instructors, most of whom were black, commanded the full attention of students. There were none wandering around aimlessly as had been reported in the past. Colwell also found that the hospital, an adjunct to the campus during the Hubbard years, was becoming the essential place of learning and an important health center for the surrounding community.[5]

As one of his first acts, Dr. Mullowney hired sufficient staff to keep Hubbard Hospital open at all times. It had formerly been closed from June until October 1, while students were on vacation, in an effort to save money. Each fall students and faculty had to campaign throughout Nashville seeking sick people who would admit themselves to the hospital. Each spring there was a general clearing out, every patient having to be discharged before the close of the spring term. There was, Mullowney noted, "a woeful lack of continuity of service for the community and in the training of young medical people."

But where was the money to come from for the additional four months of service—for surgical supplies, drugs, bedding, salaries? As they often had in the past, the alumni provided the answer and the wherewithal. On a long, exhausting tour among them, Mullowney raised $200,000 for Hubbard Hospital.[6] With a part of this largess, he directed improvements in the hospital's outpatient services.

Throughout its first half century Meharry had opened its doors without charge to patients who were able and willing to present themselves for treatment before medical students. Since the founding of Hubbard Hospital they had been received in an area designated as the "dispensary." The reforms instituted by Dr. Mullowney, under the dispensary's director, Dr. John Henry Hale, included new examining rooms, laboratories, and, later, specialty clinics.[7] Meharry opened an additional dispensary and dental operatory in north Nashville in 1923.[8]

For those who were homebound and also indigent, a Social Service Department was established in Hubbard Hospital in 1927. Under the direction of Miss Grace Harrison, it identified to welfare agencies, public and private, persons throughout the city who were in need of financial assistance and made known their need for medical attention to Meharry physicians and nurses.[9]

Significant reforms in Hubbard Hospital's bed services were undertaken at the same time as the new initiatives in outpatient care, beginning with the reorganization of six disciplines into three units: Diagnosis and Internal Medicine, Surgery and Gynecology, and Obstetrics and Pediatrics. Upon admission, patients were assigned to one of these departments for treatment by a physician and study by medical students. In order to isolate those who might have an unsuspected communicable disease, wards in each department were no larger than five beds.

A division of labor and an equitable distribution of patient fees among the resident physicians raised morale. With the recruitment of a new superintendent, Dr. Paul Dietrich, who succeeded the late Dr. Josie Wells, the changes most urgently needed at Hubbard Hospital were complete. They had not cost a great deal of money, but neither had they solved all the problems. The hospital still needed more space, scientific stores, and support staff, and these things would be expensive. With the cash and pledges from the alumni in hand, Mullowney appealed to the foundations and churches for still more money. Dr. Wallace Buttrick, president of the General Education Board, answered the plea with a personal visit to the Meharry campus and a survey of its needs. He agreed that Hubbard Hospital required additional space and new equipment. The board would underwrite the costs, he told Mullowney, and authorized him to proceed.

In July 1923 construction was begun on a third story to the hospital. When it was completed the departments of obstetrics and pediatrics and surgery were relocated there. Accompanying the enlargement were many other improvements, including additional beds, new X-ray equipment, and a morgue with autopsy rooms. Elevators, call systems, and private facilities for the medical staff completed the amenities. The total cost was $88,000, over three times the amount required to build Hubbard Hospital in 1910. It was paid in full with $83,000 from the General Education Board and $5,000 from the Julius Rosenwald Fund.

The most important measure of Hubbard Hospital's value, its capacity to care for patients, was greatly increased by the reforms of 1921–23. A total of 140 sick people could be accommodated in the hospital, and the outpatient department was now staffed and organized to treat thousands annually and to continue that treatment over a period of time when necessary.

The medical course was strengthened by other gifts. Meharry built a new chemistry laboratory for the students of Dr. T. H. Elliott and a new pathological and bacteriological laboratory for those of Dr. J. H. Holman.

There was still the matter of the "A" rating from the American Medical Association. One last, seemingly insuperable barrier stood in the way: the AMA's accrediting rules required top-rated schools to have an endowment of $1 million. "A cool million!" John J. Mullowney wrote. "The vastness of the sum frightened me. . . . Where could I ever raise ONE MILLION DOLLARS? . . . That is what the pessimists bellowed at me."

The pessimists would be proven wrong. The endowment of Meharry did attain that sum, though not for several years. Meanwhile, Meharry's oldest friend, the Methodist Church, provided a plan and the means. The Church's Board of Higher Education for Negroes (originally, the Freedmen's Aid Society) approached the AMA and inquired if it would award Meharry an "A" provided the board made a grant each year equal to the interest on one million dollars. The proposal was approved, and the "A" was restored.

Praise rained down on Meharry's president, its faculty, and its students. The college's diplomas would henceforth be accepted by every state, and in England, as a sufficient credential to apply for a license to practice. Amid the general celebration, however, Meharrians were aware that even more

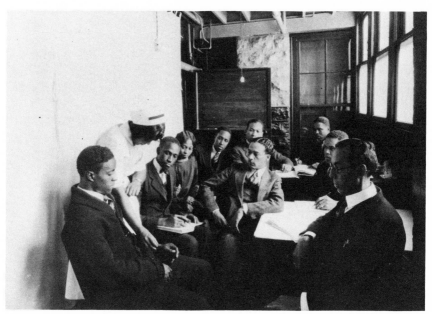

Third-year class in history and diagnostics

needed to be done. The improvements that had been made were partly makeshifts and stopgaps.[10]

The administration building, raised in 1880 as the original home of the medical department of Central Tennessee College, had come to be the outward symbol of Meharry. Inside it was blackened with the smudge and smoke from the soft coal that belched from Nashville's chimneys. A single naked bulb lit the landings, and high under the old roof Meharry's twelve poorest students were given tiny sleeping rooms—a firetrap of a dormitory—in exchange for maintenance work around the campus.

A barnlike auditorium, erected in 1908 by revivalists for the purpose of conducting evangelical worship services among Meharry students, was solidly built. So was the Dental-Pharmaceutical Building, dating from 1889. But inside, classrooms were fashioned from cheap partitions and workbenches were made by nailing planks to the walls.

In the north section of Nashville, Fisk University also needed new buildings. Fisk and Meharry had both been founded during the Reconstruction era, and many Meharry alumni had received their baccalaureate degrees from Fisk. The General Education Board, which supported the aspirations of both schools, had been reflecting for a time on their similar problem. Its members raised the question: What if Meharry could be moved from its original site and reestablished in a new physical plant near Fisk? Thereby the schools could share certain facilities.

Most members of the board probably favored the actual merger of Fisk and Meharry. Since its separation from Walden University in 1915, Meharry had been one of the few medical schools in the United States not affiliated with a university. Most medical educators clearly thought that their schools derived intellectual advantages from a university milieu and financial benefits from its access to money and other development resources. Since the first surveys of medical education by the American Medical Association in 1901, and particularly after the Flexner Report in 1910, the majority of independent medical schools had merged with universities.

The faculty and other leaders of Meharry very much wanted the new plant. Its students could imagine the opportunities it would open to them. No member of the college was willing to surrender its separate identity, however, regardless of the incentive. In February 1928 the Meharry Board of Trustees formally requested the General Education Board "to provide a modern, adequate plant . . . and the additional finances necessary to maintain the same." In a strong caveat they chose the single road, in behalf of all Meharrians: "It is understood that the proposed project does not require the losing of the individuality of Meharry Medical College, nor the loss of its corporate existence."[11]

There would continue to be a liberal arts college and a medical college, rather than the one university envisioned by the Rockefeller Foundation. The officers of the General Education Board were disappointed, but they were no less interested in helping Meharry gain a first-rate plant for its hospital and classrooms. To that end, the board appropriated $1.5 million toward the cost of a new campus. Large amounts were also given by George Eastman of the Kodak Corporation, by the Julius Rosenwald Fund, and by the Edward Harkness Foundation. A campaign among the citizens of Nashville and among Meharry alumni raised $50,000.[12]

The trustees purchased six acres on Eighteenth Avenue, North, a mile northwest of Tennessee's capitol and the heart of downtown Nashville. The site was bounded on the south by Albion Street, on the north by Heffernan Street (later called Meharry Boulevard), and on the west by Twenty-first Avenue, North. Across Eighteenth Avenue, the new campus's eastern border, stood Jubilee Hall, built with funds raised by Fisk University's famed Jubilee Singers.

This part of north Nashville, like Meharry's first neighborhood in the southern part of the city, was heavily settled by black people. They or their immediate forebears had come for the most part from a sprawling ghetto lying between the railroad tracks and the foot of Capitol Hill in the old central city. Known as "Hell's Half-Acre," it had persisted since Recon-struction, when many destitute freed people had settled there. In the last decades of the nineteenth century, many of the male residents of "Hell's Half-Acre" were intermittently employed as unskilled laborers in the fac-tories and foundries nearby. Black women found jobs as domestics in the fine homes along Vine and High streets, or as maids in the hotels and eating places that served the passenger depot.

The desertion of the downtown area by the well-to-do and its conversion into retail stores, office buildings, and boarding houses displaced many of the residents of this ghetto. Between 1890 and 1920, Negro settlement rolled away toward the northwest, through the wards of the city divided by the railroad tracks. The growth of this black neighborhood was rigidly constrained by German settlements north of Jefferson Street and the white corridor of West End Avenue. Over each succeeding decade, Nashville's black people became increasingly concentrated in this northern tier of wards and in south Nashville. But whereas the latter area, Meharry Medi-cal College's original neighborhood, was a mixed community, north Nashville did not attract many white people.[13]

The particular parcel of property that Meharry acquired was a densely populated block of residences, owned for the most part by their occupants. The first task facing the college was to provide for the resettlement of these families. Although it was accomplished with as little difficulty as possible, the change in the character of the area was resented by many residents. Meharry came into its new home suspected, distrusted, and disliked by many of its neighbors.

Construction began in 1930 and continued throughout the following year and a half. Meharry's students and faculty were cheered by every new level that the carpenters and engineers raised. Everyone was eager to make a new beginning in a new place, believing that the old troubles—factions, personal quarrels, perpetual shortages—would be left behind.

At the beginning of the fall term of 1931, Meharry occupied its new quarters, three modern brick buildings. The main building housed vir-tually the entire college and hospital, including the schools of medicine, dentistry, pharmacy, and nursing. The second building was a dormitory for nursing students and the third, a power plant. Attached to the main build-ing was an auditorium, the Public Health Lecture Hall. Besides being available for Meharry assemblies, this facility was open to public lectures on community hygiene.

The main building, executed in a simple modern style, was faced with red brick of local manufacture and trimmed with native limestone. From its core, cubical in shape, four wings projected north and south. The George W. Hubbard Hospital was located in the two southern wings in order to provide as much sunlight as possible to its solaria. Separate rooms,

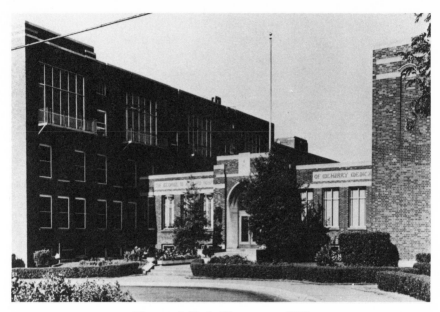

The north Nashville campus, 1931

arrayed throughout the four floors, were assigned to outpatient clinics and to the departments of roentgenology, surgery, obstetrics, and pediatrics. There were beds for 185 patients.

The outpatient department had its own entrance from Eighteenth Avenue, North, above which its name, Dispensary, was carved in stone. Obstetrical and pediatric cases, diseases of the eye, ear, nose, and throat, and genitourinary ailments were received and treated there on a round-the-clock basis.

In the north end of the main building was the dental department, which had been constructed and equipped with the funds provided by George Eastman. Both adults and children could be treated by dental students and their teachers in its forty-two dental chairs. An important feature of the new department was a large room for the teaching of dental hygiene. Here, beginning in 1931, students were taught to do prophylactic work in dental offices, industrial establishments, and schools. The gleaming new dental complex also contained extraction, surgical, X-ray, and ceramics rooms, a technics and prosthetics laboratory, and a prosthetic clinic.

Between the dental department and the hospital were the classrooms and teaching laboratories for botany, dentistry, biochemistry, physiology, phar-

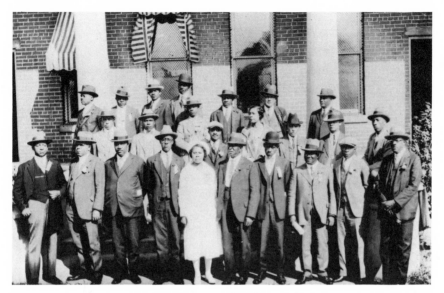

Faculty members of Meharry, 1926

macy, bacteriology, pathology, and anatomy. Each department had office rooms and private staff quarters. There was also an amphitheater two stories deep. These facilities were supplemented by the new library at Fisk University, which was opened to Meharry students. Besides providing them with a richer collection of scientific books and periodicals, Fisk's library made available collateral texts in public health, biology, and chemistry that were required outside reading.[14]

Even more crucial than bricks and mortar to the greatness dreamt of by Meharrians were teachers. By 1920 age had impaired many of the second generation of faculty members, those who had been serving since the 1890s. As they retired, Dr. Mullowney was faced with the task of recruiting new teachers to take their places. Dedication would be the first requirement sought, for Meharry's salaries remained very low. Scientific training in medicine would be another.

Between 1919 and 1948 thirty Meharry graduates obtained fellowships, mainly from the General Education Board and the Julius Rosenwald Fund, for study at leading eastern and midwestern medical schools. Many of these postgraduate students were on leave from the Meharry faculty during their work. George Hubbard's principle of selecting new teachers from among the best Meharry graduates had not been effaced. But by urging them to work in other settings after winning their degrees, Dr. Mullowney hoped that institutional habits at Meharry would be defeated by the fresh observations and latest scientific knowledge brought back to the campus. Pursuing these things, the postgraduate fellows of this period did advanced work in public health, radiology, urology, psychiatry, neurology, psychology, and other new disciplines of medicine.[15]

The superior record compiled at Meharry by William S. Quinland (Class of 1919) won him the first Rosenwald fellowship for postgraduate study in pathology and bacteriology. At the end of his work at Harvard Medical School, his major professor importuned him to remain there as a member of the faculty, but Quinland declined the offer, saying that Meharry had greater need of his services. His ceaseless labors for the next quarter of a century brought national recognition to the college's pathology department. Dr. Quinland became the first black scientist named to the American Association of Pathologists and Bacteriologists, the first black diplomate of the American Board of Pathology, and the first black Fellow of the College of American Pathologists.

Sent to Columbia with a General Education Board fellowship, Dr. Michael J. Bent (Class of 1921) returned to Meharry in 1924 as head of the Department of Microbiology and Parisitology. He served the college for nearly three decades as a research scientist, as a teacher, and, beginning in 1941, as the first black dean of the School of Medicine.[16] His scholarship included the first detailed study of the housing, living conditions, food, sanitation, and diseases of Tennessee's rural black people. Studies by Dr. Elbridge Sibley of Columbia, by Fisk University sociologists, and others had already shown that the differences in death rates between whites and blacks persisted to a striking degree in Tennessee.[17] Despite the labors of Negro health workers, a black baby born in 1935 was twice as likely to die before he was a year old than a white baby. A black adult was from three to five times more likely to contract tuberculosis as a white adult. A black man could not expect to live as long as a white man. Black women fared somewhat better: their life expectancy came closer to that for white women. If a black woman chose to conceive a child, however, the odds on her life plummeted. She was twice as likely to die during pregnancy or childbirth as a white mother, and several times as likely to develop hypertension.[18]

The findings of Dr. Michael Bent and his survey team indicated that social and economic disparities between the races and not biological differences, as some had asserted, were responsible. Where black men and women had the opportunity to live under good economic and sanitary conditions, the incidence of disease tended to approach the same level seen among white people. The remaining difference in morbidity and mortality appeared to be a matter of education—of teaching black children and their families about proper diet, personal hygiene, and sanitation.

Leaders in education and health in Tennessee read Dr. Bent's conclusions and agreed that a teaching program directed toward black youngsters in their schools might help to reduce the rates of illness and untimely death among Negroes. To discover precisely what young black people did and did not know about diseases and their transmission, Dr. Bent surveyed the health knowledge and health habits of pupils in three rural elementary schools. He and his assistant, Paul T. Jessen of George Peabody College for Teachers, found that many did not know some of the simplest health rules or had strange notions concerning them. Their knowledge of food and of balanced diet was most deficient. Bent and Jessen also examined the hygienic assets and liabilities of the homes of forty-six families whose children attended the schools. This survey revealed that the parents knew little more than their children about proper food. The interviewers also noted unprotected water supplies, inadequate heating for cold weather, filth, and overcrowding in the homes in the community.

With the grave dimensions of the problem made clear, Dr. Bent enlisted Ellen F. Greene to develop a health education curriculum to be taught in the three schools. Courses were designed in food, clothing, and personal and community hygiene and placed in the hands of the teachers. Bent visited the schools each week, giving lectures and demonstrations and showing the teachers how to use the course materials. He also tested the students from time to time. Their scores showed that they were gaining in health knowledge, but the gains were small. The key was in the teachers, who themselves needed more and better training in how to include health education in each basic classroom subject.

To help them Dr. Bent, together with Paul Jessen, prepared a health education course built around textbooks being used in Tennessee schools. The subjects covered included personal hygiene, the dangers of self-medication, nutrition, physical exercise and recreation, home and school sanitation, first aid, and the prevention of disease. The teachers were shown how to encourage pupils to prepare balanced meals and to investigate ways in which food, milk, or water might become contaminated.

Bent and Jessen's course was promptly included in the teacher-training curriculum at Fisk University and at Tennessee A and I College. The syllabus was also sent to teachers throughout the state. In 1936, five years after the pioneer study, Dr. Bent and his team conducted another health knowledge test in the three schools originally selected for the experiment. This time they found an encouraging improvement in the scores. There was also evidence that the learning program had been beneficial beyond the confines of the classroom. The new health studies in the schools had drawn the interest of parents and, despite the severe unemployment caused by the Depression, dietary habits in the children's homes had improved, especially in the use of milk, fresh green vegetables, and cereals.

Using these findings, Dr. Bent prepared an address, "A Definite and Practical Health Program for the School, the Home, and the Community." In behalf of the State Department of Education, he traveled throughout Middle Tennessee, delivering the speech and teaching young audiences the protective sanitation, hygiene, and dietary measures that the rural health experiment had proved to be effective.[19]

Complementing Dr. Bent's work were studies of health conditions among black people in the cities done by Dr. Charles Roman. In a series of papers delivered before the Southern Sociological Congress, Dr. Roman described how racism, alcohol, prostitution, and the public squalor resulting from private greed led to untimely deaths for Negroes from filth diseases, syphilis, and, especially, tuberculosis.[20]

Meharry redoubled its efforts in the fight against this last plague with the opening, in February 1926, of the first chest clinic for Negroes in the South. Its director, Dr. William A. Beck, was one of the region's leading authorities on the disease. Born on a farm near Gainesville, Alabama, he received his premedical education at Homer College in Louisiana and graduated from Meharry in 1921. He subsequently served as an instructor of anatomy and physical diagnosis and as professor of internal and clinical medicine. At the Meharry Chest Clinic, Dr. Beck and his associates treated thousands of sufferers annually. They also trained each year scores of medical students and many Negro physicians who returned to their alma mater to learn how to combat tuberculosis.

Dr. Beck was one of the pioneers in the use of ambulatory pneumothorax in the South, a procedure for tuberculosis victims who were unable to gain admission to hospitals due to the highly contagious nature of their illness. Between 1925 and 1946 he maintained an office in downtown Nashville to dispense this therapy, which consisted of pumping air into the victim's lungs.

The continuous flow of patients to his clinic and consulting room revealed as no statistic could the calamitous extent of the disease among black people. Accordingly, Dr. Beck for years urged the Tennessee Department of Public Health to build a public hospital for Negro tuberculosis victims. Although failing in this campaign, he continued his labors in preventive education by lecturing throughout the South under the sponsorship of the National Anti-Tuberculosis Association.[21]

No preventable deaths were more alarming in general than those of infants or their mothers in childbirth. Natal and prenatal causes, such as premature birth, congenital debility, injury at birth, congenital malformations, and syphilis were the leading causes of black baby deaths in the mid-1930s, with respiratory, gastrointestinal, and epidemic diseases also taking a heavy toll. The great killer among newly delivered black mothers was puerperal septicemia, an almost totally preventable malady.[22] All these

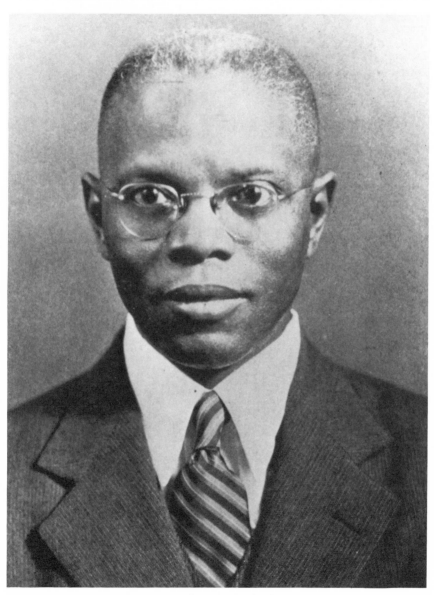

William A. Beck

illnesses associated with pregnancy and childbirth were responsible for the deaths of more Negro women than any other cause except tuberculosis.

In 1917 Meharry's medical students began working in one of the outpatient Well-Baby Clinics operated by the City of Nashville. By the early 1920s beds for sick youngsters had been specially set aside in Hubbard Hospital; yet the fear of hospitals in general on the part of many black parents left Meharry's first pediatrics ward empty.

The healing of one critically ill baby, brought to the hospital by its mother after she had abandoned hope for its life, gave the Negro community a blush of confidence in Hubbard's staff. When Meharry relocated to north Nashville, the number of pediatrics patients gradually increased, and the service grew in proportion. Meharry enlisted in the fight for improved health among mothers and children by establishing the first prenatal clinic for black women in the South. It instructed and cared for hundreds of pregnant women. Undoubtedly, the clinic saved many lives by encouraging women to give birth in the hygienic setting of Hubbard Hospital rather than at the hands of a midwife. Obstetrical patients who could not come to the clinic were often attended in their homes by Meharry staff and students.[23]

At still another pioneer facility for blacks, the Children's Venereal Clinic, future physicians were drilled in the causes, scope, and effects of congenital syphilis. To identify venereal diseases in their earliest, most treatable stages, Meharry made the Wasserman Blood Test a routine part of the admissions procedure to Hubbard Hospital after the newly systematized record-keeping revealed a horrifying incidence of syphilis among new patients and, by implication, among black people of the city and region.[24]

As with strictly organic diseases, mental illness occurred more frequently among Negroes than among whites, according to statistics from state institutions. Moreover, the evidence showed, its incidence among the black population was increasing. Some types of mental disorders among Negro men and women could be linked to poverty. The migration of many thousands of black people from the rural South to the cities of the North after World War I probably contributed to the rise in rates, when Negroes generally found themselves on the economic margins of urban society.

Psychoneurosis and its origins in the patient's basic home and work environment were becoming increasingly important concerns of preventive medicine. At Meharry studies in mental illness grew out of the courses in anatomy, histology, and neurology taught by Dr. Rafael Hernandez.

Dr. Hernandez (Class of 1928) received postgraduate training at the Presbyterian Hospital of Columbia University. In 1930 he returned to the Meharry faculty. After service as a major in the United States Army during World War II, Dr. Hernandez became head of the Department of Anatomy and special consultant in neuropsychiatry. By this time there was general agreement that medical schools should provide every prospective physician a sound foundation in diagnosing and treating mental illness. Meharry's third-year students received a clinical and demonstration course in the major types of neurosis and psychosis. In their senior year they spent three weeks at Homer G. Phillips Hospital in St. Louis for intensive training in neuropsychiatry.[25]

From preventive strategies in patient care, it was a logical step for Meharry to offer formal study in the social aspects of medicine and the place that it occupied in the community. In the Department of Preventive Medicine, seniors devoted several weeks to studies in public health. They visited the Nashville health department, analyzed milk and water samples, and examined the vital statistics of the city. Required to conceive and carry out original sanitary surveys, they identified some of the chronic health problems in the neighborhoods of north and south Nashville where black people mainly lived.

Following receipt of the doctorate in public health from the University of Toronto in 1939, Dr. Thomas LaSaine (Class of 1935) returned to the department to extend the range of courses. His seminars considered the functions and problems of community health and welfare services. Students were encouraged to "develop a tolerant appreciation for those agencies seeking 'equal distribution of medical care.' " They were assigned to patients whose health problems arose from living or working situations. Under the guidance of LaSaine and the social service staff of Hubbard Hospital, students gave counsel and medical treatment in the manner of family physicians.[26]

Some Meharry students in preventive health worked as clinicians at the Millie E. Hale Hospital in south Nashville, whose teaching programs for black nurses emphasized social service. Hale Hospital was founded in 1916 by Dr. John Henry Hale and named for his wife, a Fisk University alumna and registered nurse.

Nurses from Hale Hospital, together with a corps of women volunteers, assisted the black people of Nashville through bedside care in the home, recreation, and relief for the desperately needy in the form of food, coal, bedding, and money. They also conducted health meetings and worked in Hale Hospital's outpatient clinics, which were operated in various parts of the city.[27]

An emphasis on the community service aspects of medical practice distinguished the careers of many Meharry alumni of the time. Dr. R. D. Douglas had been born near Jefferson, Texas, in 1904 on land that his grandparents settled when they were freed from slavery. Following his graduation from Meharry, he returned to the tiny town and opened an office. "I started off with a maternity ward," Dr. Douglas recalled nearly a half century later. "During those days, most babies were delivered at home, and sometimes babies were stubborn—they made the doctor wait awhile. So I figured I'd save time and help the mother too by bringing her here," he continued. From one bed for expectant women grew the twenty-five–bed Douglas Memorial Hospital. In time Dr. Douglas and his wife opened a nursing home adjacent to Memorial. When he finally retired in 1976, 500 of his fellow citizens of Jefferson, black and white, honored him with a testimonial dinner.

One of thirteen children, Archer A. Claytor was born to parents who had once been slaves in Virginia. He graduated from Meharry in 1934 and became the first black doctor ever named Year's Foremost Physician in Saginaw, Michigan. As a general practitioner, he delivered more than 1,000 babies over a three-year period and eventually prevailed against segregation in medicine to become a staff physician at all four hospitals in Saginaw. The Claytor family would be represented for generations in Meharry's student body.

In 1905 at the age of sixteen, Daniel S. Malekebu walked out of Nyasaland (Malawi) and worked his way to New York washing dishes aboard ship. Having learned English from a missionary, he entered high school in Selma, Alabama, and eventually obtained a medical degree at Meharry. In 1920 he returned to Africa and rebuilt the mission in his native village. Forty years later it had a school for 660 students, a hospital, and a church that seated 1,500 worshipers.[28]

Meharry alumni who practiced in the South were perhaps the most representative of all. Surveying those who lived and worked in rural west Tennessee about 1920, one student found that, in this period of enormous black migration to the North, black physicians were permanently settled in their communities. In general they occupied well-located and -appointed offices, read widely in current medical literature, and participated in classes and clinics on the rare occasions when these were available. Their economic position, apparently related to the length of time in practice, was about equal to that of the average black college graduate in the United States.

These west Tennessee alumni did general practice among Negro people. Their services were sought most often for tuberculosis, venereal disease, and maladies of the throat, lungs, and stomach. In one locale, kidney troubles were prevalent; in another, typhoid fever; in still another, neurosis.

The writer noted that about half the medical attention given black people came from Negro doctors. He concluded: "The growth of the percentage of Negroes served professionally by members of their own race seems to be only a symptom of a comprehensive growth of race pride, which is becoming manifest in other important ways."[29]

Because they could depend only upon each other, black doctors were inclined to unite ever more strongly as a group. "The Colored Medical

Profession has about reached the limit of uncoordinated individual progress," wrote Dr. Charles Roman in 1934. "We must now integrate our efforts, fellowship our desires, and evolve our leaders." Many of Dr. Roman's colleagues came to similar views as the legal system of segregation was perfected by statutes prohibiting public accommodation, integrated schools, and equality of political participation. In their opinion, if the lot of black people was to be improved—in health, in education, in economic position—it was going to have to be done by black people themselves.

In Nashville a group of well-educated, articulate young blacks reacted strongly against the repressive measures taken by legislatures and courts. In outrage and opposition, Joseph Oliver Battle, Henry Allen Boyd, and Dock A. Hart founded *The Nashville Globe,* which began publication in January 1906. Their editorial page stood for economic separatism and a broad range of racially independent goals for the black people of Nashville. It argued that, since blacks were not going to be wanted in the white system for a long time, the only alternative was to build a black system, with its own self-sufficient businesses, its own schools, its own parks, and its own racial pride. The *Globe* encouraged the study of black history and the exclusive patronage of black enterprises. It advocated a voluntary end to interracial marriage.

The *Globe* thought that these goals could best be achieved through local initiative and action. In 1912 it supported the formation of the Nashville Negro Board of Trade. The board in turn sponsored several health projects, including a cleanup campaign in the black business district and the appointment of a Negro nurse in Nashville's health department. In vigorous editorials the *Globe* crusaded for reforms in the adverse social conditions present in the city's black neighborhoods. Sanitation was a chief concern. In cooperation with the interracial Nashville Public Welfare League, the newspaper attempted to remove peddlers of "tainty meat and rotten fish" from Negro communities, sought a free milk dispensary as an aid to lowering the incidence of infant mortality, and called attention to antiquated public sewage disposal facilities. It assisted the league in disseminating knowledge of recent findings on hookworm and typhoid fever. It also gave extensive publicity to National Negro Health Week, an annual event begun in 1915 by the National Medical Association and other sponsors.

The migration of many Negroes from rural areas into the cities and successful programs of civic reform, such as those carried out in Nashville, contributed to the new sense of group consciousness in the years after World War I. In such a fertile soil the seeds of black rights, black economics, black politics, and black education sown by the *Globe* began to sprout.[30]

"Efficiency" had always been a key word in the lexicon of the young progressives in Nashville's black community. They and the atmosphere they helped to foster encouraged the important reforms at Meharry Medical College and at Hubbard Hospital in the early 1920s. Also strengthened was the wish among many Negro Nashvillians that Meharry might have a black president. When Dr. Charles Roman, speaking at Dr. Hubbard's investiture in 1916, told of his hope that the president's mantle would, upon Hubbard's retirement, fall on "some worthy alumnus of Meharry," he received tremendous applause.[31]

Black desire for greater autonomy in the schools and colleges that had for a half century been conducted for them was dramatically expressed at Fisk University in 1925. The university's white president, Fayette Avery McKenzie, had suppressed the student newspaper and student council, refused to allow a student athletic association, censored all student orations and debates, and instituted a rigid dress code.

Some of the male students at Fisk had served in the armed forces in World War I. They, in particular, resented the restrictive conditions and autocratic administration. In January 1925 the students called a general strike to persuade the university's trustees of the need for a new president. Their leaders made it plain that they were not demanding a black president, but merely one "in sympathy with the institution, regardless of race, color, or creed." Nonetheless, the reasoning expressed in their resolutions left that prospect open.

Black opposition to McKenzie grew rather than diminished throughout the winter, and in April he resigned. The unspoken hope of Nashville blacks for a Negro administration and the opposition to that prospect by most of Nashville's white leaders were carefully weighed by the search committee. Although it eventually selected a white man, Thomas Elsa Jones, as the new president, the repressive measures that McKenzie had instituted were soon lifted. Northern philanthropy continued, white Nashvillians made good the pledges of financial support they had previously given to Fisk, and working relations were reestablished between the university's administration and Nashville's black community.

Several Meharrians played a role in the tumultuous events at Fisk. Dr. Charles Roman and Dr. John Henry Hale, although sympathetic with the students, doubted the wisdom of a strike and worked behind the scenes to persuade them to put an end to it. Another Meharry alumnus, Dr. W. W. Sumlin, bitterly attacked the students and won lavish praise in the white press. But his stand soon made him so unpopular among his medical colleagues that he was ejected from his post as president of the Rock City Academy of Medicine and, by its resolution, banned from the organization.[32]

In the aftermath of the Fisk strike, Dr. Mullowney and the black community of Nashville traded uneasy glances. Mullowney shared the paternalistic ideas toward black education of many of his fellow whites. His writings and speeches were replete with adult-child imagery. From his point of view Meharry's new physical plant was the latest of many gifts from the white race to blacks. What blacks made of these opportunities so generously given was entirely up to them, he insisted time after time. Yet, relying upon racist notions and stereotypes, he denied firmly that black people were ready to lead at Meharry:

> Negroes have not yet developed many good disciplinarians or administrators, nor do they seem, as a general rule, to be as dextrous or as able to coordinate highly skilled actions with thoughts, nor are the majority of them blessed with impelling energy. . . . The white men will need to act as heads of nearly all branches of clinical medicine for at least ten, possibly twenty years longer.[33]

Mullowney saw his views confirmed in the "experiments" he allowed in Negro leadership at Meharry. Whenever a black man or woman proved to be an outstanding administrator, he simply failed to observe it. He constantly exhorted faculty members to find ways of saving money. He depended upon them to set examples for students by attending college religious services. He expected them to pledge a portion of their modest salaries to the fund-raising drives. He even permitted them to formulate academic regulations, to pass upon candidates for graduation, and to review student disciplinary cases.[34] But, based on his foregone conclusions, he declined to give the predominantly black faculty a substantive role in governing Meharry.

Because Meharry remained the province of one man, the postgraduate fellows had little incentive and less power to implement the progressive ideas they gathered at other medical schools. The subordinate position of the faculty, along with the low salaries, discouraged some men and women of wide experience and knowledge from coming there to teach or remaining for long if they did.

As Dr. Mullowney constantly sought financial support for Meharry in Nashville, his views became known among its black citizens. Many of them in north Nashville had not yet become reconciled to the presence of the college and as its president held forth in public forums, their confidence in the institution dropped still further. So many began seeking treatment at Vanderbilt University's hospital or at Nashville's General Hospital that the sparkling new Hubbard Hospital operated at only about half its capacity.

In 1937 Meharry was placed on probation by the American Medical Association, following an evaluation by its Council on Medical Education and Hospitals. The council's report cited grave weaknesses in organization and administration and noted especially the paucity of teachers with postgraduate training or specialty attainments. Accreditation was not entirely revoked, but the council clearly believed that Meharry did not present standards that it prescribed for the best medical schools. In the aftermath of the report, the General Education Board reviewed affairs at the college and concluded that Meharry would have to create more opportunities for faculty members to prepare themselves in medical specialties, provide them a chance to implement what they had learned in such preparation, reorganize departments, and increase the output of research.[35]

The loss of Meharry's "A" rating twenty years before had revealed the failing capacity of Dr. George Hubbard. This second reversal showed that the college's leadership was faltering again.

In the spring of 1938, Dr. Mullowney retired, ostensibly for reasons of health. To succeed him as president and as dean of the School of Medicine, the Board of Trustees elected Dr. Edward Lewis Turner. Dr. Turner, who was a white man, had been brought to Meharry as head of the Department of Medicine in 1936 to help implement Dr. Mullowney's announced plan to begin preparing faculty members to succeed to department chairmanships at some future time.[36] According to the General Education Board and the American Medical Association, such preparation had already been delayed too long.

By training and temperament Dr. Turner was well suited to advance this critical work. A man of diverse interests and accomplishments, he had been born in Alton, Illinois, on August 9, 1900. He received a bachelor's degree from the University of Chicago in 1922 and a master's degree the following year, whereupon he became an instructor in anatomy there. In 1928 he earned the M.D. degree from the University of Pennsylvania. From that year until 1936 he served at the American University in Beirut, Lebanon. There he was adjunct professor of physiology, associate professor of medicine, and finally head of the medical department. From this base in the Middle East, he traveled throughout Europe, studying in schools of medicine in England, France, Germany, and Italy. He was the first president of Meharry to be an active research scientist, contributing papers on immunology to numerous journals. Out of his years on the Meharry faculty came additional studies on premedical education and on the characteristics of successful medical students.[37]

Dr. Turner agreed with the findings of the medical educators and philanthropists about the state of affairs at Meharry. He was also sensible of the widespread desire, developing out of the progressive independence movement encouraged by *The Nashville Globe,* for a greater black role at Meharry. Accordingly, within the first years of his administration, Negro men and women of the faculty assumed a more visible role in the college than they had ever had. Dr. Michael J. Bent was named associate dean of the School of Medicine, and Dr. John Henry Hale was appointed chairman of the Department of Surgery, in which post he served until his death in

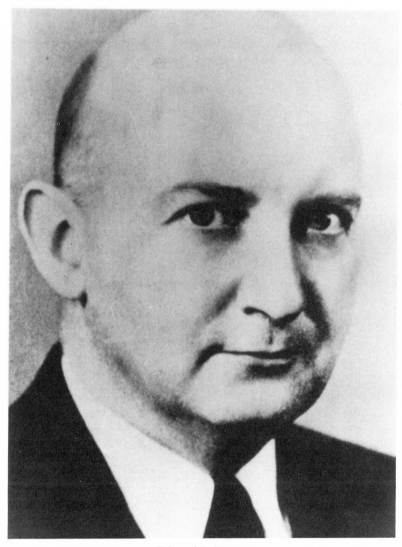

Edward L. Turner

1944.[38] Dr. Daniel T. Rolfe became chairman of the Department of Physiology. They were eventually joined by other black department heads, including Drs. Harold D. West in biochemistry, Walter Maddux in pediatrics, and William H. Grant, director of the pathology laboratory.

To provide the means for greater faculty participation in policymaking, Dr. Turner increased the number of college committees and appointed a black teacher to head each one. To these panels, he announced, he would delegate as much authority as possible.

The new president moved quickly to carry out his predecessor's declared intent to increase the number of black faculty members in leadership roles. He encouraged the heads of departments who were white to employ one or more black understudies. These junior faculty members were then helped to obtain fellowships for study under a leading authority in another institution.[39] As they received specialty training, young Negro doctors were assigned to relieve the burdens of aging teachers, some of whom had been educated in the era before laboratories and X rays.

External reorganization of certain departments, revisions of the content and methods of teaching particular courses, and a new emphasis on clinical instruction utilizing a growing hospital census were three further priorties of Dr. Turner's administration. Specialized courses in cardiovascular diseases and metabolic disorders were added to the medical curriculum, the scope of studies begun earlier in the dermatology and syphilis clinics in Hubbard Hospital was expanded, and a school of clinical laboratory technology was opened.[40] To increase the quantity of instruction in these and other relatively new fields, Dr. Turner recruited additional part-time teachers, most of them from the Vanderbilt University School of Medicine.[41]

Meharry's new leaders insisted that all teachers include time in their schedules for original investigation. "Efficient and progressive teaching obtains only when scientific activity is in progress," wrote Dr. Michael J. Bent. It was the first time that such impetus had been given to research at Meharry, and dividends were forthcoming almost immediately.

Because of racial discrimination, however, many black doctors were not able to obtain money for their projects. In 1946 Meharry embarked upon a program to raise research money for Negro scientists throughout the United States. The faculty Committee on Research, under Dr. Harold D. West, headed this effort. Four pharmaceutical houses gave the initial funds, which were directed to Negro doctors in biophysics, physiology, and biochemistry.[42]

Another objective of Meharry under the new leadership was improvement in the quality of the student body by selection of freshmen who had already proved themselves equal to a modern education in medicine, dentistry, or nursing. Soon after World War I Meharry had begun to require from prospective students scores on the Medical College Aptitude Test

offered by the National Board of Medical Examiners. Additional requirements were also imposed at the behest of the National Medical Association: all candidates for admission were required to have completed their
premedical studies in a college approved by the American Medical Association and to have acquired a thorough grounding in the basic sciences.
Chemistry, physics, and biology were the chief prerequisite courses, and
English composition, Latin, and a modern foreign language rounded out
the list. But students were strongly urged to elect zoology, psychology,
logic, and mathematics and to earn more credits in chemistry and physics
than were strictly necessary before coming to Meharry.

Prior to 1938 large first-year classes had been admitted to all three
schools with the expectation that forty to fifty percent of those entering
would fail during the first or second year. In Dr. Turner's view this policy
worked to keep morale low among students and faculty alike. Early in his
administration he placed the responsibility for admissions wholly in the
hands of the newly constituted admissions committees and charged them
with assuring that every young man or woman admitted to Meharry had
the qualifications stipulated in the catalog, which indicated a reasonable
chance of success.[43] As a result the freshman student of the late 1930s and
early 1940s entered the college better prepared for a rigorous course of
study than his counterpart of any previous generation. The ink was scarcely
dry on his matriculation forms before he was plunged into a life of continuous learning.

Anatomy lay at the foundation of all that he would study over the next
four years. Through hundreds of hours in the dissecting room he mastered
the gross structures of the body and then examined them in microscopic
sections. He and his laboratory partners were furnished with human
brains, which they first dissected, then discussed in detail. They studied
the development of the embryo, from fertilization through the appearance
of the organs.

For two years the medical student's life was an endless round of laboratory work, demonstrations, lectures, and original investigation, as he completed the rest of the required basic science curriculum: physiology,
chemistry, pathology, bacteriology, parisitology, and pharmacology. There
were also courses in medical jurisprudence, professional ethics, and the
new sciences of the mind. The vocabulary of his medical course would have
amazed and mystified his predecessor of a half-century before: "enzymes,"
"pathogenic organisms," "culture media," "alkaloidal assaying," "tox-
icological action," "psychosis." At night he bent over his notes and sketches,
making them his own.

It was not until his fourth semester at Meharry that he was deemed ready
to begin the study of physical diagnosis. Instruments in hand for the
examination of the body, the third-year student was drilled in their use

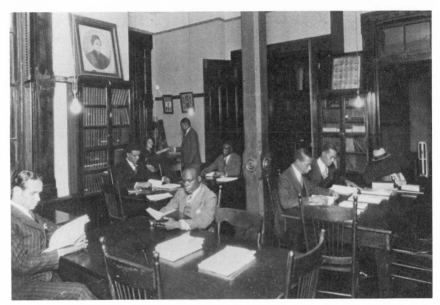

Mastering the texts

during rounds in Hubbard Hospital. In dermatology and "syphilo-dermatology" he wrote prescriptions, which were reviewed by his instructor. These advanced courses were specifically designed and conducted not to fit the prospective doctor as a specialist but to assist him as a general practitioner.

The outpatient clinics conducted by the faculty at Hubbard Hospital were a highlight of the junior and senior years. Clinics were held in general medicine, surgery, obstetrics and gynecology, tuberculosis, venereal diseases, neurology, and diseases of the eye, ear, nose, and throat. Third- and fourth-year students spent several weeks in each clinic, observing the therapeutic strategies of the residents and assisting them in limited ways.[44]

Advanced studies, in particular, were improved by the pedagogical reforms encouraged by Dr. Turner and implemented by the faculty. Prior to 1938 clinical teaching at Meharry had been conducted largely through methods in vogue in former years, when the description of a disease was the sole means of identifying it and differentiating it from other diseases. In that interval, however, researchers had discovered many new physiological, biochemical, and pathological mechanisms. Dr. Turner and Meharry instructors recognized that this growth in knowledge was bringing about a

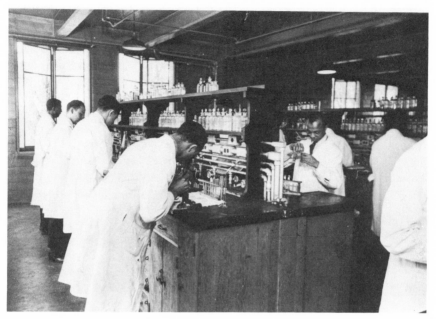

Exploring the fundamentals

transition in medicine from an empirical to a rational therapy. Accordingly, they ceased to emphasize the fact that a certain combination of drugs compounded in a prescription would reduce fever or some other abnormal symptom, and began to teach, first, the way in which the abnormality might develop and, second, the pharmacological action of each drug. With this innovation students of the 1940s gained a greater versatility in diagnosis and treatment, one that would accommodate the constantly advancing content of medical knowledge.[45]

The low tuition charged at Meharry and the lower cost of living in Nashville when compared to the cities of the North and East were two features especially attractive to many applicants. Despite the increasing rigor of medical studies, many Meharry students continued to have to work during the school year to pay all or part of their expenses. During the Depression, enrollment plunged sharply in medicine and dentistry as jobs that students depended upon disappeared or were given to heads of families.[46]

With the national recovery, the number of applicants began to exceed the places available. The committees on admission found their jobs difficult under such circumstances. They performed so well, however, that the percentage of withdrawals from Meharry dropped from almost 60 percent in 1940 to about 20 percent in 1943. In the same period there was a consistent increase in the number of graduates. By the end of the 1940s care in student selection and the emphasis laid upon faculty excellence produced a spectacular drop in the failure rate of Meharry graduates before state and national licensing boards.[47]

No amount of sacrifice or excellence, however, guaranteed the Meharry graduate the rewards that society normally paid to the white physician, dentist, and nurse. A study by Dr. Paul Cornely published in the *Journal of the National Medical Association* showed that the Negro doctor practicing at the end of World War II was in most instances a private physician without any other source of income; that he generally had an office alone, with equipment costing less than $5,000 and an office staff of one other person; and that he lived in a home for which he paid between $5,000 and $10,000. His annual gross income was $10,267, but he collected only 80 percent. He saw 155 patients a week and spent seven hours a day in his office, with additional hours given to hospital visits and house calls. Although his patient load might be greater than that of his white colleague, his income was likely to be 25 to 30 percent lower.[48] This was true in part because the overwhelming majority of the black doctor's patients were poor people. Most of them were black, although where race prejudice was less intense—in upland areas of the South and ethnic communities in northern cities, for example—a few Negro physicians had a sizable white practice, usually among low-income persons.[49]

Trained nurses from Meharry faced not only the barriers of segregation but also prejudice against their sex. Even at Hubbard Hospital prior to the reforms of the early 1920s, nurses were sometimes regarded as a kind of domestic servant. In addition to carrying out physicians' orders and keeping medical records, nursing students were expected to clean the entire hospital, from top to bottom.

Beginning in 1921, the nursing course was revised in the interest of matching nationally accepted standards. Practical and theoretical courses were combined so that, for example, the unit on typhoid fever included bacteriology, pathology, laboratory analysis, dietetics, hydrotherapy, and the bedside care of the patient. Members of the medical school faculty were appointed to assist with the teaching program.[50]

At about the same time entrance requirements were made more stringent. By the early 1930s all Meharry nursing students were high school graduates, and many had some college work. The nursing course consisted of three years of twelve months each. Besides the classical scientific subjects, the nursing student in this period first encountered courses that reflected a new identity and respect for the profession. Among these were "Modern

Health and Social Movements," "Public Health Nursing," and "The History of Nursing and Medicine." At the end of the three-year period the graduate was given an examination by the nursing board of her home state and, upon receiving a passing score, was awarded the title Registered Nurse.

Meharry took a further step in 1938 by changing the name of its nurse education program from Training School to School of Nursing. Applicants were required to have one or more years of college. Encouraged by the Turner administration to increase the scope of clinical studies, the nursing school faculty began to give ward assignments to first-year students and arranged for seniors to study communicable diseases for two months of the year at the Isolation Hospital in St. Louis. Dr. Turner himself announced his intention to develop a program of public health nursing at Meharry; and in 1939 the Board of Trustees approved a plan whereby a student might pursue two years of undergraduate courses at Fisk University, study for three years in the School of Nursing at Meharry, and receive from Fisk the bachelor of science degree in nursing.

In recognition of her achievements as a nursing educator and hospital administrator, Hulda M. Lyttle was appointed dean of the school, the first Negro dean of nursing in the United States. In 1943, after thirty years at Meharry, she retired, to be succeeded by Rebecca T. Clark for the 1943–44 school year. During Mrs. Clark's period of service a United States Nurse Cadet Corps was established at Meharry as part of the national war effort. All of the student nurses enrolled in the program.

In 1945 Mrs. Clark yielded the deanship to Alma E. Gault, under whose administration Meharry's program leading to the bachelor of science degree in nursing was established. The School of Nursing was accredited by the National League of Nursing Education in 1947 and was named to membership in the Association of Collegiate Schools of Nursing the following year. By the time baccalaureate degrees were awarded in 1950, Meharry's nurse education program was ranked among the top 25 percent in the United States.

In the autumn of 1947 Meharry's nursing students commenced leaving the campus during part of their day to give care in the homes of indigent patients. The program of home visits extended Meharry's aid to those who needed medical attention but who were too ill to come to Hubbard Hospital. It also helped student nurses to understand the role that social, family, and economic conditions played in health.

Deep-seated racial fears, suspicions, and distrust led Nashville officials to refuse the nursing students permission to work in the city schools. Industrialists likewise denied them access to factory infirmaries and, thus, experience in the increasingly important area of occupational health and safety.

A number of health agencies, public and private, did open doors for the black field nurses, however. The Davidson County Health Department provided them "observational experience" in a few schools. But no organization would admit the program to formal affiliation, which made it unacceptable to national nurse education accrediting bodies.[51]

Matters were more favorable on the national scene, as Meharry nursing graduates found increasing opportunities to serve in public health careers. In 1947 27 percent of Negro graduate nurses were working in public health positions, compared to 10 percent of all graduate nurses in the United States. In that same year about two-thirds of all black nurses were employed in hospitals or other institutional settings. A third of these held administrative, supervisory, or teaching posts.[52]

Like the nursing program, the School of Dentistry sought and found new reason for existence during the difficult and challenging time between the wars. As the American army began demobilizing after World War I, the trains to Nashville filled with black veterans eager to enroll in dental studies. Dr. L. H. Jenkins (Class of 1924) recalled how scores of prospective dental students formed a line at the office doorway of Dr. John A. Lester, the registrar, before dawn on the opening day of school.[53]

Although classes of the early 1920s were large, the number of freshmen became smaller each year as entrance requirements were raised, first to one year of college, then to two. For a time the same qualifications would admit an applicant to medical studies, and many were diverted into that course. Finally, the onset of the Depression led to a further sharp decline in enrollment, so serious that the dental school was threatened with closure. Dr. Mullowney and the faculty aggressively recruited students by circulating figures showing that there were far from enough dentists to supply the demand and by describing in detail the gleaming new equipment that George Eastman had presented to Meharry.[54]

When the Turner administration assumed office in 1938, Dr. Donley H. Turpin was one of the first black members of the faculty to whom the new president turned for advice. A native of Piney Point, Texas, Dr. Turpin received the degree of Doctor of Dental Surgery with Meharry's Class of 1918. He immediately joined the faculty as chief demonstrator and was soon promoted to assistant professor of operative dentistry. Subsequently, he was named to the post of professor of prosthetic dentistry and supervisor of the dental clinics. Upon President Turner's accession, the dental department became the Meharry Medical College School of Dentistry, and Dr. Turpin was appointed dean.

Many of Turpin's colleagues credited him with preventing the closing of dental studies when the enrollment ebbed in the 1930s. Despite that triumph, the program had not advanced because of its small income. The opportunities for students to work in a clinical setting and to care for patients under their instructors' supervision were insufficient. Moreover, the faculty remained deeply ingrained. Its full-time members were themselves Meharry graduates, and few had the advantage of a fellowship to study elsewhere after graduation.

During the first year of the Turner administration, the faculty was augmented by several part-time teachers, mostly white practitioners in Nashville, who gave their services without pay. Nevertheless, new sources of income for the school eluded the administration and the prospects for satisfactory development of studies in dentistry at Meharry appeared bleak. In August 1941 Dr. Turner assumed supervision of the School of Dentistry and prepared to recommend to the Board of Trustees that it be closed.

Before taking irrevocable steps he put a final, desperate appeal before the W. K. Kellogg Foundation. His request was for funds for the salary of a director of dental education who would reorganize the school, for fellowships, and for money for new faculty members who could teach disciplines never before offered at Meharry. The foundation approved Dr. Turner's proposal in March 1942 and provided funds for strengthening the School of Dentistry as part of a larger grant for the improvement of undergraduate teaching.

Dr. Turner immediately approached his old friend and colleague, Dr. M. Don Clawson, formerly director of the dental school at American University, and explained Meharry's need for new directions. A dentist of international stature, Dr. Clawson had just returned to the United States from the Middle East and was being actively sought by many faculties. However, the ties of old friendship and the challenge of the situation at Meharry prevailed over larger financial inducements offered by other schools. Dr. Clawson accepted the offer of the trustees to be Director of Dental Education, commencing his duties on May 1, 1942.

Dr. Clawson, working alongside Dean Turpin, enlarged the faculty and assisted several of its black members in obtaining stipends for postgraduate study. The success of this team was reflected in a number of major events that occurred in 1945. Student enrollment attained a 200 percent increase over its level three years before, and the School of Dentistry was granted full approval by the American Dental Association. Omicron Kappa Upsilon, the national dental honorary society, established a chapter at Meharry—the first time its charter had come to a black school. Finally, Dr. Clawson succeeded to the top leadership post of the college. His tenure as Meharry's fourth president is the subject of a subsequent discussion.[55]

Aware of the need voiced by alumni for competent chairside assistants, Dr. Clawson took steps to revive and expand the training that Meharry offered in the auxiliary branches of dentistry. In the autumn of 1944 a new two-year curriculum leading to a certificate in dental technology was of-

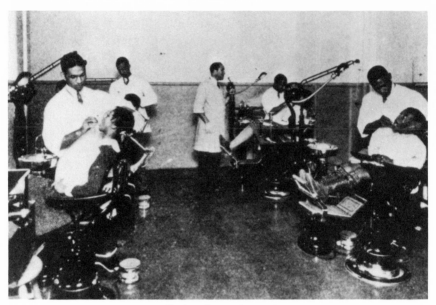

Caring for patients

fered. This course was the first one in the United States to be established as part of a dental school. In 1946 it was expanded, the most significant addition being the rotation of each student in a dentist's office or technics laboratory.

The School of Dentistry was also pioneer of another important development in dental education at the end of World War II. Courses in dental assistance, hygiene, and technology were conducted in the same classrooms and by the same teachers as the courses for Meharry dental students, while in the clinics the future dentists and future technicians worked side by side at the patient's chair.[56]

The new leadership at Meharry was determined to confront some of the dental health problems of the people who lived in the environs of the campus. By the spring of 1943 the dental school's four clinics had been renovated and modified to accommodate more patients. In the admissions clinic the patient was examined by students under the supervision of an intern. Following the latter's diagnosis, he was referred to the operative clinic for routine dental work, or to the prosthetic or dental surgical unit in the case of a more serious problem.

With the cooperation of the Nashville school board, clinical dental students began a public health field program in black primary and secondary schools to teach children proper methods of tooth care. Besides providing demonstrations in oral hygiene, the dental health team examined every student. One of the clinicians recorded a history for Meharry's records, while another demonstrated the correct technique for brushing. After this demonstration each brush was placed in a sterile test tube bearing the child's name and returned to Meharry. Each child was then given a letter to carry to his parents, asking that he be permitted to visit the dental school for a complete examination and corrective work. All children who did so received a complete oral prophylaxis—and the toothbrush in the test tube.[57]

Due to the declining health of Dean Turpin, the School of Dentistry came largely under the direction of Dr. Clawson, who served simultaneously as president of Meharry, Director of Dental Education, and "administrator" of the dental school. When Dr. Turpin died in 1948 the dean's post passed to Dr. Clifton O. Dummett,[58] professor of periodontics. Dr. Dummett left Meharry in 1949, to be succeeded by Dr. William H. Allen, a Meharry alumnus (Class of 1943) and professor of prosthetic dentistry.[59]

In the age of scientific medicine that included complex therapeutics, the training of physicians, dentists, and nurses could not stop at commencement. Yet Meharry graduates faced special problems in obtaining the postgraduate training necessary for permission to practice and for the continual deepening of skills.

In the late 1920s only three large non-Negro hospitals—Cook County in Chicago and Harlem and Bellevue in New York—employed black interns. Of the black hospitals, including Hubbard Hospital at Meharry, only a dozen were approved and these offered just sixty-eight internships, many fewer than the number of Negro medical graduates annually.[60] The limited spaces at Hubbard permitted the selection of only a few interns each year from among the graduates with the best averages. Another small delegation was sent to work in the various clinics at John A. Andrew Memorial Hospital at the Tuskegee Institute.[61]

It was crucial that black schools and hospitals lead in establishing more internships and residences, the latter enabling the black doctor to specialize. Graduates, especially those practicing in small towns and rural areas, also required opportunities to add to their knowledge the new techniques and theories in medicine.

For years many individual alumni had been returning to Meharry on an informal basis and at their own expense to study the latest developments pertinent to their practice. In 1925 several of them proposed that Meharry offer a postgraduate course during the summer months of the year. The faculty Committee on Instruction was eager to fill the need; nevertheless it postponed any action on the grounds that Meharry lacked, for the moment, the capacity to assume the increased responsibility.

It was not until 1936 that a postgraduate seminar was offered in the School of Nursing. Within a few years nurses from throughout the South were coming to study principles of teaching, ward management, and the history of their profession. The success of this course encouraged the faculty to begin similar programs in medicine and dentistry. In 1938 the medical school began sponsoring clinical presentations open to the physicians of Nashville and the region.

That same year a formal postgraduate course in medicine was conducted at the college under the direction of President Turner and Drs. William Quinland and Michael Bent. The first participants studied recent trends in clinical laboratory methods, cardiovascular and renal diseases, gastrointestinal disorders, and infectious diseases.[62]

Soon several states of the South and the Midwest began providing scholarships for their Negro doctors for advanced study at Meharry. Graduate study in various specialties was begun in the early 1940s, with offerings in maternal and child health, surgery, radiology, obstetrics and gynecology, and anesthesia. In 1943 Meharry conducted the first extension courses for alumni and other black health workers. Held at Terrell Hospital in Memphis, they drew participants from throughout western Tennessee and northern Mississippi.

During World War II postgraduate study at Meharry was curtailed by the Army Specialized Training Program, which encouraged accelerated preparation for physicians, dentists, and nurses as part of the nation's war effort. However, these programs became an increasingly important endeavor of the college in the postwar years, when the master's degree in the basic sciences was offered. The first students enrolled in 1947 in biochemistry and were awarded their degrees two years later.[63]

Black medical students and new graduates needing clinical experience, black people in isolated communities needing medical care—each presented the other with a potential opportunity. Only the institutional arrangements for bringing the two together had to be imagined. During the war years Meharry and the people of Mound Bayou, Mississippi, began such a venture in medical education and service that was to endure and grow in significance.

An all-Negro settlement 100 miles south of Memphis, Mound Bayou had been founded during the early 1880s as a haven for black people wanting to escape the tumult and repression of the post–Reconstruction South. The Yazoo and Mississippi Valley Railroad had just completed its New Orleans-to-Memphis line, parallel to the Mississippi River. Along its right-of-way lay a wilderness of undrained land, from just below Memphis to the hills above Vicksburg and stretching eastward for some fifty miles. This steamy cypress lowland was known as the Delta, and it was here that Mound Bayou was established.

Medical knowledge of the day held that black people were better able to survive yellow fever, malaria, "swamp air," and the oppressive summers of the South. Thus, the railroad decided, the potentially rich but fever-ridden Delta could best be developed by Negroes.

Two young men—Isaiah Tecumseh Montgomery and Benjamin T. Green—who had been slaves on the Vicksburg plantation of Confederate President Jefferson Davis approached railroad officials and persuaded them to deed over 30,000 acres of Delta country. The two men then sold or leased sections of this huge tract to Negroes to start a town of their own. By 1887 a hundred black settlers were clearing the forest and building cabins. They fought insects, snakes, wild animals, mosquitoes, and the very diseases to which they were supposedly immune. As the land was cleared and put into cultivation, the railroad thrived and the community grew.

About the time Mound Bayou was founded, scores of black fraternal and benevolent organizations were established throughout the South. These self-help groups frequently combined fervent religious faith and elaborate ritual into a meaningful social outlet for poor people. One such society was the Knights and Daughters of Tabor. It boasted a mystic link with a secret organization started by blacks before the Civil War to fight for freedom and to "encourage Christianity, education, morality, temperance, the art of governing, self-reliance, and true manhood and womanhood." The Knights and Daughters also managed an insurance program. Subscribers who paid a few pennies a week were assured burial with dignity and a small death benefit to the beneficiary whom they designated.

The Mississippi section of the Knights and Daughters of Tabor was founded in 1889, and despite some early financial troubles, it ultimately prospered. Principally responsible for its success was R. D. Smith, a black man from Mound Bayou who served as Chief Grand Mentor—or manager—from 1893 to 1909. His son, Perry M. Smith, who had been born in 1876 and was an alumnus of the Tuskegee Institute, became head of the Mississippi unit in 1926. Over the next twenty years, the Knights and Daughters of Tabor grew to a statewide membership of 40,000, organized into local tabernacles and temples.

In 1939 Perry Smith began to reflect on the fact that there were practically no hospitals for Negroes in Mississippi. The only beds available to critically ill black men or women were in the basements of white facilities in Jackson, Natchez, and other large cities. What was insurance finally worth to a black Delta family who had no hospital, Smith reasoned. But why couldn't a people who built a town also build a hospital? Many of Smith's associates told him that this undertaking would be impossible. But like the black homesteaders who had cleared the Delta swamps, Smith was a man of considerable tenacity. He raised the $100,000 needed, partly from surplus funds of the Knights and Daughters of Tabor.

Taborian Hospital opened its doors on February 12, 1942. Subscribers to a hospitalization insurance plan paid a small periodic fee. In the event of illness it provided them outpatient care and thirty days of hospital stay, including medical care, drugs, surgery, X rays, and laboratory tests. Income for the hospital was provided by financial drives among organization members and by payments from the county government for the care of nonmember patients.

Mississippi had almost a million black citizens, of whom nearly 600,000 lived in the cotton-growing Delta. By the best estimates, 3,000 hospital beds were needed to take care of that number adequately. But there were not that many for Mississippi's white population, let alone the state's Negro people. As a result the demand for rooms at Taborian Hospital was roughly twenty times the supply, and the clean, lighted wards and the cream-and-brown hallways were perpetually crowded.

The need for health workers was also very great. Most black physicians found the rewards of practice in the cities more attractive than prospects at Mound Bayou.[64] In an effort to recruit professional men and women to serve in their hospital, a delegation from the Knights and Daughters of Tabor came to Nashville to visit Meharry and to talk with President Turner and with Dr. Matthew Walker, assistant professor of surgery and gynecology. The two institutions were in a natural position to help each other: Taborian Hospital needed the skills of Meharrians and the college required opportunities for its students and graduates to expand their horizons and to meet the licensing requirement of an internship.

That Dr. Walker had attracted the notice of the Mississippians was scarcely surprising. Although still a young man he had emerged as one of the new black leaders of Meharry and was rapidly gaining a national reputation as a surgeon and medical educator. Born in Waterproof, Louisiana, on December 7, 1906, Matthew Walker won a baccalaureate degree cum laude from New Orleans University and entered Meharry Medical College in 1930. Four years later he graduated with honors. With a few members of his class who had made outstanding records, he interned at Hubbard Hospital and then entered a full residency in surgery and gynecology under Dr. John Henry Hale. From 1936 to 1938 Walker also served as instructor in orthopedics, anesthesia, and diseases of the eye, ear, nose, and throat. With a fellowship in surgery from the General Education Board, Dr. Walker studied for a year at Howard University. In 1939 he became assistant professor of surgery and gynecology at Meharry. At the same time he taught pathology and physiology and performed notable research in the latter discipline.

Dr. Walker was instrumental in initiating the postgraduate program in surgery at Meharry in 1941. The ambitious training course provided for five to seven years' work following completion of the internship. The most fortunate of the advanced surgical students also had the opportunity to study at some other medical school on a fellowship, such awards being brought to Meharry through Dr. Walker's constant contacts with medical deans and chiefs of surgery throughout the United States. He became full professor of surgery and gynecology in 1944 and the following year was named chairman of the Department of Surgery. A continuous stream of honors confirmed his stature as a physician, educator, and research scientist.[65]

Dr. Walker chose to remain at Meharry rather than accept the position of chief of surgery at Taborian Hospital, proffered by the group from Mound Bayou. In his stead he suggested a number of capable surgeons who might be available. Eventually, Dr. T. M. Howard, chief surgeon at Nashville's Riverside Hospital was chosen for the post. Mrs. Katherine Dandridge, head of anesthesiology at Meharry, was named director of nursing. Hospital staff other than physicians and nurses were hired primarily from Mound Bayou and the surrounding area. Most had no training prior to their employment; many subsequently studied at Meharry for credits and certificates as medical technologists. Dr. Howard resigned from Taborian in 1947 and became chief of surgery at Sarah Brown Hospital, also in Mound Bayou. An institution of about twenty beds, it had been built by a faction of the Knights and Daughters of Tabor calling itself the United Order of Friendship.

Dr. Matthew Walker was again approached by a delegation from Taborian Hospital and offered the vacant surgical post. Unable to accept the offer due to his increasing responsibilities at Meharry, he proposed to assist the surgical service at Taborian by supplying it with qualified house staff and surgical students on a rotating basis. Hospital officials accepted the plan gladly and Meharry executed a formal agreement of affiliation with Taborian. The instrument contained a clause permitting other departments at Meharry to send students and staff to the Mound Bayou hospital in due time. Dr. Walker himself made frequent visits, traveling there for the most critical operations and to conduct ward rounds and conferences.

The arrangements between Taborian Hospital and Meharry Medical College were strengthened in the years that followed. Senior and junior surgical residents from Meharry served from four to six months each year at Taborian. As a result Taborian Hospital was able to give competent surgical care to thousands of patients from the Delta, and Meharry's advanced students received exposure to practice in a rural area, while they helped to provide valuable assistance to physicians throughout Mississippi. They also worked to educate the community of Mound Bayou in the prevention and treatment of disease.[66]

For twenty years Taborian Hospital remained primarily a teaching service for surgical students. In the 1960s, when the story of Mound Bayou and Meharry resumes, other departments began to send their staffs and students, and the joint efforts of these two neighbors was proposed as a model for rural health care throughout the nation.

The extension of Meharry's responsibilities outward from its campus to Mound Bayou and deeper into its own community made the attainment of financial stability more critical than ever. Each of its presidents had strenuously but futilely sought an endowment that would be a secure financial reserve. The college had first depended upon the generosity of the Meharry brothers and the Methodist Church. Then donations from alumni, stimulated by the tenacious personal campaigns of Drs. Hubbard and Mullowney, had won continuing support from the philanthropic foundations. Meharry's friends in Nashville continued to give privately and through community agencies for the support of Hubbard Hospital, and there was also a small amount of income from investments.[67]

Nevertheless, the budget was balanced every year by anxiously assembling just enough from the several sources and by practicing stringent economies in the laboratories, classrooms, and hospital wards. By 1940 it was clear that these revenues, even when accompanied with austerity measures, would no longer be enough. Meharry was gravely threatened by the rising costs of operations. The greatest expense, and the greatest need, was people. In order to recruit and retain men and women of experience and to develop their knowledge and teaching skills continuously, Meharry needed more money than its alumni, friends, and modest investments could provide.

President Turner renewed his efforts to gain an endowment in December 1939 when he presented a summary of Meharry's financial needs to the General Education Board, which had made gran s for the operating expenses of the institution since 1916. At the same time he initiated a national fund-raising campaign. The latter was led by Dr. Abraham Flexner and endorsed by U.S. Surgeon General Thomas Parran.

Dr. Flexner's goal was $6 million. Toward this sum the General Education Board pledged $3.7 million, provided Meharry could raise the remaining $2.3 million. Although the drive for the latter encountered numerous difficulties, it managed to collect about $2 million from alumni and other loyal friends. In the spring of 1944 the General Education Board increased its pledge to $4 million, removed all conditions, and paid over the remaining sum outright.[68] "Nothing of greater significance could have happened to our institution at this moment," Dr. Turner said in gratitude. The attainment of the goal that had eluded the college for three-quarters of a century seemed like a confirmation of the future.

This optimism was soon to be tested, however. The gift of the General Education Board brought its total investment in Meharry Medical College to over $8 million. With that, it declared, it could offer no further support.[69] Other philanthropic groups insisted that they, too, had done their share and would gradually cease making contributions for the operational expenses of the college. Nonetheless, several groups continued such grants for the rest of the decade, and Meharry officials applied them toward the growing costs of running its hospital.

The fortunes of Rockefeller, Carnegie, Kellogg, and others could not meet the continuing needs of Meharry indefinitely. As Meharry's leaders considered how to obtain the capital required for the decades ahead, the question of whether to foresake the college's independent status in favor of a university affiliation was raised anew. Dr. Turner strongly supported the merging of Meharry with Fisk University. The two schools already operated a joint health clinic for students, and when Meharry moved its medical library from Fisk's campus to its own in 1939, the two facilities continued to retain a joint director. During his first year in office Dr. Turner proposed still more areas of cooperation leading toward merger, including shared course offerings in the basic sciences, joint degree programs, and appointment of the president of each institution to the other's board of trustees. He believed that "the Meharry medical unit of Fisk University" would be greatly strengthened in the larger setting. "The position of Fisk would also be materially improved," he predicted, since, joined together, the two schools would constitute a "regional university center."

Dr. Thomas Elsa Jones, Fisk's president, was as eager as Dr. Turner to effect the affiliation of the two schools. He apparently went so far as to urge the General Education Board to condition its endowment to Meharry upon that step. Rockefeller officials did not act upon the idea, however, and when Dr. Turner proposed a resolution calling for the merger to the Meharry faculty it was defeated by an overwhelming majority. So vigorous was this reaffirmation of Meharry's independence by the teaching staff that the question of university affiliation remained closed for another twenty years.[70]

With the failure of the university plan, public funds seemed to be the only remaining source for the long-term financing of Meharry. Such support from the Federal government was unlikely. Education was not generally regarded as a proper concern of Washington. States, counties, and cities, on the other hand, already devoted a major part of their budgets to paying for public schools and colleges; however, they were frequently handicapped by narrow fiscal bases and limited taxing powers.

Southern states in particular tended to rely upon inadequate and regressive revenue schemes; their leaders encouraged low-paying, nonunion industry; and they clung tenaciously to a pervasive network of racial segregation and separation that condemned many of their black citizens to live in poverty generation after generation. By virtually every economic measure the states of the South were among the poorest in the land and consequently the most educationally impoverished, especially in postgraduate, technological, and professional studies. At the end of World War II, for example, Florida had no school of medicine, dentistry, or veterinary science.[71]

Of all the currents spilling into the flood tide of change that would overwhelm the South in the postwar years, the demand for education was among the strongest. Tens of thousands of veterans, their GI benefits in hand, were pressing for admission to colleges. If the South lacked places for them, they were prepared to take themselves and their families north, west, anywhere where American society offered the higher learning and advanced training and repaid it with jobs, increased earnings, and a larger life.

Due to persistent economic woes, few of the dozen states of the region could afford to create or develop a system of colleges equal to the demand. Clearly, however, if they could combine resources, it would be possible to support several specialty schools—in medicine, for instance, or law or library science—so that students could remain in the South and, after graduation, turn their talents and their tax dollars to the region's benefit.

Interstate support of higher education was already a proven success on a limited scale. For example, Tennessee, Virginia, and Alabama had executed contracts with Meharry in the early 1940s to pay part of the tuition of their black citizens who attended there.[72] In 1942 President Turner proposed that Southern states utilize Meharry as a regional professional school for blacks and thereby help build its endowment.[73] Were Meharry to close, the victim of its own financial difficulties, these states would not only lose a continuous flow of black physicians, dentists, and nurses but they would also have to open the doors of their own all-white medical schools to black students in order to make up the difference. The former possibility was acceptable to a few Southern politicians who were indifferent to the continued high mortality and morbidity rates among black people. The latter course they were determined to resist.

Accordingly, in 1948, Southern governors and their legal advisers proposed the Southern Regional Education Compact. Those states ratifying this agreement would be considered members of a "geographical district . . . for the establishment, acquisition, operation, and maintenance of regional schools." I plementation of the plan was placed in the hands of a Board of Control (later known as the Southern Regional Education

Board), whose members were the states' governors, educators, and private citizens.[74]

Actual joint ownership of institutions by the Southern states was one of the ideas heard in early board discussions of Meharry's precarious financial condition. Those who drafted the compact believed that the board could acquire ownership of Meharry and, with funds contributed by the states who were party to the accord, see that it remained the one medical, dental, and nursing school open to black people in the South.[75]

Some of Meharry's leaders were evidently willing to relinquish the college's legal autonomy as the price of regional support. When a committee of Southern governors visited the campus in January 1948, college authorities informally offered to place the operation of the institution in the hands of the Board of Control.[76] However, they reckoned without the alumni. When word spread of the possible subordination of Meharry to regional authority, scores of graduates demanded that their alma mater reject all support, not just ownership, by the Southern states. Like some other black leaders, these outspoken alumni regarded the compact as a device to use Meharry to preserve the all-white medical schools of the South.[77] The Southern governors, they charged, were attempting to evade recent decisions of the United States Supreme Court, notably the ruling in the Gaines case of 1938,[78] which held that laws separating the races in the enjoyment of privileges afforded by the states were constitutional only as long as the privileges were equal. *Gaines* had opened the University of Missouri law school to a black student for the first time, and in light of the decision, racial segregation in graduate and professional education was everywhere in question.

The pressure from the alumni helped to thwart the proposed transfer of Meharry into outside hands. In the fall of 1948 the Southern Regional Education Compact was amended to permit the member states to contract with Meharry, as Tennessee and other states had been doing for several years. For every medical and dental student enrolled from their state, they would pay the college, out of public moneys, $1,500 a year, and for every nursing student, $750. Admissions standards were expressly reserved to Meharry, with the Southern Regional Education Board relegated to the role of fiscal agent.[79]

Meharry received the first group of freshmen under the regional plan the following year. For the next decade the college led all other participating Southern schools in the number of contract students it enrolled. Most of them would have been denied admission to the segregated state medical schools or prohibited by the expense from pursuing education for a career in health. For conferring these benefits, Meharry realized one-third of a million dollars a year at a critical time in its financial history.[80]

For this success and others that it had enjoyed, many regarded Dr. Edward Lewis Turner's administration as among the most brilliant in Meharry's history. Turner himself was not unaware of how much had been accomplished with the help of the faculty, students, and alumni. Meharry "has her face in the right direction and her eyes focused on the stars," he said. His great enthusiasm remained the practice and teaching of medicine, however, and in December 1944 he resigned his office to resume these vocations.[81]

To follow Dr. Turner the trustees elected Dr. Mation Don Clawson. Coming to the presidency from the post of director of dental education, Dr. Clawson had the distinction of being the first dentist to serve in the top leadership position at Meharry. A white man of Dutch ancestry, Clawson had been born in Clay City, Illinois, on February 10, 1900. He was educated in the public schools of the town and went on to take predental training and basic dentistry courses at St. Louis University, one of the best-known of the numerous Jesuit institutions of higher learning in the United States. For advanced training he transferred to the Washington University School of Dentistry, also in St. Louis, and graduated with the degree of D.D.S. in 1926.

Dr. Clawson spent a number of years in the Middle East, where he met and worked as a colleague with his predecessor, Dr. Turner. Clawson served as professor of operative dentistry at the American University in Beirut from 1929 until 1932 and as director of dental education until 1934. At the same time he was director of dental services for the International Petroleum Company, traveling in its interests throughout the Middle East and Africa. Between 1934 and 1939 he was a faculty visitor at the University of St. Joseph, Beirut, and at Syrian University, Damascus.[82] His remarkable success at reviving the moribund School of Dentistry at Meharry, of which an account has previously been given, commended him to the trustees when it fell to them to choose Meharry's fourth executive.

President Clawson assured the faculty and students that there would be "no basic changes in Meharry policy." He pledged his administration to consolidate and make perpetual the gains won by his predecessor. He was particularly intent upon continuing the efforts begun by Dr. Turner to attract the finest teaching talent available and to train outstanding graduates in America's leading medical schools, who would then come to Meharry to teach. The single lofty goal of the new administration was summarized in a motto selected for the college by the faculty in 1938. "A thing worth doing is worth doing well," Dr. Clawson quoted. "Let us make Meharry a center for undergraduate and graduate professional training in medicine, dentistry, nursing, and medical technology second to none."[83]

Even before he could advance the regional plan for medical education entered upon by Dr. Turner, President Clawson was faced with another

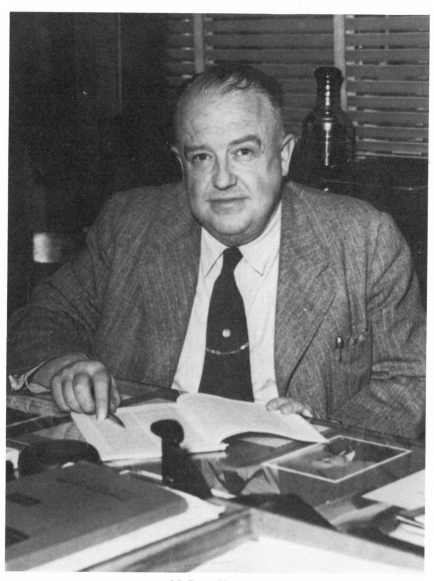

M. Don Clawson

critical financial problem. It began at Hubbard Hospital, but in threatening that facility it soon imperiled all of Meharry. Like the rest of the college, the hospital had been strengthened by the gathering of an endowment. But unlike the rest of Meharry, it had not received occasional support from foundations, nor would it share in the income from the regional education compact. Philanthropists and planners alike took the position that because its patients were primarily residents of Nashville and Davidson County it ought to be supported wholly by those governments or else by money raised locally.

Operating on the income from patient fees was out of the question. Ever since the onset of the Depression, most of those admitted to Hubbard Hospital every year had been unable to pay all or even part of their bill. As national recovery quickened in the late 1930s, the number of paying patients rose slightly, but by 1948 nearly half the hospital's beds were constantly filled by indigents. Most of all the other people treated each day in the outpatient clinic were also without means. Less than 2 percent were able to pay for all the medical services rendered them.[84]

Meharry leaders had for several years sought financing alternatives, including a public hospital for blacks or the operation of Hubbard by the City of Nashville as "the Negro division" of General Hospital. In 1942 Dr. Turner asked the Board of Trustees for authority to seek from the city reimbursement of the costs for treating indigent patients. Local support of Hubbard Hospital remained entirely insufficient, nonetheless. State, county, and city governments contributed little or nothing for the care of patients who were essentially a public responsibility. And although the gifts of charitable organizations, business firms, and private citizens of Nashville were diverted mainly to the hospital, they were not adequate to meet the expenses that Meharry incurred there for treating poor people. As a result the difference between Hubbard's income and its expenses grew year by year. In 1944 it lost $160,000. In 1947 the deficit was $300,000.

The alternatives were clear: either the local governments would have to underwrite Hubbard's operating expenses and erase its debts or the hospital would have to close.[85] Unfortunate as the latter choice would be, Dr. Clawson told a gathering of alumni in 1948, it would not affect Meharry's teaching program. Without patients at whose bedsides they might gain clinical experience, Meharry's junior and senior students would simply be transferred to other hospitals and medical schools with whom Meharry could create affiliation agreements.[86]

Nashville and Davidson County stood to lose mightily if the doors of Hubbard Hospital were shut. At least $1 million a year spent locally by Meharrians would go elsewhere. The two local governments would also have to replace Meharry's $150,000 in services to the poor annually.[87] The loss of an institution of national stature like Hubbard Hospital would, moreover, be an intolerable blow to civic pride at a critical time. Depression and World War past, local leaders were eager to make up for lost time in the growth and development of the city and county.

Nonetheless, in the spring of 1948, neither city nor county was ready to provide for the care of the poor at Meharry's hospital. As a consequence, on June 22, a committee of college officials met to draw up a schedule for closing down Hubbard by July 1. The panel determined the sequence in which services would be curtailed, wards shut, and patients transferred.

The publication of the schedules in the afternoon newspaper evidently convinced city and county officials that Meharry was in earnest. A meeting of the city board of hospital commissioners was convened that same evening, and the group offered the college a contract to keep Hubbard Hospital open. Under its terms the board would pay Meharry for services to indigent black citizens.

The commissioners refused to guarantee a certain amount of money. Instead, the agreement provided for a minimum census at Hubbard of 100 poor patients. For their care the city would reimburse Meharry at the rate of $8.50 per patient per day. So that the 100 beds would always be filled, the contract obligated officials at the city's own hospital, Nashville General, to refer indigent patients to Hubbard "when possible." As long as they did, Meharry could maintain its census, and as long as it cared for 100 poor patients a day it would realize between $215,000 and $225,000 a year from the contract. The latter was the sum required annually to operate Hubbard Hospital.[88]

By July 1949 the plan had failed. Only a little more than $100,000 had been paid to Hubbard Hospital in the first year of the agreement. In Dr. Clawson's view the cause was General Hospital's refusal to refer patients to Meharry except as a last resort.[89] Officials at General insisted that most of its indigent Negro patients could not be spared. General, they pointed out, had a teaching program of its own to maintain: many of its staff, residents, and interns were from Vanderbilt University School of Medicine, and they required for teaching purposes virtually all the poor people who came to General for care. Nashville's two medical schools faced an impasse.

In the middle stood the indigent people themselves, who had very little control or direction over what was to be done about them. As early as 1932 a national study done by the Committee on the Costs of Medical Care, comprising leaders in medicine, public health, and the social sciences, had shown that there was a direct correlation between income and all types of medical service. Nearly half the individuals in the lowest income group in America received no professional medical or dental attention of any kind. Such complete neglect was most common in the South. A specific example was a sample of 500 black patients in Tipton County, Tennessee, who suffered from syphilis: When investigated by the committee, only 3 percent had been given both neoarsphenamine and mercury, and only 14 percent had received any professional medical treatment whatsoever.[90]

By the time the Roosevelt Administration took office, health insurance as well as social security, unemployment insurance, and old-age pensions were being demanded by many private citizens and public interest groups as emergency legislation. Throughout the 1930s, health insurance grew in importance as a national political issue, and in 1936 Senator Wagner of New York introduced in Congress the first of a series of health bills. By the mid-1940s amalgamations and amendments had transformed the legislation into the Wagner-Murray-Dingell bills. They provided for medical care and cash benefits in the case of disability and applied to virtually the entire working population. The sick person was free to choose a physician, who would be paid from Federal insurance funds through fees-for-service or upon a per capita basis or by salary, the choice between these methods being left to the majority of local practitioners.

Despite widespread support from organized labor and black doctors speaking through the National Medical Association, none of these bills was enacted. The American Medical Association led the opposition to their compulsory, national features. As a result the idea of a comprehensive health insurance system supported by tax dollars was shelved for more than a decade. In the meantime the sick and injured among Nashville's poor were thrust into the ironic position of being claimed by two competing hospitals and two friendly but sometimes rival medical schools. The future of Meharry swayed in the balance.

In July 1949 a proposal was at last put forward that addressed Meharry's financial needs while guaranteeing to Vanderbilt an adequate teaching service. Drafted by Nashville attorney Cecil Sims at the request of Mayor Thomas L. Cummings, the proposal called for shifting all ward and outpatient services for indigent Negroes from Nashville General to Hubbard Hospital and, to a lesser extent, to Vanderbilt. For the care of these patients, the two schools would receive subsidies from the city and county governments. In the case of Meharry, the agreement would provide 30,000 patient days of ward service annually at $8.50 per patient per day. Hubbard Hospital would divide another $20,000 each year with Vanderbilt for the care of outpatients.[91]

Dr. Clawson's leadership, together with this commitment by Nashville officials, thus assured that Hubbard Hospital would remain open. With that achievement and the perfecting of the Southern regional education plan, Meharry's fourth president resigned to return to the private practice of dentistry.

In 1950, the year that Dr. Clawson stepped down, over half the black physicians and dentists in America called Meharry their alma mater. With the beginning of the fall semester, there entered the seventy-fourth class in medicine, the sixty-fourth in dentistry, the fiftieth in nursing, and the tenth in medical technology. American life would be fundamentally altered by the time they graduated. The movement for equal rights did not begin with *Brown* v. *Board of Education,* of course. But the new decade would see no American's life untouched by the struggle, no one's mind or spirit uncommitted one way or the other. At Meharry Medical College a new era began with the accession of the first black president in its history.

6

Yearnings for Excellence

DR. M. DON CLAWSON handed his resignation as president of Meharry to the Board of Trustees at its annual meeting in early June 1950. His departure was set for a little over three weeks, the first day of July. It was out of the question for Meharry's executive chair to fall vacant. Such short notice, however, effectively limited the trustees to choosing an administrator who was already well acquainted with the college, its problems, and its opportunities.

Money continued to be a formidable obstacle in Meharry's path. In the decades to come, medicine and medical education would be built upon a foundation of research. Such experimentation and discovery would be largely a matter of sophisticated technology—of antibiotics, isotopes, laser rays, electron microscopes—which required large outlays of capital.

Research would by no means displace bedside teaching as the essence of medical education. Indeed Meharry officials of the 1950s continued to regard training for students to be the chief reason for the existence of Hubbard Hospital. Yet throughout that decade the hospital's manifold fiscal problems would grow more and more acute, until they posed the most serious threat to the survival of the college in its history.

A knowledge of money—how it worked, its uses, its limitations—was therefore critical to Meharry's new president. Among the faculty and staff, Dr. Robert A. Lambert had few peers as financial experts. Dr. Lambert visited Meharry for the first time in 1929, as associate director of medical sciences for the Rockefeller Foundation. In charge of the foundation's programs for medical education and research in the South, he had taken a special interest in the college and had secured many benefits for it through his influence. He was particularly active in efforts to strengthen the faculty, helping Meharry teachers to obtain fellowships for further training. Dr. Lambert was instrumental in bringing to campus Dr. Edward L. Turner, who later presided over six of the most significant years in the history of the college. Throughout the administrations of Drs. Turner and Clawson, Dr.

Lambert took a leading part in Meharry's relations with the Rockefeller Foundation, its single largest benefactor. In 1949, following his retirement, he was elected to Meharry's Board of Trustees.[1]

Whoever succeeded to the presidency would also be expected to increase the scope of Meharry's research activities. A number of faculty members were well qualified for leadership by this criterion. Among them was the biochemist Harold D. West. Besides having published more than fifty papers himself, Dr. West directed the Meharry Biological Research Fund, which raised money for the support of research by black scientists throughout the United States.

It was important that Meharry's new leader be an experienced teacher, since the college's first task remained the education of physicians, dentists, nurses, and technicians. Meharry's chief executive must necessarily be sensitive to the place of the faculty at the heart of the college's life. Among the scores of teachers qualified for the post by classroom experience were Dr. Matthew Walker, chairman of the Department of Surgery, and Dr. Amos Christie, instructor in pediatrics at Meharry and chairman of that department at the Vanderbilt University School of Medicine.

With its roots sunk deep in the soil of the South—most of its students came from there, most of its graduates returned there to practice—Meharry derived important strengths from a sense of its past. As one financial storm after another shook the institution, its faculty and student body took courage from what had been accomplished in seventy-five years against great odds. In that sense, continuity was inseparable from growth. Dr. Hugh J. Morgan, a Meharry trustee like his father and grandfather before him, and professor of clinical medicine at Vanderbilt, was well acquainted with the college's history, as befitted a president.

The skill or expert knowledge possessed by each of these individuals needed only to be combined for Meharry to have the leadership it required. Accordingly, on the advice of Dr. Clawson, the Board of Trustees designated all five as the Interim Committee. Under Dr. Lambert as chairman and Dr. West as vice-chairman, the committee was directed to administer the affairs of Meharry until a new president could be selected.

Every week for the next two years, the five men—three white, two black—met on the Meharry campus to carry out the commission. Decisive choices about the immediate future had to be made, and none of the group felt compelled to dissemble his views. "There was a lot of 'give and take' in those meetings," Dr. Christie recalled. "Dr. Lambert usually activated the recommendations—but the Interim Committee as a whole made the policy."[2]

To the trustees' annual meeting in June 1951, the Interim Committee presented a balanced budget, the first at Meharry in more than a decade. A second important development at the college during the administration of the group was an increase in the number of graduate students, who enrolled to take advantage of a widening range of postdoctoral studies, from short refresher courses through specialty training.[3]

Dr. Lambert and the Interim Committee also presided over the first important expansions of Meharry's twenty-year-old physical plant. A three-story residence hall for unmarried male students represented the college's pioneer venture into student housing. Another new building, Alumni Hall, erected with money raised by the Meharry Medical College Alumni Association, served as its national headquarters and provided refectory and recreation facilities for students and staff.[4]

The ringing of hammer on steel and the whirring of welding irons evinced the beginning of a new period in the history of Meharry. It was not enough, in the words of one trustee, that the college should "stand on its own two feet." There had to be a march forward, to keep pace with new developments in teaching and healing and with changes in the aspirations and self-perceptions of black people in the United States and throughout the world.

On June 6, 1952 the Board of Trustees met in the relative quiet of the college library and elected Dr. Harold Dadford West as president of Meharry Medical College. "A happy choice . . . fitting," declared the city's morning newspaper. Because black teachers had led the faculty throughout Meharry's history and participated in the college's governance to an ever larger extent, the time was at hand for one to assume the top administrative post. Dr. West was recommended by his four colleagues on the Interim Committee, from which, in the words of Dr. Christie, he had "emerged as the leader."[5]

Like several of his predecessors, President West came from a small town in the northern United States. He had been born in Flemington, New Jersey, on July 16, 1904, to the Reverend George H. West and Mary Ann Toney West. While he was still a young man, the family left New Jersey for a pastorate in Washington, D.C. Harold graduated from Dunbar High School there and subsequently enrolled at the University of Illinois.

West received a baccalaureate degree in a premedical curriculum in 1925, but he was unable to attend medical school for financial reasons. Instead he accepted a position as a teacher at Morris Brown College in Atlanta, which had been founded in 1880 by the African Methodist Episcopal Church of Georgia to prepare young men and women for Christian and industrial work. West taught chemistry for two years before being promoted to professor and head of the Department of Science. The year 1927 was one of personal extension and commitment for the young teacher. He became professor of physiological chemistry at Meharry, beginning with the October term. Two months later he married Miss Jessie Juanita

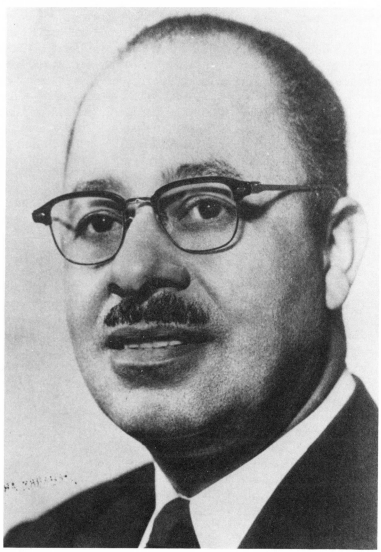

Harold D. West

Penn, daughter of Dr. William F. Penn, chief of the surgical service at Tuskegee Institute.

A fellowship from the Julius Rosenwald Fund enabled West to earn an M.S. degree in biochemistry from the University of Illinois in 1932. With another grant, from the General Education Board, West returned to Urbana in 1935. In the commencement procession of 1937 he wore the hood and colors appropriate for his new degree, the Doctorate of Philosophy in biochemistry. The following year began the brilliant administration at Meharry of President Edward L. Turner. Dr. West returned to Meharry as the first Ph.D. ever to join the faculty. His appointment as professor and chairman of the biochemistry department was part of the new administration's commitment to recognize formally what had long been true in fact—the leadership of the college by black teachers and scientists.

The high quality of medical and dental teaching at Meharry between 1938 and 1950 was nowhere more clearly demonstrated than in the increase in the number of graduates passing state examinations for licenses to practice. Because their success depended upon a thorough grounding in the basic sciences, Dr. West and his coworkers in that division shared in the credit.

West's own reputation was secured by his work on the synthesis of the essential amino acid threonine. Later, he was among the first scientists to use radioactive silver in locating infections and tumors. His research interests also included proteins, vitamins, blood calcium, and the relationship between nutrition and metabolism. His work in the field of detoxication led to important findings about foreign compounds and their role in carcinogenesis. West always acknowledged that research was his first love. Along with his accomplishments as Meharry's president, it was one of his enduring achievements.[6]

Two years' work on the Interim Committee gave Dr. West the experience in financial affairs that Meharry's president needed. His grasp of these and other issues in the institutional life of the college won him the confidence of the trustees. Their ballots were unanimous.[7]

A chilling wind whipped over the campus on the day of Dr. West's inauguration, October 20, 1952. Although the cold held down the audience in number, it was an impressive assembly, with delegates from colleges throughout the nation, including Columbia, Harvard, Fisk, Tennessee Agricultural and Industrial, Vanderbilt, and Yale. Dr. Robert A. Lambert, presiding over the ceremonies, called Dr. West "one of America's greatest scholars."

In his inaugural address and subsequent statements to the press, West defined a humane, limited, practical vision for Meharry. He foresaw himself guiding the institution through a period of "vertical, rather than horizontal development." The foremost task would be the continued growth of the faculty, in quality and in number. Meharry would have to provide fellowships to more of its teachers, pay them higher salaries, and construct additional laboratories where they could do research.

Dr. West also made a realistic inventory of Meharry's problems for the trustees. Certain departments were staffed at levels far below those in other medical schools of comparable size. Meharry desperately needed more room, notably in the obstetric and pediatric services at Hubbard Hospital. Finally, the college had to find ways to cooperate with schools of medicine in other parts of the country, to overcome the isolation imposed by its "special situation" as a black institution.[8]

One problem—lack of money—led to all the others. The endowment, student tuition, paying patients in the hospital, grants, and income from the Southern Regional Education Compact provided enough to balance the budget of the educational program. But the care of indigent patients at Hubbard Hospital, which Meharry carried on in behalf of the city, was causing the college devastating losses. By 1953 the cost of medical services had made the rate at which the city reimbursed Meharry—$8.50 per patient per day—obsolete. When Dr. West saw that the college would in that year spend $161,000 more than the city had appropriated for the program, he directed that the agreement be renegotiated. Meharry's counsel, attorney Cecil Sims, persuaded the City Council to nearly double the reimbursement rate to $15.94. But the college had long owed an overriding moral debt to its nurses, who were working for the lowest professional wages in the city. This increase in Hubbard Hospital's income was spent almost immediately by raising their salaries.[9]

Meharry was losing $11,000 a month on the indigent care program by the autumn of 1955. Rising costs—chiefly supplies and drugs—accounted for part of the deficit. The greater fraction was brought about by the failure of the city of Nashville to honor an important part of the revised 1953 contract with Meharry. The key clause obligated the local government to reimburse the college if Hubbard Hospital was required to spend more to care for needy patients than the city allotted to it in the annual budget. When Meharry presented its bill for excess costs in 1954—more than $75,000— the City Council allocated only a portion of the sum. Most council members evidently were persuaded by the argument that some of the poor being treated at Hubbard Hospital were not residents of the city.[10]

The counties surrounding Nashville that made no adequate provision for the care of their own indigent Negro patients were indeed among the contributors to the hospital deficit. These local governments regularly sent them to Hubbard Hospital where they were received and treated. Sometimes officials of these locales would give assurance that they would honor Meharry's bill, only to refuse any responsibility for it upon the patient's discharge. The government of Davidson County itself added to Hubbard's problems by paying almost nothing, even though a large percentage of indigent patients were county residents.[11]

For the year 1955–56 the Nashville City Council again appropriated less than the amount that Hubbard officials said was strictly necessary for indigent care at the hospital. When the cost exceeded this sum, the council declined to make up the difference.[12] Meharry considered a suit against the mayor and the council to enforce the terms of the 1953 contract.[13] Before taking such a drastic step, Dr. West laid the case for the college before the public. He convened scores of leaders from the education, business, and church circles of north Nashville and asked that they join together as the Meharry Medical College Community Council. This group undertook the task of making visible the plight of the indigent patients and the burden that Meharry shouldered in providing them medical care.[14]

West and other officials also pressed the argument for more public money for indigent hospitalization in every available forum. Meharry's trustees telephoned members of the City Council or sought them out in the restaurants near Fourth and Union streets, where bankers, financiers, and power brokers customarily transacted the affairs of the city over lunch. All these efforts won Meharry the editorial support of Nashville's two daily newspapers.

In the spring of 1956 the city offered to redress Meharry's grievances with a new contract. Its terms, Meharry officials were advised, were not negotiable. The city would pay eighteen dollars per day for each poor person admitted to Hubbard, but the total annual bill for all indigent patients could not exceed $500,000. It would honor a small fraction of Meharry's claims for reimbursement of its excess expenses incurred after 1954. Finally, its auditors would henceforth make a detailed monthly accounting of the hospital's expenses, and further controls would be instituted over indigency determination and length of patient stay.

"If we accept this contract, it is, in a sense, a capitulation," Dr. West told the trustees. Hubbard Hospital would continue to incur a deficit each year into the future, for its costs would exceed the reimbursement offered by the city; it would continue to bear the entire costs for needy outpatients; and it would have to absorb the unpaid deficits for the years 1954–56, most of which the City Council declined to reimburse. Despite its drawbacks, Dr. West had little choice but to sign the new agreement. "Meharry cannot operate Hubbard Hospital without the indigent patients and incurring even more substantial losses," he wrote. "Yet without a teaching hospital we cannot operate a medical school."[15]

In 1963, ten years after the city of Nashville first agreed to indemnify all of Meharry's expenses, the cost of giving medical care to the poor whom it served was still claiming three-fourths of the income from the college's endowment, imperiling support from foundations and the Southern Regional Education Board.[16] Seeing that the city government was not going to meet its obligations toward the indigent, Meharry offered to lease Hubbard Hospital to the municipal hospital authority. As an alternative it suggested that the city build a public hospital in north Nashville, leaving Hubbard chiefly private. Neither idea was acted upon, and Meharry's deficit deepened by nearly a quarter of a million dollars every year.

The consequences were endlessly destructive. Meharry had to replace Hubbard's losses with money that would otherwise have gone to hire teachers, to build research laboratories, to expand the hospital, and to provide more health services to the poor. By mid-decade Meharry needed but lacked funds to hire full-time instructors in psychiatry, gerontology, anesthesiology, and physical medicine and rehabilitation. Because there was no money to enlarge the hospital, there were too few patients to provide an adequate clinical experience for all Meharry students. Some important subjects Meharry was unable to offer at all. The college that had fostered the preventive and therapeutic work in tuberculosis of Dr. Robert Fulton Boyd and Dr. William A. Beck could not afford a full-time teacher of chest diseases. For their clinical work in this subject, some students had to travel to the University of Tennessee's medical school in Memphis.[17]

Despite efforts of Dr. West to pay prevailing academic wages, even veteran members of the postwar faculty had to make personal sacrifices to remain at Meharry. There was simply not enough money to match the salaries available at other American medical schools. Many of these teachers, believing strongly in the necessity of the college, reconciled themselves to low pay as a fact of life. Others, for the sake of their families, felt compelled to accept offers elsewhere. The resignation of several gifted teachers was the single worst reversal dealt Meharry by the financial woes of the 1950s. Their departure caused accreditation teams from the American Medical Association, the Association of American Medical Colleges, and the American Dental Association to withdraw approval of certain programs and to condition others because of the lack of a sustaining number of faculty members. A 1961 accrediting team opined that, because of inadequate operating capital, Meharry compared "very unfavorably with the average medical school in the United States." A timely gift from the Danforth Foundation in 1962 enabled the deans to hire some of the needed instructors and thus save the college's accreditation.[18]

In the School of Nursing, however, difficulties mounted until they proved overwhelming. Enrollment began to decline at the end of World War II and by 1953 there were fewer students enrolled in the first-year class than there were places available. The length of time required to graduate was probably the chief cause. For the Bachelor of Science degree in nursing, the student was required to complete two academic years, followed by three full calendar years. Most families of Meharry students, being of modest or low incomes, could not afford to support their child at the college for such an extended period. Even though Meharry managed to pay a small salary to advanced students, it was also forced, in 1958, to raise tuition and housing fees in the face of its mounting hospital deficit.

Many of those admitted to the School of Nursing after World War II did not do well in their studies. Like most Meharry students, many of them were from the South, where the legally separate primary and secondary schools for black children were extremely poor. Their records prior to enrolling at Meharry often revealed deficiencies in verbal ability, general information, arithmetic processes, and mechanical aptitude.[19]

With competent instruction they, like medical and dental students, could have overcome such handicaps. However, by the late 1950s, Hubbard Hospital had ceased to be an adequate facility for nurse teaching. Forced by its indebtedness to require a forty-eight–hour work week, it offered at the same time the lowest salaries for nurses in Nashville. As other local hospitals gradually desegregated their staffs, Hubbard lost its senior nurses who also taught in the nursing school. The resulting shortage forced Meharry officials to place licensed practical nurses in charge of various units. This action provoked the resignations of still more instructors, who doubted that their students could receive adequate training in such a setting.

When the National League for Nursing evaluated Meharry's program in 1958, it noted the serious problem of faculty turnover, and it requested regular reports from the School of Nursing. By the spring of 1960 no substantial progress had been made in recruiting and retaining teachers. In an effort to bolster the chances of keeping the league's approval, Dean Laurie Martin Gunter, who became head of the school in 1959, sought accreditation from the Southern Association of Colleges and Secondary Schools. Executives from this group had already toured the campus and decided unofficially that the nursing program did not satisfy its requirements.[20] Dean Gunter and Dr. West gambled that a formal report would be more favorable. It was not, however. Accreditation was refused by the Southern Association, then withdrawn by the National League.

In September 1960 the Board of Trustees voted to close the School of Nursing. Although Dean Gunter sought ways to prevent it, such as transferring the program to state-supported Tennessee A & I, her efforts proved futile. No more applicants were accepted, and that year's first-year class received the last degrees. Even after the closing of the school, Meharry was unable to pay prevailing wages to the nurses and nurse aides whom it hired, and it suffered a continual loss of these skilled, essential people.[21]

To meet the continuing financial crisis and prevent further adverse consequences, Dr. West sought to multiply Meharry's income and increase its endowment. Holding that the alumni represented the college's greatest income potential, he personally reactivated chapters of the Alumni Association throughout the United States.[22] Like several of his predecessors he attempted to save money by implementing commercial and financial techniques borrowed from business. (The most conspicuously successful was a personnel and fringe benefit program intended to lower the high rate of staff turnover.)[23] Dr. West also inaugurated several national fund-raising campaigns, increased the admission of paying patients to Hubbard Hospital,[24] and urged the trustees to undertake long-range financial and institutional planning.

The board in 1959 adopted a development plan similar to one that Dr. West had first proposed three years before and set out to raise $20 million over the next decade. The goals were to retain faculty members by boosting salaries and building research facilities, to increase the size of Hubbard Hospital, and to add several new buildings, including a basic sciences center.[25] Progress was agonizingly slow. By 1962 only one-tenth of the amount had been realized.[26] Dollars from private philanthropic organizations continued to be a mainstay of Meharry. Sizable gifts to the endowment fund by the Ford Foundation in 1956 and the General Education Board in 1959 yielded some additional support for teaching.

During this period, for the first time, money was becoming available to Meharry in significant amounts from the Federal government; indeed, these public funds became the largest source of revenue to the college. Grants were realized to develop courses and research programs in the great killing and crippling diseases, including cancer, cardiovascular disorders, and infantile paralysis. Studies in the basic sciences were strengthened when, with a grant from the National Institutes of Health and contributions from private donors, Meharry built a three-story addition to the west wing of the main building. These new suites, opened in the summer of 1963, were devoted to the expansion of research in anatomy, biochemistry, pathology, pharmacology, and physiology. The following October Meharry completed a 111-bed addition to Hubbard Hospital, built with money allocated under the Hill-Burton Act and matching funds from the Stanley Kresge Foundation and other sources.[27]

From one Federal research grant in 1946 the amount of such funds grew steadily at Meharry, as Congress launched national efforts against the chronic diseases. Soon the college was in the ironic position of having access to more funds than it could utilize, due to the shortage of faculty members and laboratory space. Nonetheless, scores of papers from Meharry published in the two decades after World War II testified that it was a period of unprecedented scientific accomplishment there.

Earlier and better diagnoses at Hubbard Hospital showed that cancer was more widespread among black people than had been generally believed. This finding led to the establishment of a cancer clinic and research laboratory. In 1946 Meharry scientists, under the direction of Drs. Paul F. Hahn and Horace Goldie, began experiments with radioactive gold to determine whether it could be used as a screen between diseased and healthy tissues or could even overtake and destroy cancer cells bound by way of the lymphatic system to new sites in the body.[28]

Some members of the Meharry faculty investigated the health menaces that particularly beset black people. Staff cardiologists sought the causes of the high incidence of certain types of heart disease among Negroes, including hypertension, arteriosclerosis, and myocardial infarction.[29]

Countless numbers of people in Africa, South America, the Caribbean, and elsewhere were potential beneficiaries of research into a cure for leprosy. Microbiologists directed their inquiry at cells from leprosy victims, searching for a specific antigen that would produce antibodies to ward off the infection.[30]

Preventive concepts were implicit in the hypotheses of several projects, such as a study of mental retardation in children.[31] A monograph by Fisk and Meharry researchers entitled "A Longitudinal Study of Negro American Infants and Children" concluded that physical and intellectual growth of young black people was tied to social and economic factors.[32] Dental researchers studied the effect of dietary changes on dentition and the relationship between dental caries and periodontal diseases.[33] There were scores of other projects in nutrition, pediatrics, biochemistry, and radiology.

As the number and size of Federal grants grew, so did the pressures to devote one's energy to securing them. The sponsoring agencies often favored narrowly conceived or theoretical proposals, whose purpose was an increase of scientific knowledge rather than immediate improvement in patient care. As was the case in medical schools throughout the United States, Meharry was faced with the question of how to maintain a collaborative relationship between members of its faculty engaged in the practice of medicine and those whose interest was chiefly research. The low salaries that the college paid had the hidden benefit of compelling many of the latter to have private patients as well.

The 1961 accreditation report, when it observed that "yearnings for excellence" among the faculty prevailed over discouragement, pointed to such diversity and enterprise. One physician-educator who was typical of those who worked long hours for modest remuneration was Dr. John R. Cuff (Class of 1926). Dr. Cuff was for many years Meharry's only pathologist (and hence chairman of the "department"). Besides examining all surgical pathology specimens, he performed all the autopsies at Hubbard Hospital. He was also an exceptional teacher, giving lectures and demonstrations to 100 students every week in the morgue, classrooms, and clinical pathology conferences.[34]

In 1957 Meharry was able to employ another long-sought and much-needed teacher of this discipline, Dr. Horace Frazier (Class of 1953). Besides serving as head of the Department of Pathology beginning in 1962, Dr. Frazier published significant research, took a leading role in the development of the Matthew Walker Community Health Center (see below), and served as director of alumni affairs at Meharry.[35]

While specialization was the order of the day at most medical schools in the United States, the teacher shortage at Meharry encouraged considerable diversity on the part of the faculty. Many of the college's teachers of the 1950s carried on simultaneous careers as administrators, classroom instructors, and researchers. One was Dr. Axel Hansen, opthalmologist, director of Hubbard Hospital, and that institution's historian. Another was Dr. Theodore C. Greene, chairman of the Department of Anatomy and an associate of Drs. Hahn and Goldie in their attack against cancer with radioactive gold.

The dean of the medical school himself, Dr. Daniel T. Rolfe, was at one point head of the Department of Physiology, acting chairman of the Department of Anatomy, editor of several college publications, and an active fund-raiser. Dr. Rolfe was named to succeed Dr. Michael J. Bent as medical dean by Dr. West shortly after he became president. The two retained their respective leadership posts for the next thirteen years, working virtually as a team. During West's frequent absences from the campus, Rolfe, along with Dr. Matthew Walker, acted in his stead.

Dr. Rolfe, a man of large girth, immense physical energy, and prodigious memory, was born in Tampa, Florida, on March 1, 1902. At the urging of his father, a builder, he came to Meharry about 1922 to study dentistry. Like many of his fellow students he had barely enough money to meet initial expenses. As he stood in line to register, he overheard some of them discussing the costly equipment that first-year dental students were obliged to buy, and before he reached the bursar, he switched lines and enrolled for the less expensive medical course. He was still not able to afford textbooks, so he borrowed them from classmates, read them overnight, and returned them the next morning. He did not need to look at them again.

Pneumonia—a manifestation of the respiratory trouble that would plague him all his life—caused him to put off his graduation, as valedictorian, until 1927. Following his internship, Rolfe did postgraduate work at the University of Chicago, before returning to Meharry in 1930 to teach and to conduct research in gastrointestinal physiology. As department chairman after 1938, Dr. Rolfe insisted that each instructor be capable of teaching the workings of all parts of the body as well as their interrelationships. As a teacher himself, he was extremely demanding. He considered punctuality a particularly important virtue, and he locked the door of his classroom at one minute after the hour.

Dr. Rolfe did what he could to ensure that those students who met his high standards received the awards due them. He was instrumental in establishing at Meharry in 1957 a chapter of Alpha Omega Alpha, the

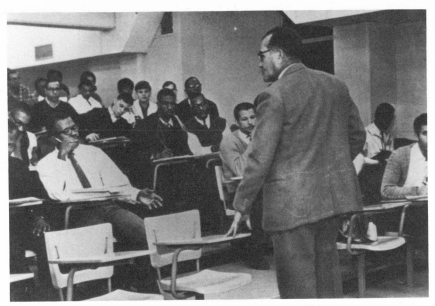

Attending a lecture by Dr. Clarence Wright

national honorary medical fraternity. He personally encouraged excellence in the study of physiology by sponsoring within the department "The Society of the Upper Tenth," which annually inducted the top students enrolled from each school.[36]

Gone were the days when a Meharry student could spare the time during the school year for an outside job. He was considered a junior member of the medical fraternity, a participant in a profession, from the day of matriculation. Such campus organizations as the Student American Medical Association, the Student American Dental Association, the Ewell Neill Dental Society, and the Pre-Alumni Association reflected the increasing self-consciousness of Meharry students.[37]

The amount of information and the number of procedures that a medical student had to master increased dramatically after World War II. To give shape and system to this multiplicity of facts, the four years leading to the M.D. degree were divided into two periods of two years each, the basic sciences and the clinical experience. During the first and second year, students were grounded in preclinical work—anatomy, bacteriology, biochemistry, pathology, physiology, pharmacology. The division between the basic and the clinical sciences was not rigid at Meharry. By the sophomore year the former subjects were being correlated with diagnosis and treatment of disease. For example, second-year students took survey courses in surgery, psychiatry, obstetrics, and preventive medicine.[38]

Upon this foundation the superstructure of clinical medicine was built during the third and fourth years. Beginning in the clinical conferences of their junior year, students took part in discussions of case histories, laboratory data, pathological findings, and diagnoses. On medical grand rounds interesting cases from the wards of Hubbard Hospital were presented to them by the medical faculty and guest clinicians. By the mid-1950s Meharry was providing its junior classes a year's didactic work in clinical psychiatry. Advanced students could also elect a seminar in psychiatry, wherein the psychosomatic approach to disease was emphasized.[39]

Third-year medical students also spent eight weeks in the Department of Internal Medicine. Here they were assigned patients in Hubbard Hospital, on whom they took histories, performed physical examinations, and did laboratory work under the supervision of faculty members. They also attended clinics in dermatology, neurology, pulmonary diseases, and other specialties of medicine.

"I learned to balance a book on one knee and a plate of food on the other," one upperclassman recalled, "to dash off a sandwich with the scent of cadaverine still on my hands. All night on the obstetrics ward—exam tomorrow—two exams the next day—three blood counts before morning—seven chapters in one book, three chapters in another book—urinalysis every four hours for two diabetics—sputum specimens—feces specimens—ward rounds—cigarettes—coffee—blood, sweat, and tears. The deafening roar became a detonating din and then a groan—a sob—a prayer. Sparkling eyes were replaced by rheumy eyes—dim, dreary, daunted, and disconsolate eyes . . . Junior year washed away all that was left of those childish, ill-conceived notions of romance which are associated so intimately with the medical profession."[40]

The highlight of the last year were clerkships in surgery, obstetrics and gynecology, and pediatrics. Each of these was intensive. During the eight weeks the student spent in the Department of Surgery, for example, he attended clinical conferences, carried out special research assignments, worked in the wards of Hubbard Hospital, served in the emergency room, and attended specialty clinics in orthopedics, urology, gynecology, and diseases of the eye, ear, nose, and throat. Seniors were also given outpatient assignments.

During the clerkships students had the opportunity to observe patients over the entire period of their illness and so gained an understanding of the natural processes of disease. They were also expected to correlate roentgenological, laboratory, and symptomatic data, which sharpened their powers of observation, recording, and comparison.[41]

Following the welcome teas and get-acquainted parties of orientation week, freshman dental students settled down to basic courses in biochemistry, anatomy, and physiology. Like their counterparts in medicine, they spent nearly two years in the study of preclinical subjects. In the second and third quarters of their sophomore year, however, textbook theory began to merge into actual practice as they were introduced to the fundamentals of diagnosis. All students were assigned to the dental clinic in Hubbard Hospital during the third and fourth years. There, under supervision of the faculty and visiting teachers, they provided treatment to adults and children, including the restoration of decayed teeth and the fitting of prosthetic appliances. Community dental health problems were the subject of an extensive lecture series in the students' last year.[42]

Beginning in 1953 a voluntary intern program for senior dental students was instituted at Hubbard Hospital. Participants were admitted to study in other areas of the hospital, where they could pose questions to the medical faculty on the oral implications of particular diseases or major trauma. The hospital dentistry program was directed from its founding by Dr. Samuel O. Banks, one of the first black dentists in the nation to be certified as an oral surgeon. In 1962 Dr. James H. Brown assumed charge of the program. Three years later, dental students began receiving academic credit for their hospital work. More and more of them began to take advantage of the opportunity, while at the same time Meharry began making a dental examination part of the care of every patient admitted to Hubbard.

The Meharry classes of this period were the most diverse, in terms of origins, in the history of the college. In the corridors of the medical and dental schools, one was likely to hear the distinctive accents of most regions of the United States. Over a cadaver in the anatomy lab, clipped Harlem street speech answered a slow, rounded Mississippi drawl.[43] Meharry was also deepening its international character. In 1964 its student body included citizens of several African nations, Bermuda, the British West Indies, the Bahamas, Jamaica, British Guiana, and Thailand. Many of them were preparing to return home to help relieve a shortage of physicians suffered by their countries.

Asked why he had chosen to study at Meharry, Samuel Sunday Ezenwa of Onitsha, Nigeria, replied that he had heard about the college from practicing physicians back home. "The study here was pressing," he said, "but this is what I was looking for—hard work. If I am ever able to serve humanity, I'll owe it to Meharry." Following his graduation Dr. Ezenwa joined a thousand other physicians in Nigeria, a nation of 45 million people.[44]

By 1957 Meharry alumni were practicing or teaching in thirty-nine states and seventeen foreign countries, mainly in Africa, Asia, Central and South America, and the West Indies.[45] Many, like Dr. George Henry Starke, had established their own clinic where none ever before existed. Dr.

Starke (Class of 1930) was a veteran of twenty-two years' practice in Sanford, Florida, when he opened his small hospital there in January 1952. He
had begun his practice in the depths of the Depression, immediately upon
graduation from Meharry. Working as a team with Seminole County's
public health nurse, he toured the countryside, treating hookworm and
giving inoculations. Although he never offered his services to whites ("I
didn't want to get into trouble," he said), many of them asked his help and
got it, free of charge. In one year, the county nurse estimated, he did
$27,000 worth of charity work. He was paid barely $2,000, plus oranges, to
support himself.

By the time Dr. Starke built his clinic two decades later, he had 5,000
patients scattered over 1,800 square miles. The two-story facility was designed to accommodate a constant flow of sick people. The forty-seat waiting room was larger than the doctor's office and examining rooms combined. There was also space for $14,000 worth of X-ray, hydrotherapy, and
physiotherapy equipment.[46] As Dr. Starke's sizable practice indicated, there
were still too few Negro health workers to serve black people. For example,
in 1961 there was only one black doctor for every 6,000 Negroes in the
South. In Mississippi every black physician had 18,000 black citizens as
potential patients.

Besides lacking enough doctors, Negroes in the United States continued
to be more vulnerable to disease and untimely death than whites. In 1960
almost four times as many blacks died from tuberculosis as whites. The
incidence of syphilis among blacks was roughly ten times greater on the
basis of reported cases. The rate of Negro children dying from whooping
cough, meningitis, measles, diphtheria, and scarlet fever was at least twice
as high as that for white children. The rate of Negro mortality from cardiovascular disorders was about three times as high as the rate for whites.
Negro women who frequently bore most of the burden of earning a living
in a black household were especially likely to fall victim to hypertensive
heart disease. The deaths of Negro mothers in childbirth and of Negro
babies in their infancy had historically been high, and such was still the
case in the middle of the twentieth century. In 1959 complications arising
out of pregnancy and childbirth resulted in maternal deaths among
Negroes four times as often as among whites. The death rate of black
children before the age of one was almost two times as high as that of white
children in the same period. Mental illness was another malady that occurred more often among blacks than among whites. In 1950 most of the
patients in mental hospitals were Negroes.[47]

These gaps between the health of white and black people were caused
primarily by two factors. The first was economic deprivation. Blacks held
the lowest paying jobs in the labor market, when they could find work at
all. Consequently they tended to subsist on less nutritious diets and to live

in housing without adequate heat and sanitation. In rural areas like the South, such a dwelling could in itself become a source of infection. In northern cities the overcrowding of ghettos and working class areas added to the likelihood of the spread of disease.

A second cause for the differences in Negro and white health in the United States was discrimination by hospitals against black patients and black doctors. Hospitals throughout the South simply refused outright to admit black people, even in emergencies. In the North and West, the sick or injured Negro man or woman was likely to have to wait for one of the few beds reserved for them. These were usually on a "colored ward" or floor, and were less desirable and less conducive to recovery than those available to the hospital's white clientele. Sometimes, local governments, with the sanction of the Veteran's Administration and the Hill-Burton Act, built "separate but equal" public hospitals. These facilities were typically small and antiquated.

Blacks who sought treatment on an outpatient basis from a white doctor might or might not be able to obtain it. Some received humiliation for their pains. Such was the case of a black postal worker in Nashville who became ill on the job one day. From a roster of doctors approved by the post office (no black physicians were listed), he chose one, and upon arrival at the clinic was made to wait in a broom closet.[48]

Even the seriously ill black person who managed to find a hospital bed might be forced to give up his doctor if he or she too was a Negro. To be appointed to the staff of a hospital or to attend one's patients there, a physician had to belong to the local affiliate of the American Medical Association. Until the late 1940s most city and county medical societies refused to let black doctors join. Negro dentists and nurses were likewise denied membership in professional groups other than those they themselves formed, the National Dental Association and the National Association of Colored Graduate Nurses.

In 1946 the American Nurses Association opened membership to all qualified nurses, regardless of race, creed, or country of origin. It thus became the first professional medical association in the United States to end discrimination in its ranks. The AMA followed suit in 1950, although less forcefully. It merely instructed all chapters to "take such steps as they may elect" to eliminate membership restrictions based on race.

A few city and county medical societies had already seized the initiative and admitted black doctors. Very slowly, after 1950, more did the same. In the South AMA affiliates generally continued to hew to a "white physicians only" policy. But even in that region there were notable exceptions. In February 1955, three members of the Meharry faculty—Drs. E. Perry Crump, Axel Hansen, and Matthew Walker—became the first Negroes ever elected to membership in the Nashville Academy of Medicine. This followed a precedent set by other Meharrians a few months earlier in Pulaski, Tennessee, and still earlier by alumni who joined AMA affiliates in Georgia, Oklahoma, and Kentucky.[49]

Among the groups that fought hard to end hospital discrimination against black patients and their doctors was "Imhotep," founded in 1956 by Dr. Montague Cobb. The name, meaning "he cometh in peace," first belonged to a physician of ancient Egypt. The tactics utilized by Imhotep in integrating American hospitals were indeed peaceful, but also relentless. Chiefly the group sought to prevent public funds from being used to construct hospitals that practiced racial discrimination.

Advances in eliminating such barriers in health were slow—internships, residencies, and staff appointments for black doctors were still difficult to obtain. Neither was progress uniform. By the middle of that decade there were still many hospitals in the South with discriminatory policies and local AMA chapters that disallowed black members.

Despite all the obstacles and the continuing differential in rates of death, black people in general were making triumphal gains in health. In 1940 the life expectancy of blacks, fifty-three, was eleven years less than that for whites, sixty-four. In 1960 the gap was just seven years, sixty-four for Negroes, seventy-one for whites. From 1900 to 1960 the lifespan of American Negroes doubled, from thirty-two to sixty-four on the average, twice the percentage gain of the white population.[50]

In addition to laboring for still greater improvement in health among black people through its dispersed alumni, Meharry began, in the late 1940s, to expand its services to the sick and injured in Nashville and the surrounding area. A crippled children's ward and outpatient clinic was opened in Hubbard Hospital in 1946. Its most prominent feature was a hydrotherapy tank that enabled Meharry's physical therapists to massage any affected area of a patient's body without entering the unit. The first of its kind in Tennessee, it was purchased by several community agencies and individuals interested in the welfare of crippled children. The new unit, together with grants from the National Foundation for Infantile Paralysis, made it possible for black physicians and graduate nurses to become specialists in poliomyelitis. At the time there was no other facility in the South where Negro children who were victims of the dreaded disease could be treated.[51]

Meharry began a pediatric care program in 1947 with annual grants from the United States Children's Bureau, an agency of the Federal government. Each year almost 2,000 black children from Nashville received medical and dental care that they would have otherwise done without.[52]

In the autumn of 1956 one wide-eyed, underdeveloped boy celebrated his sixth birthday in his room at Hubbard Hospital. Under the circumstances, the event was a triumph for him and for his doctor. Young Vernon

Donaldson had been brought to Hubbard Hospital from his hometown, Ocala, Florida, with an enormously high count of white corpuscles in his blood. The diagnosis was acute lymphatic leukemia.

Dr. Edward Caldwell, resident in pediatrics, took charge of Vernon's case. For the next thirty hours, while the boy's body cleared itself of previous medication, Dr. Caldwell and his colleagues studied Vernon's condition. The Hubbard staff then began treatment with two drugs, aminopterin and Meticorten, which destroyed the excess white cells. Slowly the boy's blood count returned to normal. It was only a stage of remission, Dr. Caldwell told his patient's parents. Vernon would have to return to Hubbard for further treatment. In the meantime, however, he could go home—and look forward to a seventh birthday.[53]

Meharry also continued to reach out to the impoverished people of the Delta country of Mississippi by sending two dozen surgical and obstetrical students every year to Taborian Hospital in Mound Bayou. "It's an old story," Dr. Matthew Walker said, "the call for help from Mound Bayou. A surgical team—anesthetist, surgeon, and a specialist—jump into a car after working all day and drive half the night for an operation." In the first twenty years after the affiliation agreement, Dr. Walker himself made the trip between Nashville and Mound Bayou more than 200 times.

Under close supervision of their teachers, Meharry students followed patients from admission to Taborian through postoperative or postpartum recovery and discharge. Few of them looked forward to their tour of duty in Mound Bayou. ("We sometimes had to draw straws," Dr. Walker remembered.) But many found the experience rewarding and were encouraged to practice where the need for physicians in the United States was greatest, in small towns and rural areas.

Like all modern general hospitals, Mound Bayou's needed many kinds of people in addition to medical specialists to carry on its work. Members of the supporting staff at Taborian—cooks, admitting clerks, social workers—were residents of the town or the surrounding area, descendents of the black pioneers who had settled there after the Civil War. Prior to being hired many of them had had no training or work experience, as such things were ordinarily measured. Once employed they were taught to do their jobs like Meharry's medical and dental students were prepared for theirs—by actually performing them under skilled supervision. A few, such as anesthetists and laboratory assistants, were sent to Meharry for short courses of technical training.

Like the officials of Hubbard Hospital, Taborian's administrator, Mrs. L. B. Griffin, was faced with a chronic shortage of money and space. By 1966 Taborian Hospital, designed for fifty-two sick people, often had twice that number, with beds lined up head to foot down the halls. There was a waiting list, never enough equipment, and little of the latest. Early in 1965

Mrs. Griffin contacted the new Office of Economic Opportunity in Washington to see if it could furnish any help. The OEO, as it came to be generally known, was the command post of the "War on Poverty," which had been declared by President Lyndon Johnson in his first State of the Union address in January 1964. His battle plan, the Economic Opportunity Act, was quickly passed by Congress.

One of the most ambitious parts of the act was the Community Action Program, which supported various kinds of social improvement initiatives directed by local authorities with "maximum feasible participation" of the people served. Community action was intended to foster better housing, wider educational opportunities, and improvements in health services for—and by—the poor.[54]

The prospect of help for her beleaguered hospital led Mrs. Griffin to present Taborian's story to OEO officials. When she explained to them that for two decades Meharry had been providing care for disadvantaged patients at Mound Bayou, the interest was suddenly mutual. Dr. Howard Brown, medical director of New York's Beth Israel Medical Center and consultant to OEO, immediately traveled to Mound Bayou to confer with Mrs. Griffin, Dr. Walker, faculty members, and students. He also examined patients in the hospital and in their homes.

Many of those admitted to Taborian Hospital suffered from gallbladder ailments, a result of the fatback that was the staple diet of many Delta people. Some of the children in the hospital showed bleeding tendencies, pot bellies, and skin discoloration—symptoms of pellagra, a niacin deficiency not uncommon among youngsters fed mainly on salt pork, meal, peas, and beans. Many of the children had from eight to fifteen cavities.

The visitor to Mound Bayou also called at hovels that were home for as many as a dozen children. At one, the father had tuberculosis. At another there was a stove that did not work, a water well on the same level as the privy, and a dirty icebox that contained nothing but a pan of mush that was the daily meal for a young woman and her ten children, aged six months to thirteen years. One was a mongoloid. They worked five acres of land belonging to a plantation owner, and the cotton crop grew up to the broken planks that passed for a porch.[55]

Appalled by these conditions, Dr. Brown was nevertheless impressed by what Meharry had helped to accomplish at Taborian Hospital. Pregnant Delta women who would otherwise have had their babies at home were examined throughout their term and delivered in safe, antiseptic surroundings. Sufferers from simple but debilitating ailments were treated and cured. Victims of serious illness often received help before it escalated into an irreversible condition.

If Mound Bayou needed anything, it was more of the same, Dr. Brown concluded. At the end of his tour, he suggested that Meharry submit a formal application for funds to expand Taborian and to augment the staff. Dr. Walker had long beheld the prospect that the visitor from Washington glimpsed, and he returned to Meharry determined, now that the means were available, to enact it into reality. Dr. West shared his senior colleague's enthusiasm. Immediately Meharry's president appointed a committee to assist him in preparing a formal proposal to the OEO. He, Dr. Walker, Dr. C. W. Johnson, and Dr. Robert S. Anderson, composed the initial group.

The four men discussed the matter at length during the spring of 1966 and concluded that Meharry must seek funds for Mound Bayou's hospital. But, they added, the college should at the same time request a grant to build a health center to serve the poor people who lived in the vicinity of its own campus in Nashville. At its annual meeting in May, the Board of Trustees gave permission to proceed with this plan. Drs. West and Walker immediately flew to Washington to present to OEO officials the draft of the application prepared by committee members.

On June 3 Meharry officials met with agency staff members, Drs. John Frankel and Joseph English, over breakfast in Nashville's Andrew Jackson Hotel. They agreed to a few refinements, arrived at a financial request, and the completed document was signed by Dr. West and Dr. Walker. The OEO representatives assured Meharry that a favorable decision would be forthcoming. However, they insisted that three steps would have to be taken immediately upon formal approval.

The first was that Sara Brown Hospital in Mound Bayou be included in the project there and that its wards and staff be opened to whites. The second was that Dr. Walker meet with officials from Tufts University and that the two colleges begin preparing to cooperate in the expanded attack upon the health problems in Mound Bayou. Tufts had already received an OEO grant to carry out a project similar to the one upon which Meharry was about to embark. It planned to locate its urban community health center near its campus in Boston. As for a rural clinic, university officials had considered several sites in Mississippi and chosen Mound Bayou because of the staff and services offered by Meharry at Taborian Hospital. Two members of the faculty of Tufts University School of Medicine, Drs. Count D. Gibson, Jr., and H. Jack Geiger, had lent technical assistance to Meharry in preparing its grant proposal. Finally, approval was to be given with the stipulation that poor people themselves be involved in Meharry's program at the new Nashville health center. It was expected that they might perform a multitude of important jobs, including assisting physicians, advising homemakers, caring for children, and dispensing nutrition advice.

On June 24, 1966, Dr. West received a telephone call from Washington confirming approval of the grant. A telegram from Sargent Shriver, director of the OEO, followed the next day. The initial grant to Meharry, in the amount of $54,000, was to be used to identify the health problems of the poor in Nashville's inner city and to evolve a plan for a facility that would attack them. When the plan was approved by the OEO, additional funds would be made available to carry it out.[56]

Nashville's indigent people were, of course, already well known to every Meharry student and teacher. Daily they crowded together on the benches in the outpatient department or gazed up from a worn mattress serving as a sickbed in their home. At Hubbard Hospital the care dispensed to them had brought the college to the edge of bankruptcy. Despite the multi-million-dollar development program of the early sixties and incalculable sacrifices and service by its faculty and staff, Meharry still lacked sufficient resources to cope with the extent of illness among the poor in its own environs. Their cramped frame houses in north and south Nashville and in the shadow of the Capitol disgorged an endless stream of misery.

The Nashville health center would mark a turning point in Meharry's commitment to the poor. It would be built with the first grant given to the college by the Federal government solely for the care of sick people. It would also reflect a reconsideration of what Dr. Matthew Walker called, in his Convocation Day address in 1966, "the high 'ivory tower' concept" of medicine that was "mainly research-centered."[57]

As Dr. Walker and scores of other Meharrians began to plan for the new facility, they often spoke among themselves of "comprehensive care" and "multidisciplinary approaches" to describe the treatment they hoped it might dispense. These were untested ideas, and their meaning awaited fulfillment in human terms. But they did point to a new understanding at Meharry of the patient and a more sophisticated effort to view him or her as a whole person whose plight was caused or complicated by a tangled skein of pathology, racism, and poverty.

Meharry's patients, these planners asserted, required a sympathetic comprehension of their powerlessness. Bereft of their health and without means, they were likewise liable to be stripped of their humanity, to be regarded as "clinical material" or "charity cases."

Meharry's health center committee had to take account, as well, of their powerlessness as citizens. It had been vividly demonstrated in the refusal of Nashville's city council to fund at an adequate level the indigent care program at Hubbard Hospital. But the black poor of Nashville had long been excluded from a role in many basic decisions that affected their lives—decisions made by government, by commerce, even by Meharry itself. And each of these institutions had contributed to the conditions that characterized the black neighborhoods of the city and kept mortality and morbidity rates within them high.

If Meharry, through the new health center, were to attack sickness among Nashville's poor in a comprehensive way, it would have to bring to the individual sufferer the finest care available from modern medicine. It would also have to move to disassemble the network of ills that brought people to the health center in the first place. That meant helping them to gain a voice—to attain "maximum feasible participation"—in the life of their city, including the health center itself.

Scarcely anyone could foresee or predict the consequences of such an undertaking. Virtually all of Nashville's black people, and particularly that considerable portion who were poor, were themselves invisible, deliberately and relentlessly unseen by the power structure of the community. But in the tumultuous decade of the 1960s, they made their presence felt, in the streets, in the courts, in unmistakable ways.

7

Time of Transition

THE BLACK STUDENTS were sitting quietly at Woolworth's lunch counter, waiting to be arrested, when the group of young white men entered the store. Some of the students were reading. Most were poised and silent. They were the fourth group of Negro students to apply for service at downtown eating facilities on that last Saturday of February 1960. More than fifty of their friends had already been led out of McLellan's and Walgreen's to the waiting paddy wagons.

When the doors opened, therefore, they expected to see the police. The gang of whites entered instead. They jostled and shoved each other as they trooped down the aisle between the stools where the blacks were sitting and the store's cosmetics display. In a moment a wad of gleaming spit flew through the air and splattered on one of the students. Another demonstrator stiffened as the heel of a boot slammed into his back. One of the whites took a cigarette from his mouth and ground its burning point into the back of a third. "Black bastard," he muttered.

A second group of Negro students was sitting at the other counter on the mezzanine. When the whites noticed them there, they clumped up the stairs. One of the gang assumed a boxer's stance behind the seated students, and his companion did a bebop dance. Suddenly the tense situation exploded. A pair of white youths grabbed Maurice Davis, an eighteen-year-old college freshman, and spun him from his stool. Another white boy slammed his fist into Davis's face. The black student did not strike back. Neither did he allow his assailants to wrestle him to the floor. "Stop, you s.o.b., and fight!" the white youth screamed, shoving Davis against the wall.

Other gang members set upon Elvin Seale of Tennessee Agricultural and Industrial College. Then they grabbed Emory Irving of Fisk University and rolled him down the stairs. When the police arrived a few minutes later, the white thugs had fled the store and disappeared into the crowds that gathered to watch the arrest of the Negroes.[1]

129

Two months later at 4:30 on an April morning, a car slowed in the street in front of Meharry Medical College. A figure slipped from it and hurried to the sidewalk opposite the campus. In his grip were more than ten sticks of dynamite, which he lit and hurled toward the dark, quiet house in front of him. The blast threw wood, glass, and smoke into the air, as the bomber fled away in the car. Although it reeled under the concussion, Meharry was not the target. The intended victim had lain sleeping in the back bedroom of the house now wrecked by the bomb.

For more than a decade, attorney Z. Alexander Looby had been recognized as one of the foremost Negro leaders in Nashville. Recently his reputation had taken on national proportions as black demand for participation in the life of the city closed with old and settled patterns of gentility, lethargy, exclusion, and neglect. Born in Antigua, British West Indies, on April 8, 1899, Looby immigrated to the United States in 1914. He received the A.B. degree from Howard University in 1922 and the LL.B. from Columbia in 1925. The following year he earned a Doctor of Juristic Science degree from New York University. Coming to Nashville in 1926 Looby served for two years as assistant professor of economics at Fisk. He was admitted to the Tennessee bar in 1929, and in 1931 he was appointed lecturer in medical jurisprudence at Meharry. Subsequently he founded the Kent College of Law, which offered legal training for blacks, who could not be admitted to the law schools of the South. From 1943 to 1945 he was president of the J. C. Napier Bar Association, Nashville's organization for black attorneys.

Looby first came to prominence in the latter years when his efforts led to the establishment of equal pay scales for black and white teachers in the public school system. Then in 1946 he won acquittal, before an all-white jury, for twenty-three black citizens of Columbia, Tennessee, arrested during a gun-blazing raid by the sheriff's department on the town's Negro quarter. In the opinion of *The Nashville Globe,* Looby's defense was "one of the greatest battles ever fought to vindicate the Constitutional rights of American citizens."[2]

As chairman of the legal committee of the National Association for the Advancement of Colored People, Looby was credited with desegregating the dining room at the Nashville airport and the city's public golf courses. He also traveled to other points in Tennessee as co-counsel with local black attorneys to challenge segregated public schools and colleges. In 1951 Looby became the first black elected to the City Council in more than forty years. His north Nashville district included Meharry Medical College.

Ten years after the dramatic trial at Columbia, Alexander Looby filed suit in Federal district court to desegregate the public schools of Nashville. A. Z. Kelley was a Negro barber whose son, like little Linda Brown of

Topeka, Kansas, was greatly inconvenienced by having to take a bus across town to attend a black school while there was a white school within a few blocks of home. Nashville's Board of Education had emphasized the adjective rather than the noun in the U.S. Supreme Court's order to admit black children to public schools "with all deliberate speed." Young Robert Kelley's litigation was the first step by blacks in Nashville on a long road toward winning compliance with the law of the land by local officials.[3]

The NAACP, under Looby's leadership, was a principal sponsor of the lawsuit, and it otherwise played a key role in nurturing a new generation of black leaders in Nashville. It also encouraged thousands of black citizens to add their names to the rosters of registered voters. As the rolls swelled in black precincts, Nashville's political leaders found it necessary to create at least the appearance of consultation. Yet only a few blacks invested by the white establishment as spokesmen for the Negro community were admitted to council and their views entertained for the record.

Despite the examples of Harold West at Meharry and Charles Johnson at Fisk in transforming "colleges for blacks" into colleges under black leadership, the traditional perception that Negro advancement took place at the pleasure of the white majority was still widespread in 1960. In this view, voting, school integration, and wider employment opportunities were benevolent grants and not necessarily rights or amenities enjoyed by black people as a legacy of citizenship. Some postwar black leaders in Nashville tried to advance black rights and opportunities locally by pursuing tactics of accommodation.

The Nashville Globe, on the other hand, while hewing to the banner of the Republican Party on national issues, offered a radical economic interpretation of the causes of World War II and struck a militant stance in favor of black participation in the shaping of Nashville's postwar future. In 1946 it successfully rallied voters against a proposed civic plaza that would have required resettlement of the principal black business district, near Fourth and Charlotte avenues. It opposed increases in fares by the city's transit company, in the interest of low-income riders. The *Globe* was also a major forum through which the NAACP conducted its campaigns to enlist members and register voters. On this and other issues, including the controversial Fair Employment Practices Commission, established by President Franklin Roosevelt as part of the war effort, the newspaper and the black rights organization spoke with one voice. The conspicuous successes of the *Globe* and the NAACP were gratifying to the rising generation of young black Nashvillians and those who settled in Nashville after the war.

In 1940 blacks showed a gain in numbers in the city instead of a loss since the previous census year. During the 1950s there was evidence that the Negro middle class was growing, however slowly, as a small number of young people moved out of traditional black occupations—the ministry, undertaking, barbering, domestic service, and manual labor—into at least entry-level jobs in various kinds of employment previously reserved to whites. The median age of blacks in Tennessee's capital also dropped as the midcentury approached, suggesting a slowdown of migration of the young from the city.[4]

All shades of opinion on the pressing questions facing black people could be found among the faculty members of the four black colleges in the city. To an ever-increasing degree, however, the conservative habits in the administrative suites were being challenged by the liberal ideas in the classroom. Even the most scholarly and objective account of, for example, the recent liberation of India from British rule, could not help but breed a certain restlessness in the black men and women students. And while the older spiritual leaders of black Nashville continued to preach the Gospel of a meek and sentimental Jesus, many young black people looked for their example to "Christ the Tiger," who triumphed by a righteousness that would not be resisted and a love that would not yield.

The Reverend James Morris Lawson, Jr., was typical of the educated, articulate members of this generation who took up the cause of desegregation in Nashville. Thirty-two years old in that winter of 1960, the Reverend Lawson was looking forward to graduation from the Divinity School of Vanderbilt University the following spring. For two years he had been immersed in intensive studies of the Bible, Christian ethics, and Western philosophy. That intellectual experience strengthened his conviction that violence was a sin. It also led him to conclude that the laws of a just God took precedence over the mundane codes and statutes of man, a view that he shared with the abolitionists, black and white, of a century before. Lawson was not content to remain a theoretician, however. It was clear to him that the progress of black Americans meant that the dispositions of the heart and convictions of the mind must be translated into tactics for the street.

Lawson admired the Reverend Martin Luther King, Jr., and was a member of his Southern Christian Leadership Conference. Ever since the refusal of Mrs. Rosa Parks to yield her seat on a Montgomery bus to a white passenger, the SCLC had been a leader of the nonviolent forces against segregation across the South. In workshops sponsored by the Nashville chapter, Lawson and other black ministers, together with scores of eager students, talked about the best ways to carry out a successful protest against the city's segregated lunch counters. Drawing upon their classroom studies and the experiences of the first sit-in demonstrators of Greensboro, North Carolina, the workshop participants drew up a set of practical instructions.

DO show yourself friendly at the counter at all times.

DO sit straight and always face the counter.

DO refer all information to your leader.

DO remember the teachings of Jesus Christ, Mohandas K. Gandhi, and Martin Luther King.

DON'T strike back or curse back, if attacked.

DON'T laugh out.

DON'T hold conversations with floor walkers.

DON'T leave your seat until your leader has given you permission.

DON'T block entrances to the stores and aisles.

Remember love and non-violence. May God bless each of you.[5]

Each of the nearly 100 demonstrators who assembled at three of Nashville's black colleges on the morning of February 13, 1960, was handed a mimeographed copy of these guides. Then they set out on foot through a falling snow to take seats at the lunch counters of Woolworth's, Kress's, and McLellan's in downtown Nashville. For five hours they sat unserved. Two days later some 200 students marched on the same establishments and added Grant's to the list. By the end of the week the number of marchers rose to 350, and Walgreen's was included. Finally, on Saturday, February 27, seventy-nine demonstrators were arrested. Seventy-four of them were black. None was from Meharry Medical College.

Four days later, Vanderbilt University gave the Reverend James Lawson the choice of withdrawing as a student or being dismissed. When he declined to leave voluntarily, he was expelled. There was no prospect that Vanderbilt's action would put an end to the sit-ins. The protest against Nashville's segregated dining facilities did not depend upon a charismatic leader. Facing the baleful stares of the crowds, the shouted insults, and the fists drawn back in rage, the individual, his courage, and his self-discipline were what counted. As the cases of those arrested in the sit-ins reached the dockets of city court, a dozen NAACP attorneys enlisted in their defense. Several, such as Avon Williams, were prominent in the black bar of Nashville. One, Robert Lillard, served on the City Council. The dean among them was Z. Alexander Looby.

Looby, although belonging to a different generation from the students and possessing credentials honored in the city's white establishment, was persuaded of their cause. The claim that a higher law mandated disobedience to state regulations requiring segregation in restaurants might be settled in some other forum. But in the court where the students' cases were to be heard, they required a skillful defense.

As the trials proceeded Looby appeared almost daily in the headlines. If his was a name that inspired admiration in some, in the mind of one it rankled. That one fashioned a bomb out of dynamite and hurled it with a rage, arising perhaps out of oppression that he himself suffered, toward the picture window of Looby's north Nashville home. Misaimed slightly—a fact that saved Looby's life—the dynamite fell to the ground, detonating alongside the foundation. The floor of the dining room took the full force of the blast and sank under the weight of splintered furniture.

Like a giant's fist the concussion slammed into the walls and windows of Meharry Medical College across the street. Blasted from its frames, the glass from the windows in the men's dormitory flew through the air, cutting several students who were asleep in their beds. It was strewn over the floors of the cafeteria and the recreation center in Alumni Hall.

Meharry students were among the first to reach the shattered Looby home. Dazed, blinded by the swirling smoke, the attorney and his wife stood miraculously unhurt in the doorway. Broken windows were all the damage done to the back room where they had been asleep. Even before the wail of sirens rose on the chill morning air, it was clear that amid the rubble lay any hope that Meharry could stand apart from the forces of change swirling around it. That afternoon the largest demonstration since the lunch counter sit-ins began wound from north Nashville's black colleges down Jefferson Street to the courthouse to demand an immediate end to segregated dining facilities in Nashville. Mingled through the line of 3,000 marchers were many from Meharry.

Imperative and troublesome, the demand for equal opportunity regardless of race agitated the campus as well as the city and the nation. Throughout the 1950s the pressure grew upon Meharry to admit white students. One source of this pressure was the beginning of the desegregation of public schools in the United States. Its slow, checkered progress was accomplished by an increase in the number of black students admitted to previously all-white colleges, including medical schools. By 1958 one black medical student in three was attending a predominantly white institution.

Meharry's charter made no stipulation prohibiting white students; indeed, whites had enrolled there in its early years.[6] But the opening of some medical, dental, and nursing schools formerly closed to blacks seemed to call for a larger, reciprocal response on the part of Meharry.

Dr. West opposed the admission of white students on any significant scale until there was a sizable increase in the number of places open to Negroes in freshmen classes at other schools. At the same time, he opposed segregation at Meharry in perpetuity. Following the decision of the United States Supreme Court in *Brown* v. *Board of Education* in 1954, he ordered dropped from the college catalogs the word "Negro" whenever it was used in reference to Meharry students.

Other Meharry leaders stood forthrightly in favor of admitting students without regard to race. In December 1955 the faculty of the School of Dentistry declared in a resolution that it would not "exercise the act of racial proscription" in selecting students, and that henceforth applicants for admission would be considered "on the basis of educational qualifications and character." Prior to that step, the Interim Committee had established a policy that "opportunity for training" would be granted to "non-Negro applicants," providing qualified black applicants were not displaced.[7]

The difficulty was that most of the whites applying to Meharry did not meet the entrance requirements: at least three years of acceptable college credit (two for dentistry), with a heavy concentration in biology, chemistry, and physics, and a satisfactory score on the Medical College Admission Test. Many of them were unqualified for any medical school; yet they assumed that standards were lower at Meharry than at other colleges and, therefore, that their chances for admission were better. Some had actually matriculated elsewhere, then failed. In 1955 there were thirty-four white applicants in medicine and sixteen in dentistry, but not one of these fifty met Meharry's minimum standards.

In 1957 three young white people—two men, one woman—presented credentials acceptable to Meharry's admissions committee, and they were invited to enroll for the fall semester. Although the action broke all recent precedent, the committee (comprising the deans of the three schools) did not trouble to inform anyone in the administration.

When Dr. West learned that the white students were expected to begin classes, he anticipated some adverse reaction and took steps to see that no public mention was made of their arrival. All three registered quietly on schedule—the two men in medicine and dentistry, the woman in nursing. A full year passed before the press discovered that Meharry had integrated its classes. The reaction that Dr. West feared did indeed occur—not from the public or alumni, but among members of Meharry's Board of Trustees. In November 1958 the board's Executive Committee ordered that no more white students be admitted. Meharry's precarious financial state may have prompted the moratorium in part. However, a third of the board members were over seventy years old, and many among this senior group believed that the chief reason for perpetuating Meharry was to prevent the integration of predominantly white medical schools.

To dampen the internal controversy, a three-member ad hoc group was appointed from the Board of Trustees to study the question. Its recommendation, approved handily by the full board in May 1961, was simple: all admissions policies were to be decided by the admissions committees of the schools, which comprised members of the faculty. The resolution declared it to be the position of the trustees that black applicants should be given preference. Under its terms, however, the board would henceforth exercise no role in decisions as to who should study at Meharry.

Throughout the early 1960s the number of white applicants increased. This was accompanied by a decline in the number of blacks who sought admission. (The drop in Negroes seeking to study medicine was a national phenomenon, experienced by virtually every school that admitted them.) By 1964 the ratio of whites to blacks applying to Meharry was two to one in medicine and three to one in dentistry.

Some of the white students presented more impressive undergraduate records than some of the black students. The latter were, nonetheless, usually awarded the places in the first-year class. As a rationale Dr. West cited extensive documentary evidence showing that the health of the Negro population was still largely in the hands of Negro professional people. The accreditation committee of the American Medical Association did not find this fact compelling. Its report following its 1961 inspection strongly urged Meharry to accept only those students who would be qualified for admission to any medical school in the United States.

The policy that Meharrians themselves shaped was one that avoided extreme positions. It rejected the view that the college should admit only the "best qualified," which would effectively assure its becoming a majority white school, given the educational advantages that white students had in undergraduate training. At the same time, competition for the privilege of attending was again opened to whites. In the short term, their numbers would be relatively high, both because of the diminished number of black applicants and because Meharry was obliged by accreditation agencies to align its admissions standards with the prevailing ideas of adequate preparation. After 1965 white students made up almost one-fifth of Meharry's first-year class. To many it seemed that diversity of people, complementing and increasing the diversity of ideas that was the essence of college life, provided greater stimulus to learning.[8]

There were other long-standing institutional habits at Meharry that were destined to be overthrown by new developments in medicine, by the public's growing demands for its services, and by the aspirations of black people. World War II had profoundly affected the expectations of 15 million Americans who served in uniform in regard to doctors, hospitals, and the care provided by them. From induction to discharge the soldier or sailor usually received medical attention superior to what he had known at home.

Television and picture magazine coverage of the latest "miracle drug" or complicated and costly therapeutic device contributed to a rising expectation on the part of Americans about what medicine could and ought to do for them. Many considered that its goal should be to assist them in attaining a full and robust state of health equal to any required or contemplated task. In an important and influential definition put forward in the late 1940s, the World Health Organization declared: "Health is . . . a state of complete physical, mental, and social well-being, not merely the absence of disease or infirmity."[9]

By this concept the test of one's condition would not be a textbook standard but, rather, what one was able to do and to accomplish. The concern of contemporary medicine was the capacity of human beings for the "prodigal expenditure of energy" that Dr. Alan Gregg of the Rockefeller Foundation denoted as the sign of well-being.[10]

The role of the physician, laboring under such a standard, would likewise undergo significant change. As one observer wrote, the modern doctor "must consider the overall performance of the individual according to his position in life . . . to correct and amend what impedes [him] in his adventure of living."[11]

As the popular expectation grew that medicine could supply answers to a broad range of problems, the health questions brought to the doctor's consulting room increased in number and diversity. They ranged, according to one authority, " . . . from sagging anatomies to suicide, from unwanted childlessness to unwanted pregnancy, from marital difficulties to learning difficulties, from genetic counseling to drug addiction, from laziness to crime."[12]

Common to these and other problems in which the patient's personal and social environment was implicated was a role for him in his own care. As he assumed responsibility for helping to maintain his state of health, his presence in the process seemed natural, obvious, and essential.

The nation's chief soporific agent, television, hastened the expansion of the sick person's role in decisions that had a bearing upon his health. While insurance promotions and fund drives against cancer or heart disease emphasized the precariousness of health, the image purveyed in prime-time programming made no place for illness or even serious bodily discomfort. On the contrary, members of typical television families seemed to feel good all the time. Allergies, high blood pressure, and the natural problems associated with aging rarely figured in the plot lines.

The nation's large pharmaceutical houses were among the chief sponsors of these shows, and their commercial messages continued the theme of the needlessness of disease, given the existence of their products for the relief of aches, pains, and stress. Implicit was a certain amount of blame for the sufferer. But on the positive side, with important consequences for medical care generally, such advertising emphasized what the layman could do for himself to better his condition of health.

By 1950 that included assuming a role in the allocation of resources at the local level for its protection and advancement. Two years earlier the National Health Assembly had declared:

> Professional leadership can create a continuing demand for good health services in a community by raising the level of the public's understanding of its health problems and how best to meet them. This leadership must be

exercised in such a way that the individual accepts responsibility for his own, his family's, and his community's health. If the people of a community feel that garbage removal is the most important health activity in that community, then the health program should stress garbage removal until such time as people have been educated to emphasize some other and much more important phase of community health activity. The important thing is that the people themselves, and not solely the professionals, should be involved in determining where their interests lie.[13]

Following the triumph over fascism, it was popular to frame "democratic" solutions to large numbers of national problems. The entry of lay people into health planning was initially an effort to perpetuate the camaraderie and effective cooperation of wartime. Only a few locales implemented to a decisive degree the ideal of the National Health Assembly, that agencies making official plans for health resources should include representatives from all the people affected. But even this degree of public participation helped to reveal the natural communities that had unique or serious health problems and the leaders in them who could organize their neighbors in bringing about change.[14]

The first concern of many local health leaders was the problem of means: how to assure that the sick man or woman had access to medicines, therapeutic devices, and the skills of doctors, dentists, and nurses. Such particular and specific help for illness resembled the serums and vaccines that had reduced or eradicated infectious diseases during the era of medicine just past. Continued progress against untimely death and widespread morbidity logically appeared to be a matter of distributing the newest equipment and guaranteeing adequate numbers of hospital beds.

By midcentury, however, medicine based in specific therapies had apparently reached the point of diminishing returns. There was little likelihood that high-cost, short-term institutional care would significantly extend life expectancy. Most of the prevalent, persistent health problems that remained after the antibiotic revolution could be traced to willful or innocent misuse of one's body, such as smoking, or else to defects in one's condition of living and in the whole environment through which one moved.[15]

Practitioners of medicine therefore depended upon the knowledge of and vigilance by their patients and upon public policies that would deliberately improve housing, nutrition, and occupational health and safety. Before the gravest health perils of the age—cancer, heart disease, cerebral hemorrhage—medicine was fairly limited; it possessed no "magic bullets." Still, it enjoyed unprecedented public confidence, deriving from its triumphs during the past three quarters of a century, and it was expected to provide help for pain and illness that worked.

The larger role being assumed by the lay individual in health care involved, in essence, the practice of preventive medicine. The concerns of that venerable discipline paralleled the emerging ideal of health as a positive state of being. They addressed virtually every aspect of one's mental and physical condition. And they depended upon the individual's acute self-awareness and rigorous attention to the factors in the environment that threatened one's well-being.

During the era when medicine had been based chiefly in chemistry and technology, the practitioners steeped in preventive philosophies had stood in the shadows. The threats of chronic illness, however, laid renewed importance upon their key concept—that distortions in the victims' physical surroundings or practices of living caused, exacerbated, or originally left him vulnerable to his illness.

The challenge to the medical practitioner and the patient persuaded of the usefulness of prevention was to promote health. Such a strategy obliged them first to understand and to cooperate with the human organism's spectacular armada of natural defenses. Good nutrition, regular, sensible exercise, and proper rest had long been known for their efficacy in assisting these natural bodily processes and thus in staving off disease. Applied as preventive measures against such contemporary health banes as cardiovascular trouble, they assumed a new relevance. Like other regimens of preventive medicine, they proceeded from capabilities and potentials that the patient possessed for maintaining and advancing his own health.

From the point of view of poor people, black Americans, and other minority groups, social injustice was a fundamental hindrance to realizing that state of health contemplated in concepts such as "complete state of well-being" or "prodigous expenditure of energy." Thus it was scarcely surprising that the demand for adequate medical care should be joined to those for school desegregation, public accommodation, fair employment, and an adequate standard of living.

To be sure, wide differences continued to exist among groups and individuals in perceptions about illness and demands for service. Yet there was virtually common agreement that all Americans, regardless of race, economic status, or place of residence were entitled to the best health care available and that if new institutional forms were necessary to ensure this benefit, they would have to be created.[16]

Ever since the Flexner Report of 1910, medical education in the United States had been concerned with quality—excellence in teaching, first-rate physical plants, a depth and breadth of "clinical material" so that students might have an adequate observation of disease. Thus preoccupied with "better," few medical schools were prepared to deal with "more," just as the sheer quantity of service was what increasing numbers of Americans decided that they needed.

How the nation was to be supplied with physicians, dentists, and nurses sufficient to the demand was a question being asked with particular urgency by 1960. The existing shortages seemed likely to grow more serious in the period just ahead. Moreover, whether an individual victim found a doctor available often depended upon his ability to pay, the accessibility and attractiveness to the medical graduate of the place where he lived, and the complex of clinics and health services located there.

The demand for more health workers by citizens from all economic strata and the less visible but demonstrably critical need of the country's poor and minority people were two factors exerting pressure upon medical schools to multiply their numbers of graduates. But larger enrollments would tend to produce only more specialist practitioners for the suburbs unless accompanied by basic reforms in teaching. And more specialty care was no answer to a population who thought in terms of degrees of health; to sufferers, such as cancer or cardiac patients, who required rehabilitative as well as acute care; nor to citizens who because of racial discrimination or poverty lacked ready access to medical attention. Specialist medicine, moreover, failed to preserve the quality of intimate, personal attention that in popular mythology, at least, was the trademark of the family doctor. Consequently, the specialist's workplace, the hospital, was challenged to provide more distinguished and humane service.

Continual adaptation had long been required of the hospital. Originally small in scale, catering chiefly to charity patients whose illnesses served medical teachers and their students, it had gradually opened its doors to various classes of people. Moreover, it had moved from the fringes of medicine to its center, as the rise in the numbers of people who required or wanted services made necessary large-scale organization and financing.

In the summer of 1948 the management journal *Modern Hospital* predicted that in the future, "the greatest change will be the metamorphosis of the hospital . . . into a community health center."[17] A decade later the larger role played by lay individuals in their own care, the lay worker's importance in the hospital's daily operation, and lay leaders' roles in its administration were hastening this transformation. The problem of chronic diseases also meant that the hospital was having to expand its traditional role—providing short-term care to the acutely ill—to accommodate patients who needed long stays and social and rehabilitative services.[18]

The costs associated with these alterations were fierce. Already the expenses to the hospital of giving inpatient care were high and rising, and many institutions were forced to prefer patients who had resources to pay for their care and to allow beds to fewer numbers of sick people who did not. Fiscal constraints also compelled hospitals to consider other settings where the patient could be treated equally well but at less cost. Home care—one of the earliest extensions of the hospital beyond its grounds—was one such means. It had the further advantage of permitting the practitioner interested in prevention to view the surroundings where the patient lived.

As insurance plans were extended to cover at least part of visits to the emergency room, it too became an alternative site for treatment, even in cases that were only mildly serious. A more likely one, the outpatient clinic, also received those charity patients who could not be accommodated in rooms or wards of the hospital.

Still visible in the outpatient clinic was the hospital's centuries-old legacy as a dispensary of care to the poor, less for their benefit than that of the institution. Neglected as a matter of policy and financial exigency, the outpatient clinic frequently provided medical services that were unstable, disorganized, and notoriously impersonal. Assigned a low priority among institutional concerns, it afforded little prestige to the practitioner and was not considered a learning experience of great benefit by the medical student.[19] As might be expected, therefore, it was not held in high regard by the many poor people who came to it for care. Any gratitude that the ambulatory patient might otherwise have had for the hospital was likely to be withheld in resentment at the indifferent treatment received there.

As the 1960s began, the concept of unlimited quality care was leading to experiment and reform throughout the hospital. The outpatient department would be one of the first places where an institution's professed commitment to serve the community was tested. In time, wherever the hospital stood apart—with primary allegiance to staff, science, and management—its purposes would be questioned. Gleaming equipment and an armada of skilled givers of care were unacceptable ironies as long as there lived just beyond the doors tubercular victims without antibiotics, children who went without vaccinations, and expectant mothers approaching full-term without having had prenatal care.[20]

In the absence of private philanthropy or underwriting by state or local jurisdictions, the extensive changes that would extend the hospital's mission required support from the Federal government. The Hill-Burton program of hospital construction was the first major step since state funding of public health departments in the direction of a redress of the inequities in health services that mere wealth accorded to certain localities. A second boon of the program was to medical education, where it availed new teaching hospitals or improvements in older ones.

By the close of the 1940s, many medical schools also needed funds for general operations, capital expenses, and student aid as state or regional funding faltered and foundations selected other interests to support. As sponsorship of medical and biological research by the national government increased throughout the next decade, some schools succumbed to the temptation to organize themselves so as to be favored in the awards competition.

By 1963 the public's demand for more medical service had found political expression in the Federal law that gave financial support to students in the health professions. Limited grants were made available for undergraduate study, while more liberal ones could be had by graduate students or practicing physicians who sought further training in a critical area. That same year Congress passed the Health Professions Educational Assistance Act that authorized money for construction of medical education facilities, for the relief of schools in financial distress, and for expanded enrollments.[21]

With the enactment of Medicare two years later, the Federal presence in health took a further step. In this progress could be seen a deepening belief that the health of the whole people was a proper concern of the government elected by all of them. Thus in the century after the Civil War, the responsibility for making available resources needed by the sick person had passed from private hands through philanthropies and charities to public policymakers.[22] At the time of Meharry's founding, society had borne no responsibility either for contributing to ill health or assisting its victims. By 1960 it had been assigned a place in both, as social and environmental factors in disease were revealed and as millions of people looked to government to help pay for the costs of medical care.

In the same interval the medical school acquired a host of new responsibilities. Originally expected to prepare physicians competent to care for the sick, it was lately called upon to train its graduates to be research scientists as well. It was also the natural place for them to receive graduate education as interns or specialists and continual renewal of their skills over a lifetime of practice. Finally, as proprietors of hospitals, medical schools were being asked to balance service to the sick with commitment to education and research.

To realize the ambitious agenda demanded by the needs of the times, the medical school minimally needed a high ratio of teachers to students. Each department required a core of full-time faculty members with access to ample classrooms, fully equipped laboratories, and hospital patients. To achieve its maximum potential—the wholeness required of modern health services—the medical school had to take cognizance of the growth in research in the basic sciences and the demand for graduate education in them.[23]

The general public expectation that there would be restored to the examining room and the hospital ward a unity, thoroughness, and completeness of care also laid new challenges upon medical education. Some proportion of graduates would, of course, continue into research fields. But medical schools were expected to furnish a larger number competent in and intent upon general practice: doctors who considered the patient a whole person from a unique environment; who were capable of treating most major medical conditions and minor surgical and psychiatric ones; and who could take charge of rehabilitation in times of serious illness so that the patient could be returned to participation in the community, the workplace, and the family.[24]

In 1960 a curriculum devised even a decade earlier would no longer serve to impart these skills to the student of medicine, dentistry or nursing who aspired to a generalist's practice. Nor would it answer in a timely way the popular need and desire for more physicians, more attention, more "health." Cluttered with courses that emphasized immense amounts of detailed knowledge from recent research findings, it was likely to be a stumbling block between students wanting useful, practical skills and the sick man or woman, languishing in need.

Deletion of superfluous material would permit addition of courses in epidemiology that emphasized the origins and etiology of chronic diseases and other modern health menaces, including occupational illnesses, emotional distress, and alcohol and drug dependency.[25] Studies in physiology and its constituent basic sciences could be expanded to include consideration of how bodily systems collaborated in health. Across its face, down into its depths, a reformed curriculum would also emphasize growth and development, stages and processes, maintenance and increase.

As medicine began to reconsider illness in relation to specific environments, the social sciences were recognized as a necessary part of health studies. New graduates especially required knowledge of the methods and major findings of behavioral science. As they left the hospital they put behind them medicine that concentrated on the care of acute illness, precise diagnosis, and the administration of highly specific therapies. In the communities where they practiced they would encounter less readily described conditions of partial health that might preface serious illness or simply draw a circle of disability tighter and tighter around the victim's life. To develop modes and methods of inquiry into such complaints, they would need the tools availed them by such disciplines as sociology, economics, psychology (especially family dynamics), mathematics, and even history.

The practitioner concerned with prevention, general care, and rehabilitation needed to be a manager of resources who could locate or organize the counseling, educational, or social services that might be required to sustain the patient in the condition of health that the two of them had worked to restore. With the prospect of an increasing role by government in medicine, the future physician also needed an understanding of competing interests and constituencies who would influence the allocation and distribution of such resources.

Finally, having bred students of previous generations for careers in research or lucrative specialist practice, the medical school of the late twentieth century had the task of imbuing future graduates with a sense of the patient's individuality, an appreciation for the uniqueness of the situation that contributed to his illness, a tolerance for his culture and community, and, above all, an empathy with him in his plight. The sum and substance of the postwar changes in medicine prescribed this role for all who provided treatment to the sick. Detachment might still be a necessary virtue in one's role as a planner or coordinator of service, but it could no longer be synonymous with indifference or a mask for curiosity whose first object was the testing of hypotheses in vivo. As care came to be dispensed with regard for the patient's assessment of his needs, his active role in prevention, and his responsibility for the maintenance of his health, the physician recognized himself as a participant in a shared experience.

Students at Meharry Medical College had available in the history of their school numerous accounts of alumni who engaged in such practice. Its graduates who worked in the poor areas of the nation's cities or countryside had never abandoned the precepts of preventive medicine, since these were a constant necessity in such environments. Because their patients could not afford to consult with specialists, they had charge for complete care from birth to death. With minimal technical tools and a marginal relation to large medical centers, Meharry graduates necessarily relied upon the body as a positive force against morbidity. And as witnesses to the social aspects of major illness and minor but disabling complaints, they were in a position to observe closely the dislocation in economic status and personal identity wrought by disease. As access to and participation in the nation's institutions and political arrangements became an issue in their patients' lives, they were challenged to extend their healing role to social as well as biological pathology.

Many who attended Meharry in this period of ferment and change would testify later that their lives had been touched in a special way by Dr. Harold West. Through his personal help, some said, they had eluded the failure that appeared inevitable, as they sought to master tens of thousands of textbook facts, lab procedures, and healing skills. It was as if they had entered not a professional school but a family. "Get to be a Meharrian," President West urged new students, and he advised them to inquire how they could make better what the college already had to offer. It wasn't a revolution that was needed, he said, but their contribution.[26]

Dr. West recognized that Meharry had historically provided opportunities for young people that existed nowhere else and that it had to increase the number of its graduates in the face of the persistent health deficiencies among Negro people in the United States and the paucity of medical career opportunities for promising black men and women. Accordingly, he enlisted Meharry in the national drive for more black physicians and dentists. A 25 percent increase in graduates was a leading objective of the development plan.

In late 1962 the West administration began to institute curriculum changes that would hasten graduation and the entrance of the new physician or dentist into practice. In the School of Medicine some clinical courses were consolidated, junior and senior students were given greater latitude to pursue subjects that interested them, and department heads were encouraged to introduce a degree of unity into the discrete and specialized courses that students faced in the last two years. Comparable reforms were being studied at medical and dental schools throughout the nation.[27]

Uneven and unequal opportunities for preparation had placed a career in medicine or dentistry beyond the reach of many young black people. Others who were well grounded in the fundamental studies had interests in different directions. But those from both groups might still be qualified for and recruited to careers in scientific fields that supported and complemented medicine and dentistry.

Graduate study in the basic sciences and clinical fields had become one of the most rapidly accelerating areas of medical school enrollment in the United States. There was, moreover, a critical shortage among predominantly black colleges of science instructors holding the doctoral degree, which not only forced black students seeking a scientific career to enroll in white institutions but also depressed the quality of premedical and predental training. Therefore, in 1963, Dr. West asked the Board of Trustees to allow Meharry to begin offering the doctorate in certain basic sciences.[28] Subsequently, he applied for Federal funds to construct a building devoted to teaching these subjects. Lack of such a facility restrained enrollment at Meharry. The number of students who could be admitted to the first-year classes was limited to the number of spaces in the chemistry and biology laboratories; as the latter was small, the former was depressed.

In the autumn of 1964 Meharry's president recounted to the trustees the previous decade's progress. There had been a doubling of the endowment and a tenfold increase in grants for training, research, and service. A wing of laboratories and another for patients had been added to Hubbard Hospital, and the medical school had gained three new departments, Dermatology, Psychiatry, and Rehabilitation. Despite this growth and a 400 percent increase in Meharry's budget, Dr. West's report concluded, no additional administrative officers had been added to the payroll.[29]

The chance for financial stability would be increased as Meharry accommodated in the expanded hospital more and more patients who were able to pay their own medical bills or who had health insurance that did. As early as 1959, two-thirds of Hubbard's census was so classified. This propor-

tion fluctuated, but as development officers went among Nashville blacks
capable of contributing to the college's fund-raising campaign, they could
point to Hubbard as an institution that served them and their families.[30]
"Middle-class medicine," some Meharrians called it, half in jest.

The addition to the hospital also enabled the new Department of Psychiatry to open an outpatient clinic there in 1964. Hailed as a pioneering
facility that would chart the mid-South's course in treating mental disorders, the service included several features that would eventually be
adopted elsewhere at Meharry. It emphasized, in the words of Dr. Lloyd C.
Elam, first chairman of the department, "the family constellation" and the
"patient in the community." To the extent that neurosis and psychosis had
sources in or were aggravated by these settings, it became part of the
therapist's strategy to reconcile the patient and his surroundings so that
they could support him in his recovery, permit him to remain outside an
institution, and thus keep down the cost of his treatment.

Locating and bending to the patients' use the array of human services
already available from private charities and public agencies, the psychiatric
outpatient clinic led in calling attention to the neighborhoods of Nashville
where health needs were greatest. Open twenty-four hours and serving
populations that had been previously neglected, it early inscribed in the
Meharry story two signatures of contemporary medicine: comprehensiveness and continuous availability.

In the summer of 1964 the Department of Psychiatry began organizing
its staff and course offerings so as to stress a "holistic" approach in caring
for patients who suffered mental illness. Those who advocated that health
services be arrayed according to this concept believed that specialist medicine failed to give adequate attention to the interaction and interdependence among the biological, social, and environmental aspects of patients'
difficulties. In place of its fragmented approach, they proposed renewed
attention to the individual's personal, characteristic way of thinking, acting, and relating to others and detailed inquiry into his history and home,
family, community, and vocational background.

The departmental reorganization was specifically intended to bring to
bear on psychiatric patients' needs the helping skills of as many of the
college's faculty and staff as possible. As other Meharrians who had been
isolated in narrowly conceived technical specialties began to participate in
its work, the Department of Psychiatry became a source of ideas and
proposals for new arrangements in medical services throughout the college.[31] From these successes of the West administration, little was left, in
either money or energy, for more such innovative programs. Only the most
clamorous, immediate needs—in facilities, in equipment, in salaries—received the closest attention.

A preliminary effort to consider broader questions, including a new definition of Meharry's mission, was made during the early 1960s in surveys of the institution initiated by the American Medical Association and the Association of American Medical Colleges. The first objective of the authors, who were mainly faculty members from other institutions, was to bring Meharry into conformity with the prevailing concepts of what medical education ought to be. They commended the college on its progress in areas where their wealthier, better-known institutions already excelled. And they urged it to aspire to minimum, fixed standards at a time when they and their colleagues were experimenting with curricula, considering ways to teach comprehensive care, and reflecting on the frenetic emphasis being given to research.[32]

Very little in these consultants' reports betrayed any understanding of Meharry as an institution with a unique role, such as envisioned by Dr. West and others who were determined that it must increase the numbers of black graduates working in the health sciences. Seeing only that Meharry had the least operating capital and the smallest endowment of any medical college in the United States, they took little account of its powerlessness to recover its expenses for indigent care from the city of Nashville and surrounding communities. As for Meharry's practice of admitting some students who could not meet requirements at a majority of the predominantly white medical schools, these officials were not in a position to consider the opportunity thus given to educationally disadvantaged youth. Instead, they were impelled to stress the cognitive, quantitative, and general information that Meharry had to convey to students if it were to remain an accredited institution. Tactfully, earnestly, with the best of intentions, they thus extended to the college a subtle invitation to apologize and to account for deficiencies.

In keeping with a Meharry tradition, many of its alumni stepped forward to support the development campaign that was designed to carry the college into the channel marked in the surveys and averred to be the mainstream of American medical education. Nonetheless, a sizable number remained unconvinced of the need to recast Meharry in the image of more affluent, research-based schools. The view was widely shared that, whatever its problems and difficulties, Meharry had provided them the opportunity to learn medicine and dentistry when the doors of other colleges had remained shut.

Among all Meharry supporters, it was these alumni who felt most ambivalent about the desegregation of the institution. When a place in the first-year class was given to a white student, it meant that a Negro candidate with potential had not been recruited or provided the means to come, that he had turned to another profession or that he had enrolled in a predominantly white institution where he would likely lose any identification with the problems of Negro Americans. When openings at Meharry went unfilled by blacks, however noble the goal, it seemed to these alumni that an opportunity was lost for the education of a doctor who was likely to practice where the need was greatest.[33]

Some of Meharry's veteran faculty members also had a large psychic investment in the status quo. Dedicated to the college's survival, they had made considerable personal sacrifices to help assure it. Until very recently they had had a dearth of opportunities elsewhere, opportunities which Meharry provided through years of crisis. As a consequence, they developed an unshakable loyalty and an espirit de corps that, in turn, helped to sustain the institution as it teetered on the edge of bankruptcy. Simply holding fast under such adverse circumstances bred commitment and a slowness to yield in the face of challenge.

As doors elsewhere were slowly opened, it was the younger members of the Meharry faculty in general who felt most strongly the need for change and reform. Many of them felt personally implicated in and challenged by the civil rights movement. When Dr. Thomas W. Johnson (Class of 1957) returned to Meharry in 1962, following specialist training in dermatology, he remarked that the most overt aspects of racial discrimination had been overcome by the campaign begun with the lunch counter sit-ins. Except for housing, it was possible for a black man to "go wherever his money would take him," Dr. Johnson recalled later. Had conditions not changed, he added, he would not have returned to Meharry.[34]

The very increase in opportunities for themselves was a second cause of restlessness among some younger faculty members. The internships and residencies that were rare privileges for a previous generation were now available to them. Having the chance to work for a livable wage and for broader professional horizons that were available at solvent medical centers, they found themselves in a frustrating situation at Meharry.

Meharry, they saw, was uniquely situated, as their senior colleagues pointed out; but, they asked, was it enough, in an integrated society, to train blacks for medicine and dentistry with traditional methods and curricula? Like the consultants, these younger faculty members believed Meharry capable of excellence in teaching, learning, and research. But how were these programs to be conducted in keeping with medicine's oldest effective mode, prevention, and a concern for the whole person, both of which were absent from specialist practice? An expanded campus indeed meant more opportunities, but did greater service to the relatively affluent imply abandonment of Meharry's relationship with Nashville's poor, just when the nation was mounting a "War on Poverty?" Finally, many felt the moral and intellectual claims in favor of a racially diverse institution; but to what extent did this mean that fewer students would be encouraged to work in minority communities, where Meharry alumni, but few other practitioners, had traditionally gone?

"There was a great deal of talking in the hallways and at the water fountains," Dr. Robert Anderson recalled of this period, "and all of it was griping." Chairman of the Department of Medicine and an internist, Dr. Anderson frequently overheard his colleagues' views about affairs at Meharry, the quality of education and health service that it was providing, the place that the faculty had been assigned, and the prospective future. It would have been easy to dismiss all of it as natural resentment on the part of people who faced twelve- to fourteen-hour days for wholly inadequate compensation, who were often jealous of their limited perogatives, or who were discouraged from stepping across rigid boundaries. Instead, Dr. Anderson thought about some of the problems being discussed.

In July 1965 he flew to Boston to attend the Endicott House conference on the status and future of medical education in the United States. For ten days some of the most prominent teachers and practitioners in academic medicine deliberated its strengths and shortcomings. In this vigorous exchange of views, it soon became clear that all of the changes that were occurring in medicine meant a continually expanding need for more physicians, surgeons, and dentists, more paramedical staff, and more technicians. The burden to provide them fell, of course, on the nation's medical schools.

If these institutions were to meet their responsibilities, the Endicott House conferees decided, they would have to streamline their curricula to sharply reduce the amount of time required for graduation. In the future they should depend upon undergraduate colleges to prepare students in physics, chemistry, mathematics, and biology. In addition to eliminating superfluous work in these subjects, medical educators should reconsider requiring students to memorize vast amounts of facts that would be of little use to them in their later practice. It would be better to introduce the student as soon as possible "to the facts and atmosphere of disease," to patients and the settings where they received care.

An education that prepared graduates for a diversity of roles—from research to general practice—would be the goal of a curriculum reformed in such a manner. Those attending the conference acknowledged that the innovations they proposed were far-reaching. Yet, they insisted, such changes, coupled with imaginative, conscientious teaching, were strictly necessary if the demands of the nation's people for increased services from doctors and hospitals were to be met. In an allusion to the dramatically influential Flexner Report, the conference concluded that medical schools "must face a new orientation as radically different as 1910."[35]

Dr. Anderson returned to Nashville deeply troubled. It was apparent that Meharry's long-standing mission, however significant, was too limited to justify or sustain its existence. For nearly a century, the college had trained black physicians and dentists to serve the Negro members of a segregated society. Discrimination had virtually compelled them to work among the poor. Now the inroads being made against racial proscription in general and the opening to black students of formerly all-white medical schools in particular meant that neither of these facts would hold true any longer.

Meharry's long experience as a teacher of health workers for the nation's disadvantaged people and its location in the midst of an inner-city ghetto nonetheless qualified it to assume a leadership role in assisting the poor to realize their claims to equality in health care. To undertake such a burden, Dr. Anderson foresaw, Meharry would have to take cognizance of the new opportunities drawing black medical scientists to other locales. The college also had to acknowledge that many young Negro men and women qualified by aptitude and training for medicine and dentistry were being diverted to other vocations where the need for them was less acute. Perhaps most unsettling of all, in terms of the institution itself, Meharry needed to recognize that some who completed medical or dental school found the rewards of research overwhelming the impulses toward helping and healing that had originally brought them to Meharry.

A major first step in leading a national assault against the health problems among the nation's poor would be to do more of what for a hundred years Meharry had done well. Its graduates—about seventy-five each year from medicine, dentistry, and technology combined—were significant beyond their numbers. Yet those numbers had to be increased. With that objective in mind, Dr. Anderson believed, Meharrians needed to give thoughtful study to the ideas and proposals made at the Endicott House conference. Instead of planning only for short-term needs, the college should be looking ahead across at least a decade. Finally, there would have to be more organized activity for improving conditions, enlisting the energy being dissipated in gloom and discontent.

In his office, Dr. Anderson shared these tentative conclusions with several of his colleagues in the School of Medicine. Eliciting their ideas and general agreement, he began to approach others throughout the college. Let's meet and talk about Meharry, he suggested. What are the problems? Where are we headed? In all he enlisted about a dozen of his colleagues to take part in the discussions and urged them to bring anyone else who might be interested or helpful. For several who eventually came, it was the beginning of a leadership role at Meharry. Members of the administration were also invited to take part. Dr. Matthew Walker, assistant dean in the School of Medicine, was the only college officer who did.

In order not to seem to compromise their responsibilities to Meharry, Dr. Anderson proposed that the meetings be held off campus and on the participants' own time. For the first one he offered his own home, on a Saturday evening in the early autumn of 1965. At the outset he suggested two rules: no griping and no limits on ideas. Every positive proposal for working improvements at Meharry should be heard, even if it were not immediately feasible. At first the Saturday night group met once a month. Soon the urgency of the issues being raised seemed to demand more frequent gatherings, and they were convened every Saturday evening. Others besides Dr. Anderson opened their homes, and the sessions moved from one living room to another.

At each meeting small subgroups (and sometimes only a single member) would report on a topic of general concern. One was finance. Another was the college's standard, formal curricula, whose organization and content still required students to absorb large amounts of unintegrated material while postponing their experience with patients. The relations between Meharry and the surrounding community, especially the largely black and poor population of north Nashville, proved to be an important concern. The degree to which the faculty ought to participate in the governance of Meharry was also raised.

The one great matter was Meharry's mission. Was there even a need for a black medical school, given the gradual desegregation of institutions that had been exclusively white and given the recent decline in applications on the part of young Negro men and women? If so, how must Meharry change to take account of these two developments? And what role should it play in the community and in the nation?

The answers were suggested in the surveys of the racial composition of students then pursuing doctorates in medicine in the United States. When it examined these figures, the Saturday night group saw that there were fewer Negroes in medical school than there had been a decade earlier. The chief cause was the small number of qualified and motivated black applicants who felt that they and their families could afford a medical education.

Although raised by about fifty dollars every two years through Dr. West's administration, tuition at Meharry had been kept relatively low so that as little obligation as possible was imposed upon students and their families. A large fraction of the $20 million that Dr. West hoped to raise was earmarked for residence halls, the cost of renting off campus being a major liability against student budgets.

But a second factor depressing black enrollment in the nation's medical schools—and one that was decisive at Meharry—was the difference between Negro and white students in the thoroughness and quality of preparation. The majority of young black men and women who applied to Meharry came from colleges that were historically black. Though by no means inferior in the quality of instruction, in some cases, because of inadequate endowments or public appropriations, they lacked adequate laboratories and other facilities that premedical and predental students needed to gain competence in fundamental studies.

The gap between applicants to Meharry who had had sufficient opportunities and those who had not was wide, and it contributed to pressures upon the college from accreditors to alter admissions policies in favor of the former. Instead, Dr. West recommended more sophisticated efforts at recruiting the top black students from the nation's undergraduate colleges. However, Meharry was not initially well situated to meet the competition from predominantly white schools, and one of the last reforms proposed by Dr. West was a change in the calendars of the admissions and financial aid officers so as to extend early decisions and secure acceptance from these front-ranked black scholars.

This pool of exceptionally qualified black applicants was very small; indeed, in the view of the Saturday night group, there were far too few to make enough difference against the health deficiencies of black Americans, even if every one had an exclusively black clientele. There were not enough to provide physicians and dentists for the poor of the nation, even if every black graduate had service among them as a vocation. There were too few to contribute significantly to the general nationwide demand for more medical service and the skilled people to provide it. Finally, there were too few young black men and women whose ability had been sharpened with adequate preprofessional training to maintain Meharry as a predominantly black institution.

Although the doors of some formerly segregated medical schools were opening to Negro applicants, only the fortunate few and favored ones would gain entrance. It was unlikely that in such settings they could retain an identification with the health problems of black people in America and disadvantaged persons in general. And if Meharry were required to admit students who met only certain national standards, there might, despite the beginnings of integration in medical education, be fewer black physicians practicing where the need was greatest than ever before.

It was eminently clear to the Saturday night group, therefore, that not only was there a definite need for a black medical school, but Meharry would be required to begin assisting young black men and women who gave promise of being good physicians and dentists to overcome such deficiencies in their previous studies as might impede their progress through the rigors of a health sciences education. As an alumnus trustee, Dr. Maurice Clifford, wrote:

The door of opportunity must be open not alone for those whose combination of ability and aggressiveness enables them to overcome the hardships of a system of education never intended to prepare them for competition in the major community. The door must be open here at Meharry for those large numbers of fully capable individuals whose potential has been obscured.[36]

Identifying and stimulating such untapped human resources among young black men and women would be a continuous theme in the planning for Meharry's future. The Endicott House conference had proposed curriculum changes to speed future physicians toward graduation. The Saturday night group urged that some of these changes be adapted to reinforce basic skills, enabling more students to succeed at Meharry from the start.

Nothing in this and other suggestions that emerged from the Saturday night meetings was critical of Meharry's administration. "We sought positive recommendations," Dr. Anderson said, "ones it would have trouble disagreeing with." Perhaps the most influential were in regard to Meharry's mission. The group's two key points—"partnership with the community" and the demonstrated need for a black medical school—would become the heart of the detailed blueprint for reform drafted over the next three years.

"The Saturday night group proved that all levels in the College could provide a continuous reexamination of Meharry's work," Dr. Anderson said in summary. Its recommendations were placed in written form before Dr. West, but it did not act as a source of pressure. Despite this positive thrust the group was not viewed without suspicion by Meharrians who were more conservative. "The young Turks," the participants were sometimes called. Among themselves and those in sympathy with their purposes, it was a light touch amid serious deliberations. Spoken by those who looked toward them balefully, it sounded at times like an epithet.[37]

The momentum for change, once begun, proved irresistible. In June 1966 Dr. West and officials from Vanderbilt University School of Medicine signed a request for a planning grant that would enable the two institutions to commence a cooperative attack upon heart disease, cancer, and apoplexy. This joint work would be carried on as part of the Tennessee Mid-South Regional Medical Program. Authorized by Congress in 1965 and funded through the National Institutes of Health, regional medical programs were designed to bring to bear against chronic illness all of the institutional resources for health within a given geographical area.

Through these programs, Congress intended to encourage medical colleges to plan in terms of a surrounding area. Some institutions saw them primarily as a way to provide continuing education for physicians and dentists. Some viewed them as the mechanism by which Federal funds for health could be channeled to community-oriented hospitals. Still others regarded regional medical programs as a means for medical schools to serve the rural areas that lacked facilities and practitioners. In their joint request, Meharry and Vanderbilt proposed to meet some of these needs in central and eastern Tennessee, northern Alabama, and southern Kentucky.[38]

The grant request agreed to by Dr. West projected a significantly larger role for Vanderbilt than for Meharry. Vanderbilt was designated as the applicant agency, and both in terms of responsibility and finance, it appeared likely to have the dominant share of opportunity under the program.

Through friends in Washington, this aspect of the planning grant proposal and the fact of its approval by Dr. West in the name of the college became known to Meharry's faculty. To a number of its leaders, swift action seemed imperative. By night letter they contacted the office at the National Institutes of Health where review of the request was under way and urged that it be rejected. In a general meeting, the faculty held firm to this position. Dr. C. W. Johnson, who presided at this assembly, afterwards conveyed to the president word of the faculty's refusal to recede.

Perhaps the disagreement would have been of less moment were it not for the question of confidence in Meharry's leadership that had recently moved from hallway conversations into the center of college affairs. A universal admiration and affection for Dr. West was tempered by chagrin at Meharry's posture of concession, its self-limited aims, and its closed and centralized governance.

Although the controversy over the Regional Medical Program may have influenced the timing of Dr. West's departure from the president's office, he had already, of his own volition, determined to take that step. The hard intellectual labor and the constant physical battering required to keep Meharry solvent, open, and accredited were taking their toll upon him. Hospitalized for a brief period during his last year in office, he had mortgaged his health to the pressures of his position. In May 1965 he asked the Board of Trustees to allow him to retire and resume his work as a research biochemist at Meharry. In the letter of resignation, he agreed to serve until a successor was selected.

Speaking to the press following Dr. West's announcement, Victor S. Johnson, board chairman, reaffirmed the trustees' confidence in Meharry's president. Given his willingness to continue temporarily in the post they proceeded slowly in their search, which was, in any case, a formidable task. Only in the aftermath of the controversy a year later did Dr. West insist that his resignation take effect at an early date. With no new president in the wings, he recommended that an interim committee be appointed, with Dr. Robert Anderson as chairman. The trustees concurred in this plan and chose as other members Dr. William H. Allen, dean of the School of Dentistry, and John M. Sharp, comptroller of the college. The three men would serve, beginning October 1, 1966, on the second such governing body in Meharry's history.[39]

Dr. West foresaw many of the changes that were about to come to Meharry, and he had fostered aspects of them. But grappling with seemingly insuperable problems, he tended to favor procedure and centralized decision-making over personal initiative, selflessness in service to an established plan over participation in formulating it, and moderate, short-term success to large risk for distant gain. Meharry's goal, he told a reporter in 1962, "is to be as good as the average medical school in the United States."[40]

Clearly Dr. West believed that Meharry's persistent problems would eventually yield before his tenacity and careful management. In the meantime the college, in his view, required the stability that strong, undelegated authority gave. In the end, he had neither time nor energy, inclination nor resources to convey the persuasive details of his programs to some whose support was crucial.

As a man who inspired strong personal loyalty, Dr. West often won the kind of unquestioning commitments that he asked. The vision that he reaffirmed for Meharry—providing the physicians, dentists, and health workers who were needed by black people in the United States—had never lost its relevance since the founding of the college. Its special appeal was undeniable as the civil rights movement turned attention upon profound and enduring expressions of inequality, notably poverty.

Only through massive new investment would Meharry be able to extend to poor people who sought attention in its outpatient clinics the same quality care it gave patients in Hubbard Hospital who had personal resources or insurance protection. However precarious Meharry's financial footing, such a step was imperative. In the words of Dr. Maurice Clifford, "the distinction between ward and private care and between clinic and office practice must and will be diminished by the political pressures of democratic philosophy."[41] As the new wing of Hubbard Hospital was opened for the service of larger numbers of middle-income people, the outpatient department, where the poor were directed for care, presented a stark, inhumane contrast.

Organized by service, the outpatient clinics required patients to present themselves for different complaints at various hours and days of the week. A person with a severe cough who saw the doctor on Monday perhaps would have to return again on Thursday if he also had a skin lesion that needed examination. In both instances he was likely to be seen by teachers and students who had little time and to be sent away following treatment feeling physically better but mistreated. There was not a great deal of interest in him or his problem, except insofar as the latter served to illustrate a point that had been made in a lecture. A general complaint, however serious and foreboding, was likely to get cursory attention, while an exotic or elusive ailment provided a more interesting kind of clinical experience.

Implicit in the application for money to plan a neighborhood health center were the possibilities of ameliorating Meharry's financial woes and of bringing "middle class medicine" to the poor. (The story of the beginning of the OEO-sponsored health center is given in the previous chapter.) Pursuing this service ideal, Meharry might be expected to extend its capabilities in research, encouraged during Dr. West's administration. At the same time, by addressing the teaching issues raised by the Saturday night group and the revived precepts of comprehensive care and preventive medicine, the college could aspire to a new unity in its institutional purposes. Meharry would, in the future, not simply train more doctors; as it undertook to provide a quality of ambulatory care and service equal to that available in the private rooms of its hospital, the college would also attempt to imbue them with a sense of the special needs of economically disadvantaged people.

There were two ways to grasp the meaning of being poor. Both were valid, and both came to be regarded as essential in the new era that was opening at Meharry. The first was with the mind. The tools of social science were the means to this kind of understanding. They could show where poor people lived, what income they earned, how the facts and the patterns of their lives related to disease: stress and hypertension; poor diet and susceptibility to infection; marginal employment and on-the-job injuries; social discrimination and neurosis. Such facts were needed to organize health services that would meet the needs of the people that Meharry served.

In the fall of 1965, a few months after he joined the faculty of Meharry's Department of Psychiatry, Dr. Ralph H. Hines assigned his sophomore medical students to survey the social characteristics of black Nashvillians. Dr. Hines, a sociologist, was also interested in comparing the medical services they received with those available to the general population of the city. Before their investigation was concluded, students called at more than 400 homes, which was about 2 percent of all the black households in Nashville. A majority of the wage earners in them were laborers, semiskilled persons, or unemployed at the time of the interview. More than half of the homes had incomes below $4,00 a year.

Consistent with studies conducted in other locales, respiratory diseases cut a wide swath through this portion of Nashville's poor people. Commonly, they also suffered maladies of the bones and joints, legs and feet. Circulatory problems and allergic, metabolic, and nutritional defects occurred with high frequency. In a subsequent survey focused on mental illness, Dr. Hines and his students discovered that nearly four residents in ten in poor neighborhoods presented themselves as being in unstable or neurotic categories.

Children born in the neighborhoods of the survey—the blocks in north, south, and east Nashville that Hubbard Hospital's outpatient clinic chiefly served—often began life with serious health handicaps. Eighty percent of women pregnant and delivering in 1965 had seen a physician only during the last month of their term or just before the baby was born. The special requirements of many preschool youngsters were unattended or underattended.

The Meharry sophomores discovered that most of the people whose illness had forced them to enter a hospital lacked the personal means to pay all the costs of treatment or an insurance policy that would meet at least a part of their bills. Whether they received care depended upon whether they could avail themselves of the philanthropic services at Hubbard Hospital and other agencies in the city.

About half the households in the survey lacked a family physician. When queried on the matter by Meharry students, many people named the doctors who worked in the outpatient clinics at Hubbard Hospital. "Identification of the hospital clinic as a 'family physician,' " Dr. Hines concluded, "is indicative of increasing identification of people with community resources for medical care."[42]

The other way to grasp the meaning of poverty was through the senses. It was, after all, a physical, tangible thing. In making their survey that autumn, Meharry students walked through the parts of Nashville that were blasted, junk-strewn wastelands. They made their way past vacant lots choked with weeds and abandoned storefronts where plywood was nailed over windows. Going door to door they apprehended in a critical way— through the fingertips and the eyes—what it was to be poor.

Poverty was the slink and skulk of a rat attracted by the spillings from a garbage pail. It was a rusting tin roof and a listing chimney and wallpaper streaked from leaking rain. To be poor was often to endure Nashville's bone-cold winters in a room where an unshaded bulb gave off part of what heat the house had. It was the hacking cough felt as well as heard through the wall from the rooms of other families who shared the house.

Poverty was the face of official Nashville: the juvenile court judge, the welfare worker, the ward boss cruising the streets on Election Day. It was lacking the skills to read street signs or to understand the transfer instructions on the city bus. Poverty was the enforced regimentation of the housing project, which led many people to pay more for less substantial private dwellings where one could at least be free from arbitrary rules.

In time of illness, to be poor meant delaying the visit to the doctor in the hope that the symptoms would allay. When they did not, it meant a trip to the outpatient clinics at Meharry, the hearse of a local undertaker carrying the sufferer there for fifty cents a trip.

To be poor was having a child who was "slow," who remained small for his age, who had trouble learning to read and to add. Poverty was the butcher's parings and leavings, gizzards, giblets, backbone of beef. It was potatoes and dried beans and wilting vegetables that were sold more cheaply after their third day in the stall. It was being able to give one's children only an orange for Christmas.

Poverty often meant sharing a room with several other people. The median number in the households visited by Meharry students that fall exceeded the figure for the whole of Nashville, despite the fact that the homes where the poor lived tended also to be smaller. Many dwellings still depended on surface privies, nearly a century after the city's first board of health deplored them as a gross violation of civic decency and a grave menace to public health.

The health surveyors from Meharry glimpsed another face of poverty that fall. Suspicious and distrustful, many people in the poor neighborhoods slammed shut their doors, stopping the students in midsentence. There had already been plenty of studies of how bad things were in the neighborhoods, they grumbled. Nothing had ever come of any of them.

"Sargent Shriver was catching hell," Dr. Matthew Walker recalled. Speaking of the director of the Office of Economic Opportunity and its early days, he continued, "People were saying that the War on Poverty was a lot of talk and no action."

When the OEO grant to Meharry was announced on June 15, 1966, it released a storm of pent-up energies, and the campus became a continuously shifting scene of meetings. Responsibility for detailed planning of the centers was lodged with Meharry's OEO Committee, appointed the previous year by President Harold West when he and Dr. Matthew Walker, at the behest of poverty program officials, proposed that Meharry seek a grant. During the summer and fall of 1966, the panel accomplished several important preliminary tasks.

Dr. Ralph Hines, Dr. Walker's deputy as project director, was sent to Boston, Denver, and New York City to study neighborhood health centers already in operation. A subcommittee, charged with proposing a program for the Nashville facility, surveyed the departments of Meharry and the services provided by Hubbard Hospital to determine what extensions of them should be located in the neighborhood health center. Plans for preserving outpatient records on computer were made; Nashville's health and social welfare agencies were solicited for their cooperation; and consultants were recruited to help complete the planning.[43]

The health survey that had been conducted in north Nashville by Dr. Hines's classes was soon supplemented by more studies of the community, which aided in the center's design and provided supporting data for the planners' funding requests. In cooperation with Meharry, investigators from George Peabody College surveyed some 200 blocks in Nashville's innermost city, which the neighborhood health center proposed to serve. The summary phrase "hard-core poverty" might have been formulated for this area lying north of the central business district between the Cumberland River on the east and the interstate highway three miles to the west. Eight out of every ten residents were black, and only one in three over the age of twenty-five had more than an eighth-grade education. Nearly half of the occupied dwelling units were dilapidated or deteriorating. More than 60 percent of families in the area had incomes of less than $3,000 a year. The Peabody investigators noted that nonwhites worked longer hours for lower wages than did whites. "Underpayment for services," said the report, "may represent the general occupational picture."

On the basis of interviews with health, welfare, and education workers, the investigators derived a disturbing picture of life in this ghetto in the shadow of Tennessee's capitol. One veteran social worker in the area said that hypertensive cardiovascular disease was the leading cause of disability in the homes at which she called. Tuberculosis and alcoholism (and the two in combination) were also common among adults, especially elderly men. Ailments of the feet and legs, including bone disorders and arthritis, hobbled large numbers of people whose income had been from laboring jobs that they reached by walking or by city bus. (Nearly two-thirds of the families surveyed had no car.) Older people of the area generally regarded the loss of their teeth as part of the natural course of aging, so commonly did it occur. Mental illness and mental retardation was another plight that beset poor families in the survey area out of all proportion to their occurrence in the general population.

The tangible, extreme conditions of living to be found across the threshold of these slum dwellings were revealed in an especially tragic fashion by the health problems found among the children. Infectious and parasitic diseases were a quiet, insidious presence in the schools of northwest Nashville. The surveyors' statistical findings that a bathroom might be shared among up to four families took on human meaning when public school nurses told about treating skin and scalp diseases among first and second graders.

Impetigo, ringworm, diarrhea (due mainly to salmonella from food contamination) were often responsible for adding names to absentee rolls. Anemia afflicted children from the very poorest families, who fed them milk but little else. Malnutrition imperceptibly insinuated itself in the young sufferers' bodies, unobserved by teachers and undetected until the next school physical, perhaps several years away.

Pupils with vision problems for which their parents could not afford eyeglasses became discouraged and fell behind. Inordinate restlessness, abbreviated attention spans, and hostility pointed to unsettled home lives. Peabody statisticians working in slums observed a "noteworthy absence of nonwhite males at the age when they are most frequently the parents of young children." Separation without divorce was the general pattern of broken marriages among black inner-city families of Nashville.

As the city's children of poverty entered adolescence, adversity often mounted. The gap between their scores on achievement tests and those from other schools widened so that, in terms of skills and knowledge as these were measured by the dominant culture, poor children were even farther behind than they had been in the second grade. Despite the provision of birth control information and counseling at social agencies and settlement houses, illegitimate pregnancy was closely associated with dropping out of school. (Four senior high schools in the area had less than 10 percent of Nashville's students, but in 1965–66 they contributed more than 16 percent of those who quit before graduating.) The rates of juvenile crime and delinquency among the youth of the slum outstripped those found in other precincts of Nashville. Violations of traffic or truancy laws, dismissed with a fine or a warning, were the leading offenses among all Nashville adolescents. But serious misdemeanors were the more common class of crimes in the inner city.

Organized recreational activity might have channeled some of the young persons' energies that were turned to antisocial activity. But such opportunities were limited. Minimal participation by parents and other adults in sponsoring organizations like scouting or the Parent-Teacher Association evinced not so much a lack of interest as a dearth of leadership resources and skills, which could be traced to denial of access and participation to black people in the democratic life of their city.

Similarly, securing care for themselves or their families in time of sickness was for Nashville's poor people often a matter of knowing how and then proceeding with confidence and purpose. If health, like work and play, was a prodigious expenditure of energy, none was part of the ethos of the slum, where patterns of life often blocked avenues to self-sufficiency.

Nonetheless, the Peabody investigators found that the most frequent response to illness by residents of the poor neighborhoods was to consult a doctor, visit a clinic, or go to the hospital. Although knowing clearly what to do, the people of the area were confronted with a bewildering variety of health and social agencies, each one addressing different aspects of their need.

What they required, the researchers concluded, was guidance in how to take advantage of such resources and means to overcome the impediments to using them. Asked to describe changes that were needed, most of the slum residents interviewed agreed that clinic services ought to be easier to get to, easier to use, and offer more personal attention. The costs for registration at Meharry's outpatient department and an inability to afford prescriptions were two reasons frequently mentioned by Nashville's poor for delaying a visit to the doctor when illness struck.

Meharry's health planners took special note of another finding of the Peabody study. It indicated that many families from the impoverished precincts of Nashville had multiple problems, and that they needed a facility that would serve as the single place where all their interests could be looked after and where the organized system of helping—from medical and dental care to food stamps and legal assistance—could be coordinated.[44]

Thus the earliest concept of the neighborhood health center, fixed in the first-floor plans and architectural drawings, was that it should be the site for a broad scope of services that would be geographically convenient, made available without appreciable delay, and affordable by people who were very poor. Besides providing spaces where patients could receive a thorough physical and oral examination, the planners allocating interior space set aside accommodations for medical sociologists, nutritionists, home economists, and other specialists in community health.[45]

By 1967, at the behest of the Meharry OEO Committee, the heads of all clinical departments were at work developing the program at the future neighborhood health center. Reporting on the progress, the National Medical Association's *Journal* wrote that the indigent people to be served would be offered "continuing personalized treatment and rehabilitation and preventive care for the whole family in a friendly atmosphere under one roof. There will be appointments instead of endless waits, drop-in service when needed, convenient day and night hours, and doctors on call outside these hours."[46] As he assessed achievements thus far, Dr. Walker, the planning director, declared that he and his colleagues had reached the stage where citizens from the neighborhood who were the prospective users of the health center had to be involved.

Such a step, besides satisfying the legal mandate of participation in OEO-sponsored projects by those whom they served, had other, broader implications. Involving themselves in actual direction of the health center from an early date, poor people would gain skills in the methods of social service agencies, lacking which, the Peabody studies suggested, they were hindered from taking advantage of the resources already present in their community. The presence of neighborhood residents would also be a means for disseminating information about services available at the center, another need that the surveyors had identified.

Finally, recruiting poor people to responsible work in planning for the new facility might impart the self-regard and strengths of personality that would enable them to act forthrightly in their own interests whenever they or their families suffered illness. If they were thereby encouraged to look beyond questions of physical well-being to consider other conditions of their lives, such a step did not seem outside the horizon of meaning of the term "comprehensive health."

Helping black communities to evolve their own leadership in health matters had been one of the activities of the Medical Committee for Human Rights, an association of health workers committed to the civil rights cause, whose work drew Dr. Leslie Falk to Mississippi. Dr. Falk, a white physician who was area medical administrator for the United Mine Workers Welfare and Retirement Fund, had participated in several initiatives for greater social justice in Pittsburgh, where he lived. When the MCHR began seeking staff for its Mississippi project, Dr. Falk enlisted as its first field secretary in the summer of 1964. That step would lead him to Meharry and a primary role in its neighborhood health center.

Dr. Falk's employer and some of the nation's other large labor unions had, in the postwar years, assisted many American workers in securing health care plans and benefits at the bargaining table. Les Falk himself had developed multipurpose community health programs in three Appalachian communities. But even before assuming this leadership position in the mine workers' union, he had had a scholarly and professional interest in group health movements. Following three years as a Rhodes Scholar at Oxford University, where he earned a research doctorate for work on penicillin in the laboratory of Dr. Howard Florey, the young Les Falk returned to medical school at Johns Hopkins University. There he enrolled in seminars conducted by the noted medical historian, Dr. Henry Sigerist. Of his mentor, he later said: "I had responded to the human nutrition stream in the 1930s, the 'one-third of a nation ill-fed' of Franklin Delano Roosevelt. Dr. Sigerist gave me a way to combine scientific and social medicine."

His experiences in Mississippi accelerated Dr. Falk's interest in the ways that black and minority people, generally excluded from the mainstream movements in group health care such as organized labor, had founded alternative systems. One outstanding example was the Taborian Hospital, built by the Knights and Daughters of Tabor, where Meharry had established a helping presence shortly after World War II.

Successful though many of them were, these private and voluntary modes had not won for the nation's poor and minority people the quality and range of health services that its white middle- and upper-income groups generally enjoyed. However, it seemed to Dr. Falk that the neighborhood health center concept promised to make a difference. With the Federal outlays pledged to the War on Poverty, the centers might be able to provide more and better quality services for the poor than an improvisation for that purpose yet contemplated in the United States. Moreover, by providing for lay participation in day-to-day operations, the health center carried forward the egalitarian impulses that had informed some of the earlier group health plans and schemes devised by utopian colonies, fraternal orders, and labor unions.

Soon after it opened Dr. Falk visited the first OEO-sponsored neighborhood health center, the Columbia Point project of Tufts University, located in a poverty-ridden district of Boston. In 1966 when staff members and students from Tufts medical school began coming to Mound Bayou to work alongside Meharrians, Leslie Falk's name came to the ear of Dr. Matthew Walker. Holding the view that the first permanent director of Meharry's neighborhood health center should be black, Dr. Falk declined Dr. Walker's first offer of the job. Nonetheless, he agreed to come intermittently during 1966 and 1967 as chief consultant.

Other advisers whom he recruited accompanied him into the flurry of activity surrounding the health center project. In early 1967 Victor Pasche, a Swiss-born Yale graduate who had worked in New York as a journalist, trade union organizer, and health agency executive, joined the project staff. That winter the two men oversaw the opening of a temporary planning office in a small white house on Albion Street, adjacent to the campus.

As Victor Pasche, Dr. Walker, and the Meharry OEO Committee took the first steps toward involving the people of the community in the health center project, Dr. Falk brought to Meharry another consultant, Dr. Samuel Wolfe of Regina, Saskatchewan. The trio—Falk, Pasche, and Wolfe—shared similar experiences in organized labor and health and a number of common outlooks. Gradually they composed a team upon which Dr. Walker, as planning director, could rely. The received significant assistance from the Reverend Dan Williams, a Baptist minister who was employed to assist with community organizing. The first project staff also included Clyde Wilson, a sociologist who carried out planning tasks, arranged meetings, and performed other essential duties that no one else willingly did.

A supplementary planning grant from the OEO was approved in February 1967, and the pressure mounted upon Dr. Walker and his advisers for the name of a permanent project director. Despite Dr. Falk's persistent refusals, it soon became clear that few black physicians had the requisite training and experience in public health. Those who possessed such qualifications had risen to responsibility and authority in locales more congenial to black people than Nashville. No one whom Dr. Falk approached was interested in becoming head of the health center.

More strongly than ever, Dr. Walker and other members of the project staff urged Les Falk to accept the post. Both Sam Wolfe and Vic Pasche traveled to Pittsburgh to persuade their colleague, and Dr. Falk recalled their frenetic tone: "This is the War on Poverty! And you are hereby mobilized! Hurry up! Aren't you ashamed for taking so long?" When a formal offer followed, over the signature of Dr. Robert Anderson, Dr. Falk replied with his acceptance. In October 1967 he arrived at the house on Albion Street.[47]

With this critical step behind, planners moved apace to meet with groups in the area of the city that the health center expected to serve. In addition to disseminating news about it, they commenced the formidable, long-range task of building an advisory board of community residents who could speak for their neighbors in regard to the facility's programs and policies. Whatever the setting or the occasion, they were eager to appear and describe Meharry's plans. Several long-term residents and community leaders, including Mrs. Evelyn Graves, Herschel Groves, Mrs. Edna Alexander, and William Owen, helped them gather people together.

More than a decade later, Mrs. Graves recalled the meeting she organized among her neighbors who lived in a horseshoe-shaped block of tenement houses near 10th and Herman streets. To rouse their interests, she went door to door. Getting the health center could mean a lot to the community, she told them. But first, they had to get involved. Often they did not believe her when she told them about the potential benefits. There had been government programs in the past that were supposed to improve things, they reminded her, but very little of the money ever came down to benefit the neighborhood. "At least come and hear what Dr. Walker has to say," she replied.

With as many as eight people living in one room, there was no place among the rambling houses to meet, except a large open area that served as a common backyard. When the time came for Dr. Walker to appear, some of the residents brought out old chairs. Others sat on logs that had been ranked for firewood, on rocks, or on the ground. Washing hung from the clotheslines and flapped in the wind. "Some of the men put their jugs beside them," Mrs. Graves remembered. "Dr. Walker began talking, on their level. And after awhile, they started listening." He stressed the appointments that would do away with long waits, the free care for those who met eligibility standards, and the provision of drugs at no cost if the patient lacked the money to buy medicine.[48]

Several people from the poverty area who heard the Meharry team stepped forward to express an interest in becoming involved in the health center. These volunteers, most of whom had long been acquainted with Dr. Walker, became the *Ad Hoc* Committee for the Health Center, the first advisory organization drawn from the people that it would serve. Included in this group were a political leader, a high school teacher who was a minister, a supervisor of the Mothers Patrol, and a staff member from the Methodist community center. Poor people were represented by the area residents who served on the Metropolitan Action Commission, the local agency of the Office of Economic Opportunity.[49] One of the group's first acts was election of two of its members to serve on the Meharry OEO

Committee, comprising the faculty members and college administrators who since 1965 had carried on the planning for the neighborhood health center.

Immediate decisions, such as those related to securing operational funds, continued to be made by the planning and project staff. The *Ad Hoc* Committee, however, was delegated several significant responsibilities, including sponsorship of the neighborhood meetings where Dr. Walker and his colleagues continued to speak. When in the spring of 1967 it was called upon to consider the matter of who, according to income, would be eligible for free care at the neighborhood health center, the *Ad Hoc* Committee dramatically asserted its independent character.

The center was, of course, planned to serve the poor. The question before this advisory group was: Where was the line to be drawn so that families with incomes below it were eligible for treatment at no cost while those above it could be considered able to pay a doctor's fee and the costs of prescriptions? The eligibility standards at the clinics sponsored by health and welfare agencies in Nashville offered models that might have been adapted to the health center. The OEO had a set of guidelines, too. But when both were put before the *Ad Hoc* Committee, it rejected them.

The *Ad Hoc* members recommended instead that all persons having an income of less than $3,000 a year be eligible for free services. A couple could earn up to $5,500 before their eligibility would be ended. Four dependents in a household that lived on less than $8,500 would not be charged.[50] Such a position on the part of the *Ad Hoc* Committee evinced a growing consciousness among community leaders that real need existed, that the illness observed among so many of their neighbors could not be attributed to some natural process or "time of life." As they moved from this awareness to the conviction that the health center might offer some relief from conditions, they insisted that its benefits be generally shared.

The organization of the community was a matter of building leadership as well as finding it. By 1968 Meharry had thoroughly assessed the health of its neighborhood and begun to create a consciousness of the real causes of besetting problems. The next step was to enlist large numbers of citizens for the work ahead. In the spring of 1968 health center project staff, in consultation with the *Ad Hoc* Committee, hired the first people from the poverty area to receive training in skills that would be needed in the new facility. Preference was given to those whose family income was particularly low, to heads of households with dependents, to persons over fifty, and to persons under twenty-five who lacked a high school diploma.[51]

The first task assigned these neighborhood health aides was to extend the work of informing the community about the health center, an effort that had already been begun by Dr. Walker and his associates. The Neighborhood Health Aides were also instructed to assemble the minimal necessary information about a family's health problems and its eligibility so that waiting time to see a doctor could be shortened when they came to the health center. Finally, they were to register, at no charge, area residents as members of the Community Health Association, which would assure them the right to vote in the election of a permanent Health Council to succeed the *Ad Hoc* Committee.

In a drafty storefront near the Meharry campus, the first neighborhood health aides received three months' introduction to the principles of social work. Mrs. Lettie Galloway, first director of training, geared teaching materials to the relatively low level of education that most of the aides had. Nevertheless, the work was hard. Many of the trainees came from shattered or strife-ridden homes, and they had difficulty in assuming responsibility implied by uniforms and the necessity to be punctual for class. The storefront was far from being a forbidding place, however. Derelicts, alcoholics, and the dispossessed of the neighborhood "didn't mind walking in out of the weather," Mrs. Galloway said. "They knew it as one place where they would not be laughed at, where somebody would sit and listen."[52]

In June 1968 the first group of neighborhood health aides began going from door to door in north Nashville. By the end of September, they had registered 2,656 persons as members of the Community Health Association. Of the 37,000 people who lived in the area that the health center would serve, this was a small proportion. But the diversity among the registrants in income, occupation, and other measures suggested that it was representative.

Given their classroom training and experience in the streets of the poverty neighborhoods, the health aides were deemed capable of recognizing in others the aptitudes that Meharry needed on the permanent advisory board to the health center. Thus they were asked, following their canvass, to suggest some likely leaders from among residents whom they had interviewed and to name other persons in the community whom they knew to be well regarded. The residents mentioned by the aides were among the persons asked by the health center planners to become candidates for election to the health council.

From its beginning the health council's mandate was broader than mere oversight of the neighborhood health center. The Reverend Dan Williams spoke of the council's "responsibility to the community." Meharry, he said, expected that the panel would become an advocate for the general welfare of the people who lived in Nashville's poor neighborhoods. He continued:

> Poor treatment and inadequate funds for welfare recipients, a food stamp program which denies many families the opportunity to purchase food under its provisions, the Nashville Housing Authority's decision to deny housing to families without a father, the Model Cities Program's efforts to

make decisions which would affect citizens in the community without participation of the community are a few of the basic problems to which the Council could address itself.

If the fact was extraordinary—residents of an inner city neighborhood seeking a role in decisions about the health facilities in their community—the process was a traditional, democratic one. Devised by the Reverend Williams in consultation with the *Ad Hoc* Committee, it had all the accoutrements of an election for public office. The candidates for the health council circulated qualifying petitions, which they then filed prior to a stated deadline. Forty-one people had themselves listed on the ballot for a place on the thirty-three–member council. Polling places were set up in churches and community centers throughout north and south Nashville.

On election day, in October 1968, nearly 750 members of the health association cast their votes. When the ballots were counted it was found that most of those elected would be eligible for free care at the health center since their incomes fell below the Federal government's definition of poverty. However, the most conspicuous roles in the work of the new health council would, at the beginning at least, be played by the minority of members from middle-income households.[53]

Slowly the council created its own character and identified its independent interests. On behalf of area residents employed during the day, it asserted that the health center should be open on evenings and weekends. It insisted that transportation for patients would need to be provided, both to and from the center, and clear priorties established for its use. Continuing the controversy begun by the *Ad Hoc* Committee, it demanded broader eligibility for people who stood outside the official definition of poverty but who could not afford a doctor's services. Matters of lesser moment did not escape the health center's attention: it even considered the color of bricks that Meharry should use in building the health center. This story often was told by Dr. Matthew Walker.

The hiring and firing of center employees, other than administrative, medical, and nursing staffs, gradually came to dominate every other issue before the council. For many of its members, the health center project represented, above all else, jobs for their relatives and neighbors. Said Mrs. Evelyn Graves, a member of the original panel: "Our aim was to hire people of the area who had never done anything but push a broom or a mop and to teach them something that could earn them a living. We got prostitutes and bootleggers to drop what they were doing and take a job." Any position that did not require scientific or technical skills was deemed a neighborhood position.

By 1970 the health center would employ about 200 people, three-fifths of whom were residents of the north Nashville area working in a variety of support positions. In keeping with a basic aim of the War on Poverty, project managers sought to avoid consideration of skin color in any aspect of the center; thus, while expanding job opportunities specifically for residents of a predominantly black neighborhood, the staff was integrated from opening day.[54]

Once the health council had reviewed job applicants who were hired by project managers, it turned its attention to how well the new employees dealt with patients. Occasionally it reproved center workers who, in its judgment, mistreated people who came to see the doctor. On the other hand, the council sometimes defended incompetent or disruptive employees against dismissal, knowing the difficulty they would face without a job. In addition to basic disciplinary policy, the question of which positions in the center required technical training and experience was sometimes a source of conflict. The negotiations between council members and project staff from Meharry on these two issues often lasted late into the night. Despite such controversies, the two groups agreed on a first principle: Meharry, through the employment of poor people in health center jobs, would oppose the tendency of the modern economy to exclude them from a livelihood by setting the minimal acceptable standards of training above that which they could hope to attain.[55]

In July 1968 the neighborhood health center opened in temporary quarters, the renovated upstairs rooms of the Frierson Building, a two-story brick edifice at 1310 Jefferson Street, which was also the offices of Nashville's chapter of the NAACP.

Eager that pledges being made to the community regarding good care, personal attention, and brief waiting time be kept, the temporary health center at first served only persons living in the immediate vicinity. It also limited medical services to those that Meharry was certain could be carried on efficiently with limited space, portable equipment, and a partial complement of staff. A dentist, a pediatrician, and a nurse were on full-time duty. Several part-time specialists attached to Hubbard Hospital provided consultation while also treating patients with common ailments and complaints.

From opening day, community residents came steadily to the health center, many of the first patients being children from the local Head Start program and recipients of Medicare and Medicaid. Said Mrs. Evelyn Graves: "The people were thrilled. They got appointments, and there wasn't more than a 20 minute wait. That was quite a change from the old clinics. And they got medicine and drugs at no cost."[56]

A month after the temporary facility opened, U.S. Representative Richard Fulton, whose district comprised Nashville and Davidson County, thrust a shovel into the ground in a vacant lot five blocks southeast of the

Meharry campus. When he flung aside the dirt, construction of the neighborhood health center's permanent quarters was under way.

The project staff had arranged for Meharry to purchase the site from a small congregation eager to sell its dilapidated church building located there and move to better quarters. The planners then turned to ways and means of financing construction of the health center. In a loan application to the Federal Housing Authority, they described the services to be provided there as a medical group practice. Such an application had no precedent, but the commitment by the OEO to guarantee repayment of the loan assured its being made by the New York insurance firm to which Meharry had applied. Forty-eight hours before the groundbreaking by Representative Fulton, the FHA approved a construction loan of $1.4 million.

Late on the afternoon of June 15, 1969, local dignitaries and Meharry officials gathered at the Herman Street site to lay the cornerstone. The chairman of the health council, Herschel Groves, presided as the stone, bearing the date 1969 and a cache of mementoes inside, was lowered into place.

While construction proceeded, the project staff and the health council began planning for the dedication. Among the matters in which the latter asserted an interest was the naming of the health center. Already identical with Meharry Medical College in the minds of many people, Dr. Matthew Walker had given evidence of a remarkable capacity for changing with the times. While serving as one of the executives of the college during Dr. Harold West's last years, he participated in several civil rights campaigns and subsequently took a role in the Saturday night group that first enunciated the theme of "partnership with the community." And he had led in the winning of the first funding for the Federal-sponsored neighborhood health center, the largest government support received by Meharry to that time. Bestowing Dr. Walker's name on the facility seemed only fitting to the health council. No false modesty impelled him to demur; and when Meharry officials, who were laboring to assure an early opening of the center, were advised of the council's choice, they accepted. it.

On March 7; 1970, Meharry's first major construction for outpatient care since 1931 was dedicated as the Matthew Walker Neighborhood Health Center. The two-story building contained 31,000 square feet, which was also the number of people in the impoverished community that it would serve. Family health suites—examination, treatment, and consultation rooms, including a dental clinic—were located on the first floor. Upstairs were the administrative offices, including those for the neighborhood health workers. The center's facade was beige brick with bronze aluminum trim and windows of tinted glass.

Mrs. Fannie Lou Hamer of Ruleville, Mississippi, nationally prominent

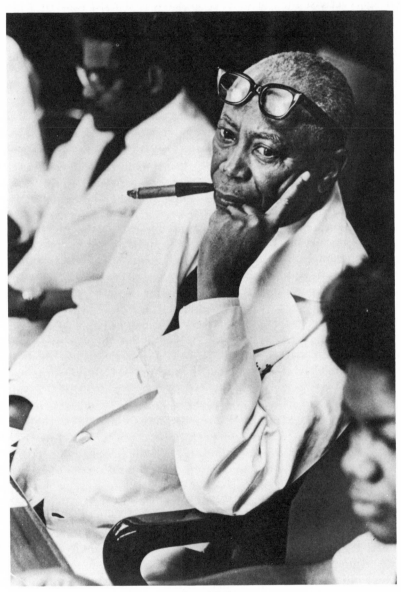

Matthew Walker

civil rights activist and consumer cooperative leader, delivered the dedicatory address.[57] Then the doors were thrown open to admit the large crowd. "We heartily welcome you!" announced the bright yellow brochure prepared for patients of the Matthew Walker Neighborhood Health Center. It continued: "Our goal is to help you and your family. . . . We wish to know you as special friends and want to keep you productive and in good health."

Past the front doors, the visitors entered the reception area. Deliberately designed to resemble one that might be found in a private clinic, it was meant also to provide an atmosphere of comfort and support that most people associated with their family doctor's office. Gone were the despised benches of the old outpatient department, replaced by comfortable chairs. Health aides, who, like the neighborhood health workers, were residents of the community served by the center, were on duty to assist patients in finding the telephone, a drinking fountain, or a restroom. Adjacent to the main reception area was a playroom for children and the nearby lobby had a color television set. The theory and design of the center anticipated that the waiting room would seldom be crowded, despite these amenities. If the patient had been registered in his home by a neighborhood health worker and if he called for an appointment, it was possible for him to see a doctor after only a brief time.

The quantity and detail of personal information to be collected, especially regarding income, had been an issue in the community meetings and in the health council. At the Matthew Walker Neighborhood Health Center, efforts were made to take only such personal information as was strictly necessary to meet OEO requirements or to help the patient qualify for various public assistance benefits. Although one's family income had to be verified, this could be done by the patient with simple documentation. The process remained potentially controversial. Nevertheless, Meharry attempted to remove the least palatable aspects from it by stressing to center staff the necessity for treating patients with dignity and assuring them of privacy and confidentiality.

Besides providing an atmosphere that encouraged people to return when symptoms first manifested themselves, the health center urged patients to regard physicians on duty there as their family doctor, just as they had done at the old outpatient department. But because the health center's organization—built around the "family health team"—differed from the clinic's, patients needed additional assistance, since it was not immediately clear how a group of practitioneers from many different levels and fields of training could be a "personal physician." Each team, assigned to one of the center's four family health suites, resembled a medical group practice. It comprised a family physician, a nurse, a nurse's assistant, and a receptionist.

Appointments were scheduled in such a way that the patient saw the same team on each visit to the health center. The theory that supported this method of organizing service held that those who came there for care would learn to regard their family health team with the trust that obtained in a private practice setting. At the same time, the family health team was a way to combine the skills possessed by several workers and thus to free the most highly specialized among them to care for greater numbers of seriously ill people.

Formally considered to be peers of the doctors and nurses, the neighborhood health aides attended the conferences of the family health team when cases were discussed. In this setting they were expected to be advocates for the patient. Having circulated through the community, they brought to the health team meetings any reports they had heard concerning the kind of attention and the degree of consideration that people were receiving at the health center. "It was a little threatening to some physicians," Mrs. Lettie Galloway remembered. "And there were enough negative comments reported about a few of them to cause them to leave."

The neighborhood health workers' unique role in the patients' behalf extended to the suite where actual care was given. There, one of their most important tasks was to try to overcome barriers to communication between staff and patient. Sometimes a sick man or woman might describe their symptoms in vernacular terms, unknown to the doctor. Often the doctor's explanation of the illness and the prescribed regimen would be in a vocabulary that the patient had difficulty understanding. In such cases the neighborhood health worker interpreted each one's meaning to the other.[58]

Even though the health center restricted itself to ambulatory care, its staff could call upon the specialized resources at Hubbard Hospital. Among the goals of the health center was a local decrease in the incidence of illness that required admission to Hubbard, which it sought to achieve by providing general, preventive care and competent treatment to arrest serious ailments in their early stages.[59] However, the institutional needs of the hospital—for the revenues represented by Medicare and Medicaid, and for filled beds for teaching increasing numbers of students—created potential tensions in these two centers of patient care at Meharry.

With the organization of the family health team and auxiliary services, Meharry was in a position to supply at the neighborhood health center a range and quality of services that aimed for the celestial standard of "comprehensive care." But the manner in which those services were rendered— the attitude of the center staff toward people who came for care—would determine whether the new community resource was regarded with trust or cynicism. If word of any discourtesy or mistreatment at the center should reverberate through north Nashville, Meharry would be accused of abandoning the trappings while keeping the hauteur that had characterized the old ambulatory clinics.

The OEO publicity in support of the center spoke of patients' "right to health care," but that was a guarantee only of quantity, a pledge that services would be available to every poor person living within certain areas of Nashville. If the center's atmosphere of welcome and personal, psychological support were to be made credible, there would have to be a vigorous, pervasive conviction among members of the staff that the proffered services would be provided with an attitude of dignity and respect toward the patient. This goal required using the esteem in which one might be held, as a health center employee, to open and extend a close personal relationship with the sick man or woman in one's care. It meant listening and acting with the outward expression and inward disposition of a teacher, a helper, a friend.

While not receding from a position of strength, staff members were also urged to recognize the latent potential in those who came to the Matthew Walker Neighborhood Health Center. They were asked to identify with the life goals of the patient, and if those goals were hindered by problems and needs that could be helped through services available at the center, the Meharrians were to bend their best efforts in the attempt. They were to gather, besides a catalog of symptoms and a medical history, a personally felt understanding of the living conditions that aggravated the complaint or illness. They were to test the usefulness of the skills mastered in the artificial setting of their health sciences course against the real conditions found in the streets of Nashville. Finally, through the health council and the neighborhood health workers, the staff of the center was to receive the views of the community regarding its residents' own interests, which on many occasions would differ markedly from Meharrians' interpretations.

By attributing worth and importance to center patients, the staff encouraged them to take that same view within themselves. Mrs. Evelyn Graves remembered the health council's advice to center workers and the response by patients: "We always told them: 'Never look down on a patient. Call them 'Mr.' or 'Mrs.' and treat them with dignity.' Then next time they came to the Health Center they would have washed their face. Pretty soon, they would put on clean clothes and comb their hair."[60] In essence the staff was to attempt to instill in patients the sense that there was something that they, with the center's help, could do about the ill health that brought them there and about other conditions under which their families struggled. Regarding its patients in this way, Meharry proceeded in the faith that reordering the institution was one means of reordering the lives of the people whom it served.

Not all the problems that patients brought to the health center were strictly clinical. Yet, lacking enough to eat, being without heavy clothing in the winter, or living in a household rent by alcoholism surely posed a threat to health. For families who needed help with such difficulties, the Social Services Department of the center was an active agent, adviser, and advocate. It sought assistance for persons who lived outside the area served by the center that would enable them to bear the costs of treatment there. Its staff aided elderly people and those receiving public assistance to verify their eligibility for Medicare or Medicaid. An office of Legal Services of Nashville was opened in the health center for indigent people who, along with the burden of illness, had difficulties that involved courts, jails, police, and the blank official face of justice. A nutritionist and a home economist were also present to consult with patients.

In another important way the Social Services Department was an extension of the family health suites. Skilled in listening, its staff members often discerned the roots of pathology in a patient's social needs. They strove to supply what had been conspicuously absent from the old clinics, the attentive ear. Together with the center's competence in assembling human resources from scores of dispersed government, charitable, and eleemosynary agencies, they sought to complete the ideal of comprehensive and preventive care. The province of the Social Services Department, like that of the family health team, was the whole person. Charged to concern itself with any issue that affected the health of the community, the health council also persisted in a broad interpretation of its mandate. When the local government threatened to curtail a supplemental food program, research by council members showing the extensive use of it by thousands of poor families led to continuance.

The violent racism that had marked the beginning of the decade in Nashville was, at the end, giving way to a polite and covert variety. Cases of blatant discrimination were still to be found, however, and the health council unhesitantly involved itself in them. When black members of the Metropolitan Police Department's fraternal organization were denied policymaking roles, the council pointed out that the group's receipt of Federal funds compelled it to lower such barriers.

Some of the health council's duties were codified and its proprietary role in the Matthew Walker Neighborhood Health Center was increased when Congress passed the Health Revenue Sharing Act in 1975. Under this law the council, as recipient of the Federal funds for the center, was designated its governing body. Henceforth it had legal sanction to establish the general policies at the facility, including the selection of the medical services to be provided and the hours that they would be made available. The annual budget would require the health council's approval, and before any vacancy could be filled in the post of health center director, the council would have to approve the candidate.[61]

In 1970, four years after Meharry received the original planning grant, it expanded the service area for the Matthew Walker Neighborhood Health Center to south Nashville, including the neighborhoods of Vine Hill, Reservoir Park, Edgehill, and Meharry's original site, Trimble Bottom. Poor people in these historically black precincts thus became eligible for medical treatment on the same basis as those who lived in the center's immediate environs in north Nashville.

In that same year neighborhood health centers throughout the nation were shifted from the Office of Economic Opportunity to sponsorship by the Department of Health, Education, and Welfare as part of a conservative national administration's strategy for ending the War on Poverty. The neighborhood health centers were also encouraged to begin striving for financial self-sufficiency and to prepare for the end of project grants.

Federal officials believed that low-income elderly patients would come to the health centers in such large numbers that the facilities would henceforth realize a substantial part of their operating cost in reimbursement from Medicare and Medicaid. These hopes were thwarted as the price of medical care continued to rise and a multiplicity of reimbursement standards under the two programs hampered recovery by providers of health services. To receive payments from other types of third parties, including private insurers, was another strategy that the Federal government directed the centers to pursue. But these also proved inadequate, since health centers from the beginning had catered to citizens who often had no insurance protection.

As a solution to the financial problems of the health center program eluded planners, Congress sought more economical means of providing comprehensive health services to defined areas or particular groups. In 1973 it authorized the first "health maintenance organizations," which were intended to provide medical care to a specific population who paid an established sum in advance of the need. As increasing sums were appropriated for HMO projects, the amount allotted in each year's Federal budget to the neighborhood health centers remained the same or decreased.

By 1976 the Department of Health, Education, and Welfare had a complicated set of funding criteria for the nation's health centers that were intended to help them effectively use the residual Federal funding sources. At Meharry the enthusiasm that had been engendered by the opening of the Matthew Walker Center crested just as Congress and HEW began to look with favor on health maintenance organizations. Even as new vistas of service opened to Meharry in south Nashville, the effects of reduced Federal support could not be entirely escaped. At the Matthew Walker Neighborhod Health Center, there were some reductions in hours of service, an end to free medicine, and the imposition of other austerities.

Faced also with financial uncertainty there, Meharry nonetheless continued its presence at Mound Bayou Community Hospital in the Mississippi Delta. In the twenty years since Meharry began its association with Mound Bayou, the United States had become the industrial, scientific, and technological leader of the Western world; indeed, a team of its astronauts was poised for the first flight to the moon. Mound Bayou, a tiny black town with a single paved street, one stoplight, a cotton gin, and a few small businesses remained a world apart.

The grants from the Office of Economic Opportunity in 1966 nonetheless increased the Delta peoples' prospects for adequate health service and their participation in the arrangements for it. Following the infusion of this Federal support, Taborian and Sarah Brown hospitals were merged to form Mound Bayou Community Hospital. The new institution sought to bring to four predominantly black, poverty-ridden Delta counties the level of care available in an urban medical center. Its own small staff was augmented by advanced students and faculty members from Meharry's Department of Surgery.

The ambitious nature of the task was shown in a 1968 census of the black population of one of the counties, Bolivar. Employed men—a majority of whom drove tractors, picked cotton, or otherwise worked as farm laborers—averaged thirty-four dollars a week in earnings. For employed women the figure was less than half as much. Nutrition among them and their families was, naturally, poor. Most housing occupied by Bolivar County's black people was wretched in the extreme, lacking piped water, bathtubs, indoor toilets, and heat. Disrepair, overcrowding, and infestation by mosquitoes, flies, roaches, and rats were typical rather than exceptional conditions. The consequence in disease and untimely death was predictable and terrible. Perhaps the most tragic example was found among the very young. The infant mortality rate for Bolivar County black babies was forty deaths per 1,000 births, twice as high as among white babies born there.

Mound Bayou Community Hospital received the unending stream of sickness from the four-county area. According to the terms of the original OEO grant, Meharry Medical College and Tufts University developed an expanded outpatient care program that provided health services throughout the 500-square-mile area. Opening in November 1967 in a former church parsonage, the ambulatory health center soon acquired its own modern new building, erected in what had been a cotton field.

Given the scope of the health problems in the vicinity, hospital- and clinic-based care was naturally less significant than prevention. Teams from the health center helped Delta residents make essential home repairs, dig wells, build sanitary privies, clean up garbage dumps, and kill vermin. Out of an organizing effort by the center also came the Northern Bolivar

County Farm Cooperative, Inc., comprising 800 poor families who pooled their labor, rented fallow land, and grew, during the spring and summer of 1968, one million pounds of food—sweet potatoes, Irish potatoes, snap beans, butter beans, black-eyed peas, and collard greens.

Consolidation of the ambulatory health center and the Mound Bayou Community Hospital was required by the Office of Economic Opportunity. The receding of Tufts University and the decrease in Federal funds created a perpetual crisis and continual prospect of closure. In 1973 Gov. William Waller vetoed the funds allocated by OEO. When agency officials overrode the action, Mississippi tried to revoke the hospital's license. Black citizens of Mound Bayou went to Federal court and won the right to keep it.

In the face of Federal withdrawal, Hospital officials sought affiliations and sources of competent management, fiscal stability, and staff that would enable it to expand to the point where it was equal to the limitless health problems of the Delta. In 1973 Meharry students from pediatrics, nursing education, and family and community health began clinical rotations at the hospital. These affiliations were not without frustration. At the centenary of Meharry, none of its students were working in Mound Bayou. However, the long association was sustained by senior consultants from the Meharry faculties of surgery, pediatrics, and obstetrics and gynecology.

When Perry M. Smith died in 1970 at the age of ninety-four, the hospital that he had founded a generation before in one of the poorest places in the nation was a strong symbol of black pride and accomplishment. Few of the thousands of patients who came there each year from Bolivar and Coahoma, Sunflower and Washington counties considered it in such a way, perhaps. They knew it primarily as a place where they would not be turned away for racist or financial reasons and where they could find an atmosphere of support in an institution managed by people of their community.[62]

To help extend the college's work at the Matthew Walker Neighborhood Health Center, in south Nashville, and in Mound Bayou, Meharry reorganized its academic program concerned with teaching and research in family and community medicine. These disciplines had been formally part of the Department of Preventive Medicine, which sat becalmed after 1964 when its chairman Dr. Thomas LaSaine suffered a disabling stroke. Meanwhile a tempest was stirring in American medical and dental education as the concerns of epidemiology were being broadened and courses in the social sciences were introduced into the curriculum.

Beginning about 1950 one school after another had created a new department with responsibility for teaching these new disciplines. A diversity of names—"Community Medicine," "Public Health," "Preventive Medicine"—indicated no consensus about the department's mission. In almost every institution the courses in public health were lodged there. Otherwise, offerings varied from laboratory analysis of local water supplies to studies in medical economics and alternative modes of delivering health services. In general, these new departments tried to provide students absorbed in memorizing anatomical structures and biochemical reactions with the tools for studying the relationships between a patient's history, his environment, and his disease.[63]

Department faculty members guided their students in projects that took them out of the laboratory and into the community surrounding the campus. Gradually, they slipped the narrowly defined bounds of public health study that limited that discipline to communicable disease. Veterans of the civil rights movement and the War on Poverty carried matters still further. The fervent and creative expressions of social consciousness in the 1960s included storefront clinics managed by students from the health sciences, located in Appalachia, in ghettoes, in isolated farm communities. Papers and academic projects growing out of these experiences were often prepared in tones of advocacy for others, rather than merely with charts and graphs. The variously named departments that took prevention, public health, and community medicine as their subject thus became a force within the medical and dental schools that inclined those institutions toward fundamental reexamination of their relations with their communities and a reconsideration of whom those communities comprised.

Meharry's Department of Preventive Medicine antedated many of the others in the United States, having been founded in the early 1920s. However, Dr. LaSaine's disability prevented it from being visible outside the classroom, and, instead, the winds of change in the college blew through the Department of Psychiatry. When the Saturday night group declared that "partnership with the community" was henceforth to be one of Meharry's missions, it virtually mandated a revived preventive medicine program with wider, more ambitious objectives.

The task for building it was given to Dr. Leslie Falk. Having as department chairman the director of the neighborhood health center would emphasize Meharry's new commitment to demonstrating that academic medicine, patient care, and concern for a blighted community were compatible and mutually sustaining. Locating the department and the health center in the same building would bind these relationships even more tightly. Finally, a new name—the Department of Family and Community Health—stated forthrightly the contexts in which students would learn and, it was hoped, eventually choose to practice.

The department taught few students at the neighborhood health center during the first three years. Wary that the latter might lapse into being a laboratory with human subjects, the Federal sponsors declined to provide any support, financial or moral, for training physicians, dentists, and nurses there. Dr. Falk was of his own volition inclined to wait until the family health teams evolved into a clinical experience that would challenge students by problems in diagnosis; then a suitable complement of courses could be offered by a faculty fully prepared to teach them. Student participation at the health center was, therefore, limited to observation at first.

But being of the generation that organized the storefront clinics and led the sit-in demonstrations, students soon exhibited a restlessness at this limited role. Shortly after the permanent health center opened, Dr. Falk urged them to enter into direct negotiations with the health council so that the community might not regard their entry as an indication that poor people were again to be regarded as "clinical material" in exchange for care.

Eager to tap their energies, Meharry also began offering elective courses in family and community medicine that included ministering to patients at the health center. In the fall of 1970, juniors and seniors joined the family health teams under the guidance of a preceptor who was a junior faculty member from the Department of Family and Community Health. These clerkships included home visits, on which the students were accompanied by a neighborhood health aide or a public health nurse. In the histories, physical examinations, and preliminary diagnoses made by the students, patients received the boon that might be expected from services of a general practitioner. The value to the students was the opportunity to see a wider range of health problems than was to be found in the hospital and to view them in the context of the contributing causes festering in a poor neighborhood.[64]

With a grant from the Carnegie Foundation, received that same year, the Department of Family and Community Health assumed a college-wide role. Carnegie's gift was used for a portion of the salaries of faculty members in almost every health sciences discipline at Meharry. Recipients in turn carried forward teaching projects in community medicine and family care.

In psychiatry the money supported work in behavioral science and the sociology of medicine. Meharry microbiologists receiving Carnegie support turned from their petri dishes to consider infectious diseases rampant in Third World nations. At the Matthew Walker Neighborhood Health Center, a survey of nutrition among residents of north Nashville was carried out by the Department of Biochemistry. In the classroom, teaching supported by Carnegie funds and growing out of such research, faculty members stressed the precepts of concern for the whole person, a preventive approach to medicine, and the importance of the patient's personal dignity.

Carnegie funds paid stipends for junior and senior medical students who, in the summers, worked for social agencies and institutions outside the college. Placements were arranged through the Department of Family and Community Health with the Medicare program, in the Tennessee and Metropolitan Nashville public health departments, and at jails and prisons.

In orientation sessions, Dr. Falk and the faculty sought to set these learning experiences in the context of needs felt by the wider community and the whole society, and the successes and failings of the prevailing system of health care.

Shadows from Meharry's previous era lingered, when pursuit of Dean Daniel Rolfe's emphasis on scholastic rigor and President Harold West's commitment to research had won students their diplomas and faculty members their professional rewards. Some of Dr. Falk's colleagues, who were conscientiously laboring in their classrooms to convey more scientific facts within a limited period, queried whether time should be allotted for community health courses as long as Meharry students were not scoring to their potential on national standard examinations. Others feared the dilution of the curriculum by what appeared to them to be subjects of dubious scientific pedigree. "What," some asked, "is epidemiology?"

Mrs. Lettie Galloway recalled the controversies aroused by efforts to engender studies in community medicine. It had been difficult for students and colleagues alike to see how such things as a seminar on communicating with patients belonged alongside an essential, traditional subject like physiology or periodontics. She pondered what answer to give. "Finally," she recalled later, "I tried to explain our goals by saying: 'If a doctor is going to prescribe medicine to be taken three times a day after meals, he should know whether the patient eats three meals a day.'"[65]

As it brought to campus scientists and scholars from a variety of interests and backgrounds, the Department of Family and Community Health acquired an interdisciplinary cast and an international character. By Meharry's centennial year, residency training in family medicine and community health were being offered at the Matthew Walker Neighborhood Health Center and other sites.

It was, however, the undergraduate courses and clinical experiences that continued to be the department's signal contribution. These made Meharry a center for training physicians, dentists, and nurses in primary care at a time when parts of the nation languished for lack of general practitioners and family doctors. A measure of the tradition that the department extended could be read in the fact that in 1976 a considerable fraction of all Meharry's living graduates were working in a field of primary care.

Meharrians who participated in the events of the late 1960s would later remember the upsurge of spirit and enthusiasm that marked the life at the college in those years. "Partnership with the community," first proposed in the Saturday night meetings, was being effected with the opening of the Matthew Walker Neighborhood Health Center. "Maximum feasible participation," a forceful paraphrase of the demand by marching students that opened the decade, was being attempted in the operations of this facility, which served the people who lived in the traditionally black and blighted neighborhoods of Nashville's inner city.

The center was seeking to remove many of the actual and intangible barriers to poor peoples' receiving medical attention, it was admitting them to a policy-shaping role, and it was lifting their expectations of themselves by treating them with dignity. Thus the center was placing an increased responsibility on the poor by implying that they had resources of individual personality and the potential as a community to take direction of their lives and the institutions that served them.

This was also the message of the new phase of the civil rights movement, which added to the kinetic energy of the times. In proposing new social arrangements designed and conducted by black people, the movement asserted that they need no longer select from a limited set of options provided by white allies nor defer to them as leaders. It preached pride and power and a sense of confidence at a time when Meharry and its neighbors were avid for confirmation of the college's new direction.

These forces raised high the expectations of college and community concerning the future. But the hopes for jobs and better housing and health facilities had been dashed before. Before the future could determine whether real change was in the offing this time, north Nashville erupted in angry and startling expressions of rage over these powerful disappointments.

8

The New Meharry

THE RIOTS IN NASHVILLE began on the freakishly hot night of April 7, 1967, with an altercation between police and black youths at a northside business. Throughout that night and the next, hundreds of black people roamed the streets around Fisk University and Meharry Medical College, throwing rocks, bricks, and bottles at police. By the third day, Fisk's campus became the redoubt from which black students kept up the exchange of blows with raiding troops.

Seeking to restore peace, a group of the city's black clergymen met with representatives from the students to hear their grievances. "If you want to know what the matter is," a Fisk senior told them, "just go downtown and look around. We are living in a city sick with segregation. Look at those white shining walls of the banks and the insurance companies and the department stores. A Negro can't get a job there unless he wants to be a porter."

Other observers would blame the arrests and injuries on Stokely Carmichael and on Tennessee State University, Fisk, and Vanderbilt, all of whom had been host to him during the previous week. The day before the general melee, Carmichael told 4,000 people gathered at Tennessee State: "You ought to organize and take over this city, but you don't do it because you don't want power. You want love. You want morality. You ought to have a black police commissioner. You ought to even have a black mayor. Dig it? That's black power."

Some white people would identify student leaders and sympathetic faculty members on the north Nashville campuses, particularly those active in the Student Non-Violent Coordinating Committee, as the cause of the disturbance. A "Freedom School" for black children that operated at Fisk University with funds from the local agency of the antipoverty program was evidence to a few observers of these leaders' malign motives.

When the Negro community assessed responsibility for the disorder, it cited instances of police brutality and the indifference on the part of white

Nashvillians toward more progress in race relations. Another analysis by a black leader noted that participants in the disturbance at least had the means to attend college, and while the episode revealed to this middle class black population the way that poor blacks were routinely treated by police, it accomplished little more.[1]

Perhaps none of these causes nor all of them together could explain the three nights of civic disorder. Conflagration was the prevailing idiom of black protest, as nonviolent resistance had been a few years before. These highly visible facts and more obscure ones were merely the tinder for the flame.

The abandonment of the inner city by white families, who took with them a personal and financial investment in its future, was a major fact of Nashville's life in the late 1960s. The trend was apparently accelerated when the Federal district court ordered an end to the last vestiges of segregated schools by means of an extensive busing plan. In the four years following the riot of April 1967, there was a 30 percent increase in what black leaders termed "second-hand schools"—those that had been predominantly white but which, as a result of the relocation of white families to the suburbs, were becoming predominantly black.[2]

The obstacles to equal employment mentioned by the Fisk student made credible the radicals' case among many of the young, who were seeking a wider future. Discrimination pervaded the workplaces of the "Athens of the South." Although manufacturing jobs increased 20 percent between 1950 and 1962, black workers held only 5 percent of the total in the latter year. Yet 80 percent of all unskilled labor in Nashville was performed by Negroes. In the city's publishing houses, where more religious literature was printed than anywhere else in the United States, the ratio of white to Negro workers was thirty-five to one. All the black employees were unskilled.[3]

In the summer of 1967 the Equal Employment Opportunity Commission found widespread discrimination in the construction, manufacturing, transportation, and retail concerns of Nashville. Black persons at the managerial level were extremely rare. Of almost 13,000 employees in these establishments, only seventy Negroes held white-collar jobs.[4]

Not only did young black men and women see themselves as barred from middle- and upper-level jobs, but they had sufficient reason to doubt that the north Nashville ghetto, which comprised 4 percent of Davidson County's land area and was home to more than a third of its population, could be made tolerable. Those who lived there did so because they had no choice, while the relative few who attained sufficient income moved out as soon as they moved up, either to the new affluent black neighborhoods on the ghetto's periphery or into expensive second-owner housing in the transitional areas west and south of the downtown area. By 1971 only one person in four employed in a north Nashville business lived in that section of the city. As their more prosperous customers relocated, these black enterprises fought to maintain a precarious stability.

The War on Poverty, Model Cities, and urban renewal all exhibited paper progress in Nashville during those years. But the effects were negligible in the black and poor districts where blighted housing, inadequate public works, and underfunded mass transit kept people as consumers of the slum. Occasionally, programs intended to help low-income persons were actually destructive. In Edgehill, the traditionally black neighborhood of south Nashville that had persisted since the turn of the century, nearly 1,300 units of public housing were planned as a single massive construction that would displace Negro families already living on the site.

The most overt and implacable insult to the north Nashville community—with whose well-being Meharry had identified itself anew—was the building through its heart of a two-deck link of the interstate highway system. Beginning at the foot of Capitol Hill (the site of one of the original black neighborhoods), I-40 cut a swath parallel to Jefferson Street. As this belt of concrete and steel and noise and stench of exhaust ran west, it isolated some 100 square blocks from stores and neighbors, the branch library, public transportation, and the public park. Only two through streets and a single pedestrian overpass were left to connect the areas lying north and south of the right-of-way.[5]

These demonstrations of the place assigned to north Nashville strengthened the militant's interpretation of events. Taken as a whole, the actions of the white community seemed to indicate that reform movements were at the very least at cross-purposes with a deeper, more enduring strain of racism and indifference. Moreover, they tended to confirm that the underlying issue was power, just as the radical black leaders insisted. Whoever could assemble the most substantial force on the side of an issue would prevail, irrespective of the merits of their argument.

Intransigence was increasingly the language of public discourse. As the Viet Nam War intensified, attitudes on both sides of that issue became firm and fixed. By the time the Reverend Martin Luther King, Jr., and other black leaders committed the civil rights movement to a posture of opposition, antiwar forces were beginning to employ forms of civil disobedience borrowed from the early days of the sit-in demonstrations. It was largely a response to institutions of government grown turgid and bureaucratic and a rebellion against the overorganization of society at every level; it was partly a genuine idealism and patriotism opposing a war widely perceived as useless; and there was a measure of self-willfulness on the part of a generation unaccustomed to inconvenience.

Each of these elements could be found in the civil disturbances that shook north Nashville in the spring of 1967. But from that time the conviction that power would be the active principle in the relation of black people to white people remained sometimes overtly, sometimes subliminally in play.

As the decade of the 1970s approached, many of Nashville's black churches were embarked upon a reassessment of their mission, which was influenced by this new phase of the civil rights movement. Like Negro congregations throughout the nation, they had long served as centers of education, refuge, community education, and social expression to people who had no such opportunities elsewhere. The stimulant to strengthen that agenda with political concerns and issues of personal development was what some ministers called a "theology of liberation" and others "black theology." The Reverend Kelly Miller Smith, pastor of the First Baptist Church of Capitol Hill, spoke to the meaning of these terms: "It is a concept of religion that sees liberation of the oppressed as the current work of God and the content of the gospel of Jesus Christ."

Like the contemporaneous student movements for social justice and against the war in Viet Nam, black theology was undergirded by profound intellectual searching. Many black ministers in Nashville had read the works of Karl Barth, Reinhold Niebuhr, and Paul Tillich. A considerable number were also familiar with writings by Malcolm X, Kenneth Clark, James Baldwin, Eldridge Cleaver, Ché Guevara, and Frantz Fanon.

Although the visibility of the black clergyman was on the decline as the number of vocational and leadership roles for black youth began slowly to widen, the black church retained a greater hold on the imagination of its community in an era of spiritual malaise than did its white counterpart. One Negro clergyman suggested that black ministration to the white churches in Nashville might include "helping them to check the frills—regalia, files, number of members, bank accounts—which kill the fire on their altars and allow racism to stalk unmercifully across this land."

In time the rhetoric of liberation theology quieted without having altered the evangelical mode that generally characterized or heavily influenced black worship. Yet its substantial presence continued to be felt to the degree that black churches remained concerned with the social as well as the spiritual welfare of their parishioners. The Reverend Andrew White, pastor of St. James African Methodist Church and longtime worker for human rights in Nashville, expressed it thus in 1971: "Black churchleaders will never separate their quest for God from their quest for human dignity."[6]

Major change was also in the offing at Nashville's predominantly black colleges as the 1970s drew near.[7] Tennessee State University (formerly Tennessee A & I) bore a particular resemblance to Meharry since it too had recently lost the services of a president to illness and had turned to a committee for transitional leadership. In 1968 the vacancy was filled by

Dr. Andrew P. Torrence, formerly of Tuskegee Institute. In his inaugural address, Dr. Torrence admonished that further civil and campus unrest could be avoided if institutions were prepared to "change from the old order" and to "take advantage of opportunities to meet special community needs."

A decade of unprecedented growth in higher education in Tennessee left this state campus little changed. While other public institutions grew in physical size and scope of programs, Tennessee State struggled to divest itself of the vestiges and atmosphere of a vocational school and to rise from the shadow of neglect where a long series of governors, legislators, and state education officials had consigned it.

The opening of a Nashville campus of the University of Tennessee in a sparkling new building seemed to some citizens, black and white, a continuation of an illegal dual system of higher education. For more than ten years, considerable energy would be spent by plaintiffs in arguing that view before the competent courts of law. Meanwhile, President Torrence and the faculty accomplished significant reorganization of the administration and earned recognition for growing strength in a number of academic and research programs. When Torrence was succeeded in 1974 by Dr. Frederic Humphries, Tennessee State had moved a considerable distance closer toward becoming a university worthy of local, regional, and national respect.

James Lawson rose from the chairmanship of the physics department at Fisk University to become president of that institution in 1968. In his first address to the community, he promised "to explore with all our might the resources of intellect and aesthetics in Negro culture, to use them to enrich new curricula, and to help devise new methods that are relevant to the unique cultural context of the Negro college." Black enterprise and achievement had indeed been memorialized by and in Fisk for a hundred years. The emphasis it gave to the distinct culture and heritage of America's Negro people became even more visible during the Lawson administration.

The musicians, writers, and other artists who had studied or taught at Fisk remained a major source of its renown. As minority economic and entrepreneurial development emerged as a theme of black advancement in the late 1960s, Fisk's esteem also grew among the relatively small number of the nation's business houses that recruited black graduates for productive and managerial jobs.

A troublesome aspect of black pride at Fisk in this period was a particularly virulent form of student activism, whose tactics included disruption of the campus. The university also encountered difficulty in translating respect won by its alumni into adequate endowment and operating capital, with the result that it found itself financially in a situation of fragile stability.

Even the transient institutions of Nashville's civic life—journalism, business, politics—were substantially influenced by the rhetoric and reality of black power. The absence of black faces from prime time local news telecasts meant one less role model for black youngsters. A threatened challenge to stations' licenses to operate in the public interest gave Negro leaders an even hand in the negotiations that led to the first visible and audible presence for young black reporters in Nashville.

In tactics reminiscent of the black Progressives a half century before, a group of north Nashville business leaders, doctors, and lawyers banded together in the spring of 1971 and vowed to deny to white merchants the patronage of black people. In politics, the 1962 statewide campaign for a seat on the Tennessee Supreme Court by Z. Alexander Looby had demonstrated the latent power of Negro voters. By 1970 organizations of the black electorate like the Davidson County Independent Political Council were a force with which office-seekers had to deal.

Professor of radiology at Meharry Medical College, Dr. Edwin Mitchell was a founder and leading figure in this movement for black solidarity at the polls. On a number of occasions, he used his considerable skills as a polemicist to attack the glacial indifference toward black people on the part of the white power structure. Six months after the disturbance in north Nashville, he stood before 400 members and guests of the Nashville Area Chamber of Commerce and called them "brave and unthinking men." Citing national statistics showing that the average lifetime income of the Negro college graduate equalled that of a white eighth grade dropout, Dr. Mitchell continued: "No, education is not the answer. Education plus opportunity is the answer! And until opportunity is created, college students will continue to pour off their campuses in protest movements."

The Meharry radiologist noted that more than a dozen years after the Supreme Court's decision in *Brown* v. *Board of Education,* 83 of Nashville's 141 public schools were still totally segregated. He attacked the failure of the many colleges and universities in the city to concern themselves with social issues; and he questioned whether the recent dismissal of several police officers for brutality against blacks represented a morale problem for the police department that exceeded the morale problem of a larger community.

Despair, frustration, and bitterness, said Dr. Mitchell, encircled the downtown business district that the businessmen had recently pledged to revive. He concluded: "We cannot imagine what manner of Negro man you feel lives here in Nashville when you continue to ignore the examples of Cairo, Milwaukee, and Louisville as though Nashville's time is not coming."[8]

In this atmosphere the second collective leadership group in Meharry's history assumed administration of the college on October 1, 1966. For almost two years Dr. Robert Anderson, chairman of the Department of

Internal Medicine, Dr. William Allen, dean of the School of Dentistry, and John Sharp, treasurer of the college, met every morning over a long list of unrealized opportunities. "We decided that we wouldn't be a 'lame duck' administration," Dr. Anderson, the Administrative Committee's chairman, recollected later. "Instead we would try some initiatives that were in keeping with the times, which served Meharry's needs and also met the desires of funding groups."[9] Some of the plans drawn up by Dr. Harold West in his last years were laid aside by the Administrative Committee, even as it reaffirmed the major ends that he had approved for Meharry: physical expansion, a radically improved financial posture, and an increase in the number of graduates.

For thirty-four years, since the relocation to north Nashville in 1931, Meharry had performed its service for the nation without significantly increasing its classroom and laboratory space. If the demands brought about by the changes in the broad popular expectation of medicine were to be satisfied, the particular health problems in minority communities addressed, and researchers trained in laboratories who would return to them to teach, then Meharry would have to grow in size, in quality of academic offerings, and in community service.

The administrative organization of the college, to the extent that it perpetuated outworn habits, was obsolete, and Dr. Anderson's committee made changes in the operation of the medical and dental schools, the admissions office, and student services. Responsibility for the last of these was assigned to Dr. Thomas W. Johnson. To succeed Dr. Daniel Rolfe in the deanship of the School of Medicine, the Administrative Committee and the Board of Trustees elevated Dr. Lloyd C. Elam, the chairman of the psychiatry department, who also continued in that post.

In May 1967 a group of faculty members led by Drs. Anderson, Elam, and Ralph Hines completed a planning document entitled "New Developmental Programs," which set forth the first steps in a new direction for Meharry. "We thought about what Meharry was, where we wanted it to go, and how to get there," Dr. Hines recalled later. Extending the resolve of the Saturday night group, the committee strongly reaffirmed that Meharry should continue to play a national role in the training of black physicians and dentists, while demonstrating a special concern for disadvantaged people of all origins, both as students and as patients.

The course offerings and the quality of teaching throughout the college were major concerns identified in the plan. It proposed renovation of both the medical and dental curricula, and it sought to deepen the preclinical experiences of students through the strengthening of the basic sciences departments. More full-time faculty members would be needed, and there would be developed more community service programs.

The plan also called for the construction of a biomedical research building, a facility devoted to fundamental and advanced studies in the basic

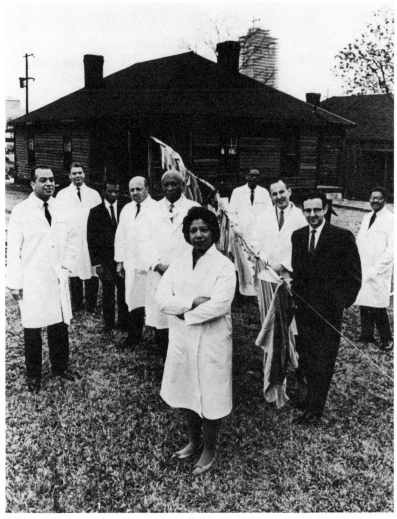

Faculty members in the ghetto (c. 1970)

sciences, and a renovated comprehensive care center adjacent to Hubbard Hospital. Ambitious, even exuberant, these first visions of a larger campus implied the acquisition of more property and the extension of Meharry's old bounds.[10]

In an innovative way the development plan addressed the unrealized possibility represented by large numbers of young black men and women who possessed aptitude for medical or dental training but whose early education and undergraduate experiences did not fit them to meet the keen competition for admission. A group of such students, registered at other Nashville colleges during the regular academic year, enrolled in the first session of Meharry's Biomedical Sciences Program in June 1969. For the next three summers they took courses in chemistry, cell biology, physics, scientific writing, calculus, behavioral science, and medical sociology taught by faculty members from Meharry and Fisk University. When they returned to their own campus each fall, they retained a counselor at Meharry who followed their work and directed them in research projects, self-instruction, and other studies.

The career paths chosen by the first Biomedical Sciences class confirmed the view that students' backgrounds did not absolutely determine the chances for success in a health career. By Meharry's centennial year more than fifty undergraduate colleges and universities were represented in the summer Biomedical Sciences classes, and the proportion of participants accepted into medical, dental, or graduate school was twice that of the national average in similar programs offered by other institutions.[11]

A second long-term effort to improve the quality of premedical and predental studies for black students was the organization of Meharry's most advanced courses into a division of graduate studies under the direction of Dr. Charles W. Johnson. Through this division, the Administrative Committee sought to meet the need of larger, wealthier institutions for more biomedical scientists to teach undergraduate chemistry, physics, and other fundamental courses. Meharry itself needed active researchers who also had an interest in extending the opportunities for laboratory work to students at all levels.

In addition to being a tool for building a stronger faculty, an accredited graduate program that loaned faculty members for undergraduate teaching would help diversify the medical and dental curricula with courses that emphasized original research and inquiry. With such preparation, students would have the option of entering graduate study following the completion of their clinical work. Those not primarily interested in careers in research would nevertheless have increased competence in its methods for whatever medical or dental practice they pursued.

As it sought to achieve its several purposes, the graduate division kept in view the ultimate aim of contemporary Meharry, an increase in the supply of workers in the health sciences, especially among groups of people who ordinarily lacked access to them because of poverty, racial discrimination, or other artificial barriers. On the hundredth anniversary of the college, Meharry had available in the graduate division courses leading to the doctoral degree in biochemistry, microbiology, or pharmacology and to the Master of Science in public health or clinical psychology. Meharry's first Ph.D. degree was awarded at its centennial year commencement to Parsottam J. Patel of Gujarat, India. Dr. Patel's research concentrated on the causes of leprosy, which, while rare in the Western world, beset thousands of people each year in his native country.[12]

A unique graduate program, through which students could earn the Master of Medical Science degree, was another tangible expression of the graduate division's accord with the institutional mission. This course allowed the student to complete all the classroom and laboratory work of the preclinical years in medicine or dentistry with a concentration in one basic science field. At the end of the second year, he or she received the M.M.S. degree and, if desired, a place in the junior class of the School of Medicine or Dentistry. As with the Biomedical Science classes, active recruitment was among students with promising records, evident aptitude, and the choice of health work as a career, but whose uneven preparation made this last an unrealistic goal. The record of the first thirty-five students who began the program in June 1968 was impressive: thirty eventually enrolled in medical school and half also completed the requirements for the master's degree in pharmacology, immunology, or another specialty.[13]

The need by Meharry students for loan and scholarship money remained critical as the cost of food, housing, equipment, books, and, perforce, tuition, continued to rise. In 1970 approximately 60 percent of all medical students in the United States came from families earning $10,000 or more, while less than one Negro family in four had an income exceeding $8,000. A sampling indicated that the family income of many Meharry students fell below even the median income of black families throughout the nation. Thus the paying of the college's bills was a burden in addition to their studies for the future dentists and physicians.

Dr. Robert Anderson's Administrative Committee sought to give relief in two ways. It committed Meharry to a student housing program, and during its period of service, a residence hall for women, named for Dr. Dorothy Brown (Class of 1948), was opened. Further projects, including apartments for married students, were contemplated in the development plan to ease one of the greatest expenses in attending Meharry. The Administrative Committee also sought to increase the scope and available capital of the college's financial aid programs. Scholarship money, which contained no obligation of repayment and thus did not influence a graduate toward lucrative practice, was the chief goal.

To try to meet the need for financial aid—for which 90 percent of Meharry students applied—the leadership group began a nationwide direct mail effort specifically aimed at expanding this budget category. As a result, between 1967 and 1970 the money available for scholarships and loans more than doubled. A secondary object of this particular fund drive was the creation of a new constituency of donors, large and small, who were involved through their gifts in the college's future.

Although they were in other ways important to Meharry, its graduates represented a large untapped resource for development and recruitment. Fulfilling an agenda of reform and expansion would require their financial support. To increase the size of the student body, they were needed to find promising undergraduates and to direct them to Meharry. Improved management, service, and communication became the Administrative Committee's objective in Meharry's alumni affairs. Narrowing the gap that neglect had opened between the college and its graduates was one of the leadership group's most important achievements.

Through a revitalized alumni office, a number of local chapters in the nation's major cities were newly organized or raised from a moribund state. There was an upsurge in the number of alumni who participated in Meharry's life by means of dues and gifts for student aid and campus expansion. Former students recruited new ones; many returned to the campus or traveled to other locales for continuing education courses; some served alumni appointments on the faculty. In "An Open Letter" to Meharry's graduates, Dr. Ralph Cazort wrote:

> Meharry is on the move. There is thrust and surge, experiment and synthesis, which will help, if diligently pursued, to keep this school to the forefront in the delivery of health care and health services research. The crown of outstanding accomplishments is to be worn not only by your alma mater but by you who have gone out into the field and proved that what was secured here . . . has stood you in good stead for whatever path you have chosen to take.[14]

In 1967 with the full approval of the Administrative Committee, the Alumni Association requested and received a larger representation for Meharry graduates on the Board of Trustees. Through all three of these councils, and others where its stronger and clearer voice was heard, it urged the selection of a black as Meharry's sixth president.[15]

By its nature, charge, and self-declared intent, the Administrative Committee was a transient means for deflecting the immediate crisis created by the departure of President Harold West. In practice, it went beyond this limited concept. Under the aegis of Robert Anderson, William Allen, and John Sharp, Meharry began gathering the energy of the times into a strategic plan for increasing its graduates, delivering broader, more humane health services to its immediate community, and raising the funds to afford these things.

During the Administrative Committee's two years the college also commenced a strenuous, long-term effort to recapture the loyalty and support of former students. A means to that and other ends was the thorough identification of Meharry as a predominantly black institution whose purpose was to prepare workers to address enduring health problems among

Negroes and other minority people. Another legacy left by the committee was its assertion, which partook of the contemporary thrust of the civil rights movement, that Meharry contained and was capable of excellence. Two other ideas were implicit in that reaction against decades of apology: the college did not exist by sufferance of the white culture, and in providing models for young black people, it bolstered the black community against forces that impinged upon its prospects.

The most marked difference between the previous administration and the Administrative Committee was the latter's determination, in Dr. Anderson's words, "to have open communication all the way down the line, to admit a continuous stream of fresh ideas." The circumstances under which it assumed the helm at Meharry and the subsequent rise to managerial posts by faculty members who had broad support among their peers marked a new direction. The office of president would not be decentralized, although power at the apex of the administration would become diffused. The faculty would not manage the institution, but the creation of college-wide advisory committees, academic tenure, and a senate gave its voice greater amplitude. Despite a stirring of activism in the School of Medicine, students would not gain a significant policy-shaping role. However, the importance of its future alumni led Meharry to give them a greater responsibility for their own education.

Although bids for power in the Meharry community were thus attenuated, the role of many members was larger than it had ever been. Such groups as the governing body for the neighborhood health center and a Meharry Employees Council, organized in 1972, acted as countervailing forces against the idea that administrators had a monopoly on leadership. For at least a quarter century, Meharry's precarious financial footing had tended to concentrate authority in the college's chief executive. That tendency would continue through the centennial year, but beginning with the Administrative Committee, a sense of autonomy and therefore of responsibility would begin to be felt and assumed by others outside the executive suite.[16]

In September 1967, Board of Trustees President Victor Johnson and two of his colleagues called at the home of Dr. Lloyd Elam to tell him of his election as president of Meharry. The choice of Dr. Elam was not made public until December, when it was announced that he would assume office in time for a new academic year.

Lloyd Charles Elam was born on October 27, 1928, in Little Rock, Arkansas. Thus he was the first president of Meharry from the Deep South, whence so many of the college's students had come and returned to practice during its first hundred years. (One of the new chief executive's youthful memories was the refusal by his father to permit the Elam family to ride in Little Rock's segregated public transportation.) With the exception of

George W. Hubbard, Dr. Elam was also the youngest president in the college's history.

Lloyd Elam's undergraduate years were spent at Roosevelt University in Chicago, where he received a baccalaureate degree in 1950. After winning the doctorate in medicine at the University of Washington at Seattle, he returned to the Midwest, to the University of Illinois at Chicago, to serve an internship. Dr. Elam's developing research interests—psychosomatic medicine and the state of mental health services in the nation's general hospitals—took him to the University of Chicago for residency training in psychiatry. Later, as a teacher there, he met Dr. Matthew Walker on one of the latter's visits to the city.

Although the existing faculty was employed on a part-time basis and money was scarce, Lloyd Elam was persuaded, following an initial contact from Dr. Walker, to come to Meharry and to increase the course offerings in psychiatry. By the time of his election as president, Meharry had a mental health clinic for ambulatory patients, an inpatient psychiatric service, a residency program in psychiatry, and a greatly strengthened research program. As department chairman, Dr. Elam recruited faculty members from many other disciplines, including clinicians who were concerned with the chemistry of aberrant neurological systems and specialists in the behavioral sciences concerned with community and society. During the transition years of the mid-1960s, creative proposals for new direction in the life of the college often arose in the meetings of the psychiatry faculty.

"I welcome the revolution at Meharry," President Elam told the sun-drenched crowd at his inauguration on June 9, 1968. Meharry's revolution, he went on to explain, included the extending of "optimal learning experiences" to students from "diverse subcultures and with widely varying interests and abilities."

Meharry would be required, the new president said, to address the most important problem in health care in the United States, which was manpower. The health services provided by the college must be expanded and accounted for in terms of actual differences they made in health conditions among the people using them, he added.

"We are using this opportunity," Dr. Elam continued,

> to respond to the call . . . for a new system of education. It is a system that is responsive to the belief that human rights include the right to health and full development of one's intellectual capacity unrelated to the ability to pay. Our response must also be to the necessity for excellence in education, quality in health care, and responsibility to the Negro community.

It was the official day of national mourning for U.S. Senator Robert Kennedy, murdered the previous week in Los Angeles, following his vic-

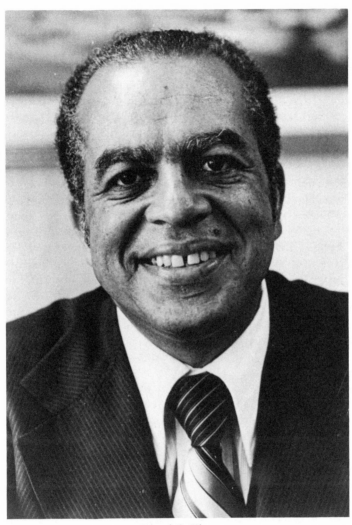

Lloyd C. Elam

tory in the California Democratic Presidential primary. Twenty-four hours before the ceremonies at Meharry, the killer of the Reverend Martin Luther King, Jr., had been captured after a manhunt that had been pursued since the assassination the previous April. For some who listened to Dr. Elam's address, the losses of the white Senator and the black civil rights leader were personal wounds that would remain open and searing for the rest of their lives. "Time is not a healer," guest speaker Carl Rowan told the audience. "But I come here to Meharry and see that time is a builder if men make it so."

After education and service to the community, such building was a third major theme at President Elam's investiture. In his speech he announced plans for $30 million worth of physical facilities, including a new Hubbard Hospital, computer center, allied health professions building, dental school, and a dozen other structures, many of which had been conceived in the ad hoc planning group. The objectives that the Administrative Committee set—an increase in the size of the faculty toward a superior academic program, more students and scholarships to support them, and a secure financial foundation for Meharry—would require an additional $20 million. The total that Dr. Elam pledged to secure—$50 million—rivaled the $58 million campaign just completed by the medical school of Harvard University. "With proper financial and moral support," Elam said in his peroration, "the energy of the revolution can be directed into channels which will cause the progress of past decades to seem, by comparison, minimal."[17]

With his colleagues who had brought about the awakening of Meharry in the mid-1960s, President Elam believed that the historical dependency of the college upon the community of people who were black and poor gave the two a special relation. The new Meharry committed itself to making that bond more equitable through increasing service to the community and helping to raise its capacity to build upon such help. This objective was advanced with the opening of three new facilities: a children and youth center, a mental health center, and a comprehensive health center for adults. Between 1968 and 1973, Meharry brought to an end its old outpatient services with their hard benches, specialty clinics, and common hours. Replacing them were these three new services, built upon the theory of comprehensive care.

Like the Matthew Walker Neighborhood Health Center, the new services were begun and largely operated with sizable Federal investment. Throughout their operations could be found the distinguishing marks that Meharry and the funding agencies were determined to introduce into contemporary medicine. Emphasis was placed upon the whole patient, including his social history and present circumstances of life, as well as the wide range of environmental influences that caused or complicated his

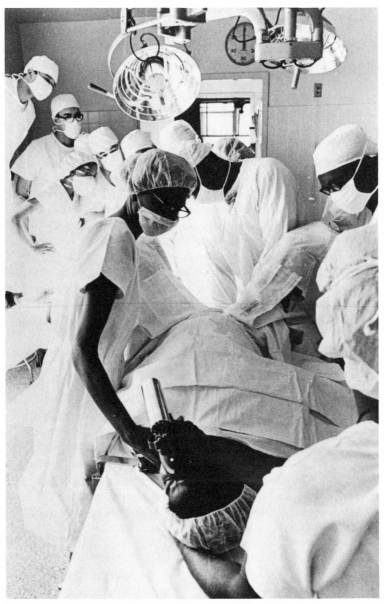

Patients, staff, and students in Hubbard Hospital

difficulty. Prevention was assigned a vital place. The role of the family and community in the illness was considered. And the needs and wishes of those served were taken into account. Each of the new centers created an advisory group comprising leaders from public and private agencies, neighborhood organizations, churches, youth groups, and community residents.

Meharry's new services for children, adults, and mentally afflicted people actually preceded in time the opening in its permanent quarters of the better-known Matthew Walker Neighborhood Health Center. One, the children and youth program, had its beginning not long after World War II. Before 1948 a black baby born prematurely in the mid-South had minimal chances to reach the age of one. In that year Meharry began a pediatric premature care program to boost the survival chances of such infants. Those whose parents lived within eighty-five miles of Nashville were picked up in the college's specially equipped ambulance jeep. As soon as the babies were out of danger, Meharry pediatricians taught the parents how to continue to care for their special problems.

Upon obtaining his certification in pediatrics, Dr. E. Perry Crump returned to Meharry in 1947 to direct the teaching and patient care program in that department. In one of the earliest attempts at the institution to address patient problems as a continuous whole with workers from several disciplines, he assembled a team of public health nurses, social workers, dentists, and physicians. Not long after becoming chairman of pediatrics in 1950, Dr. Crump received a Federal grant to study the causes of prematurity among black mothers and the relation of their income, education, and other social factors to the survival of their babies. Out of this research came strong evidence that the chances for normal full-term pregnancy and successful delivery were increased if the mother had proper nutrition and prenatal care. Refuting investigators who asserted that black babies were naturally smaller, weaker, and more likely to die after premature birth, Dr. Crump and his co-workers showed that where social and economic conditions among black and white mothers were approximately the same, so were the incidences of prematurity and the rates of survival. In a series of papers published over several years, the Meharry pediatricians explored all aspects of health among the very youngest members of the black population in the United States, about which very little had previously been known.

Some 10 percent of the children in Dr. Crump's study were found to be mentally retarded or to exhibit debilitating signs and symptoms of such retardation. A second Federal grant in 1964 brought funds to establish in the pediatrics department a mental retardation clinic, which would concentrate on case finding and detailed diagnosis. There were no geographical limits nor restrictions on sources of referral, race, or economic status. Any

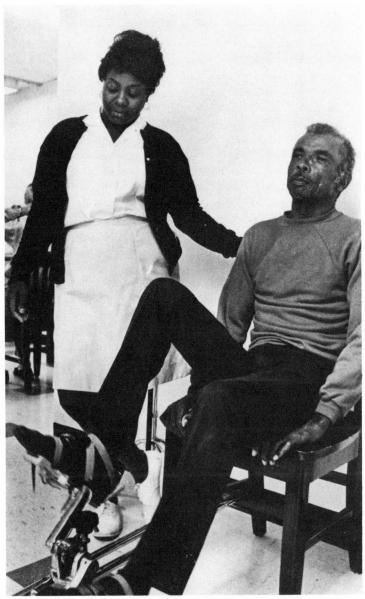

Patient and member of staff of Hubbard Hospital

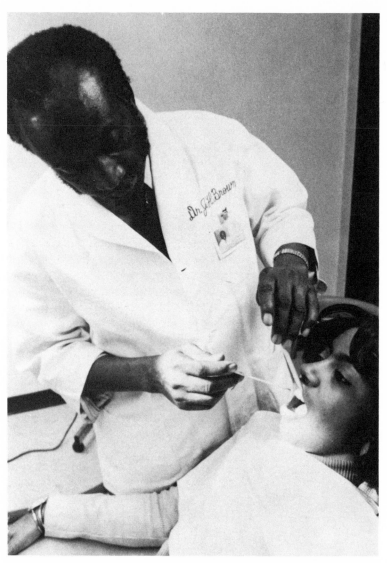

Doctor and patient in Hubbard Hospital

child who suffered from developmental problems was eligible for examination and treatment.

The Comprehensive Center for Children and Youth became the fullest expression of Meharry's oldest outreach program when in 1968 it opened in the very center of the Meharry-Hubbard complex of buildings. In the pastel examining rooms, children from birth to age eighteen had available emergency treatment, physical examinations, dental care (the reclining chairs were adjustable to any height), immunization, surgical services, and speech and hearing therapy. With parents' permission and participation, they could receive social services, a psychological evaluation, and instruction in basic health principles. Extending the team that Dr. Crump first brought together twenty years earlier were a home economist and a dietitian.[18]

Ten years after he inherited a part-time department of psychiatry, President Elam presided at the dedication of the Community Mental Health Center in 1971. There Meharry assembled the human and physical resources to treat with a variety of strategies up to 100,000 adults, adolescents, and children who exhibited neurotic or psychotic conditions. A survey of outpatients at Hubbard Hospital revealed the extent of actual need in Meharry's community. Nearly 40 percent of those coming to the clinic for care showed symptoms of anxiety, depression, or schizophrenia. As suggested in its name, the new facility gave emphasis to programs that extended beyond the campus. One such service was the crisis call center, whose telephone line was open twenty-four hours a day to persons in the throes of distress and despondency.

A major public service of the center's early years was directed to Nashville's elderly people. The geriatric section organized friendship clubs, recreational opportunities, and arrangements for treatment for those whose advancing years left them vulnerable to mental difficulties. Staff also provided training in the biological, social, and psychological aspects of aging to workers from area nursing homes. Under center auspices the Meharry Alcohol and Drug Abuse Program began in 1973, operating from a storefront on Jefferson Street in the center of a drug trafficking area. It provided behavioral and psychological therapy to patients who sought escape from the miseries of an impoverished community only to find themselves floundering in a still deeper nightmare. By the centenary of Meharry in 1976 the Community Mental Health Center was offering, in addition to regular clinical services, a foster home program for patients formerly residing in institutions and assistance to families that enabled troubled members to remain in the home setting.[19]

Transformation of Meharry's former ambulatory health services was assured with the opening in August 1969 of the Comprehensive Health Center for Adults in the renovated Public Health Lecture Hall. Together with the other new health centers, it placed Meharry in the front rank of medical schools that were leading a revival of interest in primary care and community medicine. Dr. Robert Anderson, head of the Department of Internal Medicine and formerly chairman of the Administrative Committee, was the first director.

With the center as axis, the service area inscribed an arc of 180 degrees from 18th Avenue, North, covering the west and northwestern neighborhoods of north Nashville. Thus it complemented the Matthew Walker Neighborhood Health Center, whose patients came from east and south Nashville as well as the environs of the campus. In contrast to the latter service, the Comprehensive Health Center for Adults did not at the start attempt a strong outreach program, yet it served twice as many patients. Each one who came to the Comprehensive Health Center was treated by a team comprising a physician, dentist, nurse, and social worker, supported by an array of specialists and aides. This team was considered the patient's family doctor, and it followed him through whatever treatment he received at Meharry. There was an appointment system and evening hours.

In December 1971 the Comprehensive Health Center for Children and Youth and the Comprehensive Health Center for Adults moved into a new cylindrical four-story building connected to Hubbard Hospital. Besides the Neighborhood Health Workers from Meharry who knocked at doors and counseled community residents, nurses from the Metropolitan Nashville Department of Public Health disseminated the news that the odd round wing was a place where people could obtain high quality, personal medical attention. By 1976 there were more than 50,000 patient visits a year to "Comp Health," as the combined children and adult services were familiarly known.[20]

Ironically, as Meharry gained national and international attention for programs of preventive, primary, and comprehensive care, it faced enormous difficulty in maintaining the partnership with the community represented by the several new health centers. The college's fiscal situation, described in a subsequent discussion, led the Department of Health, Education, and Welfare to direct the merger of the Matthew Walker Neighborhood Health Center and the new comprehensive health services for children and adults. Coordination or centralization of medical and administrative services and one responsible officer instead of two were among the steps taken to improve the college's financial sheet. When it became effective on February 1, 1975, the reorganization also merged the formerly separate areas of service in north, east, and south Nashville and the respective community advisory councils. Challenged to maintain the trust of these neighborhoods, Meharry had to increase its efforts to ensure efficiency and personal, attentive patient care even as fees were imposed for some services that had been free, and service hours were trimmed.[21]

To better serve these ambulatory patients, Meharry opened in 1970 an elaborate diagnostic and detection laboratory, the Automated Health Testing Service. For two hours, the person being examined walked through twenty-one stations, receiving some threescore tests that ranged from a chest X ray to vision and hearing acuity to a personality profile. All of the procedures, except the measurement of height, the dental examination, and venipuncture, were performed by machine.

Funded by the Tennessee Mid-South Regional Medical Program, the center's original object was to detect heart disease, cancer, or imminent stroke in time to prevent or effectively treat them. As the detailed profile of the patient was assembled, the health teams in each of the new centers of patient care were alerted to many other potential and actual problems. The cost for the tests was kept as low as was feasible, not only so that people from the poverty area might be served, but that practitioners from throughout the region would routinely use them as diagnostic tools. Of the nearly 5,000 people who came to the Automated Health Center in its first year of operation, some 70 percent were discovered to have some abnormality; in 40 percent of these cases, the victim had been unaware of the condition.[22]

The process of detection and analysis performed at the Automated Health Testing Service was assisted by the Meharry Computer Center, where the raw data were transmitted and converted into diagnostic information. Built in 1970 with funds raised largely by the alumni throughout the nation, the computer center became an increasingly valuable tool as the college's managerial and financial operations were overhauled in this period. In addition to critical data relating to patient care, it processed commercial transactions and made easier and quicker the formerly laborious task of student registration.

No one knew whether "comprehensive care" as conceived and carried out at the several new health centers actually made a difference in the conditions of health that had been identified by the studies of the community in the environs of Meharry in the late 1960s. To compare the results with those obtained from health services traditionally used by poor people was the assignment given to the Center for Health Care Research, established in 1969.

Describing the purposes of the center, its first director, Dr. Samuel Wolfe, wrote:

We want to facilitate the process of social change in health and welfare services through the collection of data that are relevant to the community, to its planners, to its administrators, to its teachers, to its politicians. . . . Method is our servant, not our master. People in our study areas are dying sooner than they should, their babies are less healthy, they get less care less

often. Our central aim is to focus on the differing ways to provide care, to
see if these patterns can be altered.

Center staff identified three areas of the city where poor Nashvillians
tended to live. Totaling some **85,000** people, the population in them was
mainly but not exclusively black and poor. The first area was the north
Nashville community served by the Matthew Walker Neighborhood
Health Center with its emphasis on family-centered care and a strong
program of community outreach. The second area, stretching to the north
and west of the downtown and including the Meharry campus, depended
mainly upon the Comprehensive Health Care Center for Adults. The third
area, comprising neighborhoods in south and west Nashville, continued to
be served chiefly by outpatient departments of the city hospital and by
private physicians.

Using data from a variety of sources, the center sought to determine
whether the health problems of poor people were being more effectively
addressed by one system than by the other two. A second purpose was to
determine whether the incidence of these problems was significantly reduced by the Meharry programs. For example, through long-term surveys
of hypertension in each area, it would be possible to assess which type of
service had the most favorable outcome in treating and preventing this
disease, which killed black people at rates three to four times higher than
were found among whites. Collected over a period of years, these data
would show any difference in the rates that were attributable to the presence of the Meharry programs.

In addition to physicians, dentists, and nurses, the center employed epi-
demiologists, biostatisticians, sociologists, survey researchers, and social
workers. Assembled into interdisciplinary teams, they investigated such
related questions as direct and hidden costs of the new services in comparison to traditional ones, patient satisfaction, and unmet health needs in the
three areas of the city.

Early center research confirmed previous findings regarding the serious
conditions of ill health that went unattended among Nashville's poor. They
noted, in particular, the dearth of attention to dental disease and to inter-
personal and emotional problems. Fewer than 15 percent of the patients
with serious physical and mental conditions were receiving appropriate
attention, concluded the investigators. They added:

> That which we know how to do to meet basic health and social welfare
> needs is not being applied. . . . The problems may be similar to those of
> many poverty communities across the United States. The establishment of
> health care as a priority in its own right and the elimination of pervasive

economic poverty are two key issues that must be addressed by our nation.[23]

The commitment to place more graduates into the fight against the persistent health deficiencies of poor people required the exuberant physical expansion of Meharry that took place after 1968. It was accomplished with massive injections of money realized from the development campaign that Dr. Elam announced at his inauguration. When it formally opened in September 1969 the goal of the fund-raising drive was $88.8 million. The huge sum was to be used to purchase additional land, to construct more than a dozen new buildings, to renovate other spaces, and to multiply the size of the student body and the faculty.

George Russell, vice-chairman of the General Motors Corporation, directed the development team, which included executives from other major national business houses, and faculty members, officers, and alumni of Meharry. Nashville assumed the vanguard position in the drive when graduates and friends in the college's home city announced in May 1969 their intent to raise $1.5 million locally. Fittingly, the flagship gift came from the Methodist Church, Meharry's original sponsor and continuous benefactor.

On June 30, 1971, campaign chairman Russell declared that the goal of phase one—$26 million, earmarked chiefly for construction—had been attained in cash, grants, and pledges. Meharry's budget was more than double what it was in 1964, the last year of Dr. Harold West's administration. More than 100 new faculty members had been appointed since 1968. The revival of interest in Meharry among private donors, and the stimulation of new giving by corporations, were major accomplishments of the campaign. Individuals throughout the nation, who often designated their donation for scholarships, participated in the life of the college with gifts large and small. Foundations, however, led all other private supporters.

In October 1972 Dr. David E. Rogers, president of the Robert Wood Johnson Foundation, announced the gift of $5 million to Meharry. Drawing upon rhetoric from the moribund War on Poverty, the announcement noted that the money would be used "to train health professionals for front-line service in 'under-doctored' communities." President Elam promised that with the grant Meharry would move swiftly to increase the number of physicians associated with the college's primary health care teams in comprehensive health centers. Eventually, the foundation's generosity would touch every aspect of Meharry's academic program, from supporting a program to qualify nurses for an expanded role to in-service training for faculty members in teaching methods and techniques.[24]

Another philanthropist's gift, this one in the amount of $1.5 million from the Stanley S. Kresge Foundation, helped Meharry to build one of the landmarks on the expanding campus. In the Kresge Learning Resources

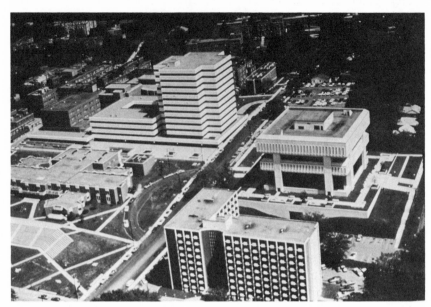

The new Meharry. The cross-shaped George Russell Tower of Hubbard Hospital
is in the upper center. To the right is the Kresge Learning Resources Center and
student housing. At left center is the Community Mental Health Center. Part of
the 1931 campus can be seen to the left of George Russell Tower.

Center, whose striking design contained elements of Moorish architecture,
were located the teaching tools of the future. They included an audiovisual
production studio, closed-circuit television monitors, and a lending library
of video-tape lectures on new medical findings from which practitioners in
the area served by the Regional Medical Program could borrow. The college library was relocated in the new center, which allowed it room to
expand its support services to the academic program.[25]

Although private support set a new record during the development
drive, funds from the Federal government exceeded all other sources of
support combined. By 1970 Meharry was receiving more Federal money
than any other predominantly black college in the nation except Howard
University, and in the centennial year, 51 percent of its income was from

Federal grants and contracts. At the same time it was not among even the top 100 academic institutions in the amount of Federal assistance, nor was its large percentage of Federal funds unusual in an era when up to two-thirds of the operating costs in most medical schools in the United States were paid by this source.

Asked at the beginning of the giant fund-raising drive about its purposes, President Elam said that it was aimed at increasing by several times the size of the student body. Beginning in 1968 about 1,400 black students a year were accepted into first-year classes in the nation's medical schools, compared to 200 a year during the century since Howard and Meharry were founded. This hopeful trend was apparently illusory, however; in 1975–76 there was a decrease in the absolute number and percentage of first-year minority medical students. A shrinking applicant pool, competition from all quarters for admission, rising costs, decreasing scholarship funds, and retrenchment of medical schools' recruiting efforts were blamed for the setback. Meharry's expansion was, in this context, highly significant. By 1976 more than 1,000 students were enrolled there, compared to half that number a decade earlier.[26]

In that same year the capital fund drive attained 80 percent of its original goal and was transforming the face of Meharry. Around three sides of the old core, consisting of the 1931 campus, was an array of new patient care buildings, classroom and research complexes, residential spaces, and the rising walls of a new hospital tower.

The building of a virtually new hospital—the third in Meharry's history—was necessary for the same reason that such a facility had originally been required. For over half a century, Hubbard Hospital had been the central element in the clinical experience of Meharry students. The new tower would raise the number of beds from about 200 to over 400, thus increasing the ratio of patients to students as required by the doubling of the enrollment. In September 1972 the Department of Health, Education, and Welfare approved $25 million in grants and loan guarantees to build the new facility. The Federal government agreed to pay the first 40 percent of construction costs. Obtaining a Federally insured loan from the Equitable Life Assurance Company, Meharry would be responsible for another 40 percent. The last fifth, some $6 million, would be sought in Nashville, where Meharry spent in capital and operating expenses a considerable amount each year.

The coming of the college to north Nashville forty years earlier had aroused the suspicion of area residents. The plans to construct a "space-age hospital" (as a local newspaper described it) required a zoning change, precipitating a controversy among property owners in the vicinity and politicians anxious to be perceived as defending the public interest. With approval finally granted by the city council, Meharry broke ground for the new hospital on November 28, 1973. A year later, the cornerstone was set in place. For another twenty-four months, construction proceeded on the twelve-story tower, whose dedication would be a highlight of the centennial festivities.[27]

Even as its potential for service to the community grew, the hospital remained a chief factor in Meharry's financial difficulties. One continuous and irrecoverable expense was the cost of caring for poor patients who had no means or subsidy. According to the way their medical expenses were met, Hubbard Hospital's patients could be divided into four groups: (1) those whose bills were paid by the Metropolitan Government of Nashville and Davidson County; (2) those who qualified for Medicare or Medicaid; (3) those who could afford to pay their own charges or who carried insurance that did; (4) those who could pay nothing for services and who had no third-party payer, either public or private.[28]

The hospital's fiscal strategy was to assist as many patients as possible to qualify for third-party payment and to realize sufficient revenues from private patients to balance the losses incurred for treating those who lacked the ability to pay their medical bills.

All insurors—Medicare, Medicaid, private policies—paid only a part of patient costs, and Meharry's ideal of partnership with a poor community limited the number of paying patients that it could serve. Nonetheless, its hospital revenues might have balanced expenses except for the staggering losses from indigent care that were not reimbursed by the city. As had been the case for twenty years, Meharry spent more than the amount appropriated by the city council to subsidize this service to patients who were essentially a public responsibility.

Seeking a more just arrangement, Meharry officials argued that the income level used by the local government to determine eligibility for reimbursement was too low, since many of Hubbard's patients who earned more than that amount still could not afford medical care. It also noted that city certification officers were on duty only eight hours a day, five days a week and thus were unavailable to establish eligibility of indigent patients who were treated at night or on weekends. As a result only one person in five who qualified for the city's subsidy was so certified. Some fifty beds at Hubbard Hospital, one-fourth of its capacity, were continuously occupied by patients who could pay nothing and who were uncertified for subsidy. Based on an average of $150 a day, the prevailing rate at hospitals in Nashville, Meharry sustained a deficit of $2 million annually for their care.

Year after year the outcome was the same. Meharry would submit a request to the city for its estimated costs for indigent care in the coming twelve months. This figure would be reduced by finance officers, the mayor, or both. When the budget was submitted to the city council, the request was liable to be trimmed still further. In the year ending June 30, 1976, for example, the unreimbursed cost to Meharry for indigent care was $2.25 million. Under its contract with the city, the hospital had been paid $600,656.[29]

In October 1975, as autumn winds whipped the plastic sheathing on the face of the unfinished tower, Meharry offered to lease Hubbard Hospital to the city government for $1 a year. The Metropolitan Government was facing an extremely expensive prospect—either to renovate or to rebuild entirely its existing General Hospital in southeast Nashville. Meharry proposed to give Nashville a new 400-bed facility, provided the city would assume repayment of the construction cost and an annual operating expense of $12 million. In return, Meharry would supply the medical, dental, nursing, and support staff.

The idea stirred intense debate. "It is a controversy of many parts," noted one journalist, "mixing medical education, public welfare, and health care with politics, money, and race." Involved was the fate of area hospitals whose applications for expansion might be denied by the competent health planning agencies as long as there were unfilled beds at Hubbard Hospital. Private and political interests would be affected by the relocation of the city hospital. The city would be required to guarantee access to Hubbard, which was often thwarted by the trains on the east- and west-bound tracks that bisected north Nashville. Objection was also heard that fewer beds would be required for indigent care in Nashville than Hubbard's new tower would make available, while the unused capacity had to be maintained.[30]

Perhaps the most complicated and difficult question was who should supply the medical talent at a new general hospital. Under the established contract with the city, written when racial segregation prevailed, Vanderbilt University's medical school had established and maintained a dominant presence there. Meharry's proposal to make Hubbard the city's primary, acute, and emergency care facility threatened to cut deeply into Vanderbilt's training program for interns and residents.

The ambivalent relations between Nashville's two medical schools threatened to ensnare whoever would enter the thicket to effect a compromise. Despite joint faculty appointments in some departments, a number of common trustees, and various cooperative endeavors, contacts between Vanderbilt and Meharry were sometimes tense and difficult. Their respective philosophies of medicine were a fundamental point of difference. Vanderbilt was renowned for training researchers and teachers, while Meharry was achieving recognition for its part in renewing American medicine's commitment to primary care and family practice and high quality health services for communities who lacked them.

The historical record included lasting contributions to Meharry's academic program from members of the Vanderbilt faculty. Times had changed, and slowly there was emerging a formal relationship of colleagues, peers, and equals. Yet a counteroffer from Vanderbilt to move the city's general hospital to its campus aroused old suspicions. And while Meharry students and residents traveled to sites as far away as New York for preceptorship and advanced training, Vanderbilt provided its postgraduate students such opportunities at General. No one denied that the result of the latter was a creditable service to the people of Nashville. The principle was whether both of the city's medical schools should not have an equal role at the tax-supported hospital.

In recommending the rejection of the Meharry proposal, the mayor's task force asserted that maintaining General would probably cost the city less than meeting the debt service at Hubbard Hospital; moreover, it noted, the status quo left the city with the option of contracting for care "from either or both medical schools." Disappointed in the recommendation, Meharrians were nonetheless encouraged by other language from the task force report. The Metropolitan Government, it said, "should undertake a mutually acceptable plan whereby medical students and physicians of Meharry and Vanderbilt in furtherance of their education have equitable access to city-supported indigent patients by rotation through the city-supported hospital or city-leased beds or both."[31]

The hope and expectation of justice at General was broadly shared among factions and diverse interest groups at Meharry in the centennial year. In October 1976 a tentative agreement between Vanderbilt and Meharry to staff Nashville General jointly was announced by the two schools. Contemplated in the protocol were cooperation in filling vacancies among chiefs of service when these occurred and a contract with the Metropolitan Government that admitted Meharry students and practitioners to the medical and teaching staff in a collegial role. The city also pledged a more just indemnity to Meharry for its expenses in caring for the poor people of the community, including assignment of certification officers to Hubbard Hospital on a twenty-four–hour basis.[32]

This last step came too late to spare Meharry a period of severe fiscal strain as its 100th anniversary drew near. In 1971 the college spent $1.4 million in excess of income; by 1974 the difference was $4 million. The cost of indigent care was the largest item in these deficits. Other factors included the escalating cost of giving health care in general, the dramatic drop in Federal student aid, and the operating expenses of the new campus buildings, as the development plan proceeded.

To meet the emergency, college officials took advantage of a new Federal law designed to assist financially troubled medical schools. Passed by Congress in 1971, the Health Manpower Training Act provided for "distress grants" to assure survival of such institutions and ensure their continuing contribution to the pool of human resources for medical care. Each year Meharry qualified for assistance under this statute, which was applied to the academic budget. In its straitened financial condition, the college was not able to make any monthly payments on the Federally guaranteed loan for construction of the new hospital.

Whether changes in the arrangement with the city of Nashville promised some relief from deficit spending and drawing upon the endowment to meet the cost of indigent care remained to be seen. As far as the people of the community were concerned, the question was moot. "Meharry has always given indigent care and not gotten paid," said Dr. A. P. Johnson, physician and faculty member, trustee and alumni leader. "You can't tell a mother whose baby is sick that you won't treat her child because she doesn't have any money."

As Meharry's new campus was built, old methods of teaching and learning were examined to see whether they served present, vital needs. By the early 1970s the student body could be characterized, in the *Journal of the National Medical Association,* as a "cultural and intellectual melting pot." Although Meharry continued to view its primary purpose to be the training of black people for careers in health sciences, the percentage of white students—about one in five—remained through the centennial year what it had been since the desegregation of the college.

The commitment at Meharry to an ethnically diverse student body, and the recent reaffirmation of its unique, historical mission of concern for the health of minority peoples were reconciled by recruiting applicants from American Indian and Hispanic citizens. By 1970 the one-fifth of the student body that was nonblack included members of these groups. Applicants for admission were placed in one of four categories: minority students from the Southeast, whites from the Southeast, minority students from other sections of the nation, and nonwhite Southerners and students from other nations. According to President Elam, Meharry "gave special consideration to admitting students based on . . . where the greatest need is." Strong preference was given to students from states that belonged to the Southern Regional Education Board, whose contract with Meharry required the college to provide a certain number of places for them. An indication that the applicant would return to practice in an area where the doctor-to-patient ratio was low also received favorable attention by the admissions committees.[33]

As had been true throughout Meharry's first century, its students came mainly from the South. In other ways the composition and character of the student body was changing dramatically. By 1970 one Meharry student in five was a woman. More undergraduate institutions than ever before had alumni at the college. Finally, student life at Meharry, as in many colleges and universities of the day, was animated by students' determination to participate in the making of decisions affecting their education.

Everyone enrolled was a member of the Pre-Alumni Association and eligible to vote for representatives to its council, the recognized student government at Meharry. The council published *The Meharrian,* which was the college yearbook, and *The Fovea,* a newspaper under editorial direction of students. Regulation of intramural athletic events, sponsorship of Student Research Day, and mediation of controversies between students and the administration were other endeavors of the Pre-Alumni Council. College committees, except those concerned with admissions and evaluations, included students as voting members. A student-trustee committee was formed to increase the exchange of views among those legally responsible for the governance of the college and those for whom it existed. When in the early 1970s curricula in both medicine and dentistry were revised, students were credited with contributing toward the final contents, notably the increase in elective hours.

Outside the campus bounds, Meharry students gave time and effort to the Student Health Coalition, whose volunteers set up free clinics and sponsored health fairs in Appalachia. Many Meharrians joined their peers throughout the nation in demonstrations against the war in Viet Nam. In 1970 the college officially observed a moratorium of classes to protest American involvement there.[34]

The simplest, rudest measure—enrollment statistics—did not count the hundreds of community residents trained by Meharry for paramedical and auxiliary occupations, whose work helped more doctors see more patients. What such statistics did show was Meharry's response to the most potent contemporary force for change in health education, the demand for more manpower.

That demand, insofar as it expressed real need, was critical among the nation's black communities. There was only one black physician for every 4,000 black Americans. In the case of black dentists, the ratio was even more adverse, with one to every 11,500 Negroes. The old problem of distribution persisted, too. Cities of the north and the west were the places of residence most favored by the relatively small number of Negro practitioners. The response to a background of personal poverty might be a ghetto, or it might be a suburban practice.

Increasing the number of students admitted each year and expanding its physical plant and faculty to accommodate them was not enough to assure more graduates from Meharry. Since the founding, students had labored to master an increasingly technical course under the handicap of undergraduate experiences at predominantly black institutions, which public policy literally shortchanged. Several educational reforms in the early years of the Elam administration were intended to turn this historical fact with its negative consequences into present, decisive advantage, both for Meharry and for its students. Among these changes were the audiovisual equipment for self-instruction and course review, the Master of Medical Science program, the strengthening of the basic sciences course, and a new flexibility in the time required to complete degrees. Formerly, such innovations might have been seen as remedial; now they were offered without stigma and indeed with reward and advancement.

Letter grades were abolished at Meharry in the fall of 1969, and students were given a "pass," "fail," or "honors" mark at the end of each semester. Through this means the college sought to encourage thoughtful attention by faculty members to the student as an individual, and in turn the student was asked to assume greater responsibility for his own learning. Without pressure to earn a grade, rote memory work became less important than a deep grasp of the material of a given course and connecting it with facts gleaned in another one. A third purpose of the new evaluation system was to prepare students to teach themselves for the day following graduation, when continual increase in their professional competence would become solely their responsibility.

Dr. Lloyd Elam was succeeded in the deanship of the medical school by Dr. Ralph Cazort, under whose administration was introduced a new medical curriculum. It sought to convey the unity of scientific knowledge in a way that had not been done at least since specialization had captivated the medical sciences. For example, "Introduction to Clinical Medicine," "Biodynamics of Human Development," "Physical Diagnosis," and "Clinical Correlation" was a coherent series of courses designed to help the student perceive the connections among thousands of seemingly unrelated facts presented in the preclinical years.

Under the new plan, the same subject was taught at the same time in each basic science discipline. For example, aspects of cell biology were discussed concurrently in biochemistry, physiology, and anatomy. And patient care was made a part of students' experience almost from their first day at Meharry. Contact with patients increased and intensified, of course, in the junior and senior years. It ranged from watching an instructor conduct a diagnostic interview to performing routine minor surgery and uncomplicated deliveries.

These last two years were divided into clerkships (or rotations, as they were sometimes called) in medicine, pediatrics, obstetrics and gynecology, and surgery. A fifth one was spent in psychiatry and family and community health. In the sixth and last period, the student could pursue an area of study that especially interested him, either at Hubbard Hospital or another approved site. Small groups of junior- and senior-year students spent a period of time, usually twelve weeks, in each of these settings.

Ward rounds illustrated the variety of learning situations in which they participated. When a patient entered Hubbard Hospital and was assigned to a department's care, a student serving rotation was included among the

team members responsible for giving care. He examined the patient, prepared a medical history, and made routine clinical and laboratory tests.
Using these findings, textbooks, and the library, he then proposed a diagnosis, a course of therapy, and a defense of these views.

During ward rounds, he, his group, and an instructor moved from one
patient's room to another. Outside the door the student presented his data,
diagnosis, and suggested treatment, quizzed at each point by the instructor. The group then entered the room, where the instructor examined the
patient. Besides refining the student's analysis and interpretation, this step
taught examination technique, and it allowed the instructor, as senior
member of the team, to provide an example of considerate and dignified
treatment.

Ward rounds were often a vigorous and exciting academic exercise. To
give a good presentation and to answer instructors' questions well, the
student was required to integrate the body of basic scientific knowlege
gained in the first two years at Meharry with information gathered by
questioning and examining the patient, conducting laboratory tests, reading the scientific literature, and observing other clinical presentations.
Before him constantly were the questions, "What does this datum mean?"
"How does it fit with the other information I have gathered?" "What
conclusion can I draw?" and "What predictions can I make from these
facts?" Most clinical departments conducted grand rounds once a week
when a problem of interest to all its students and faculty members (hence
the term "grand") was presented. Usually the patient's case was perplexing
or difficult. Sometimes prominent clinicians from outside Meharry were
invited to address the grand rounds.[35]

Educational progress of the day also included several new certificate and
degree programs that prepared students for careers related to medicine and
dentistry and required by contemporary demands for greater health service for more people. In the fall of 1972 the first class enrolled in a new
health care administration and planning program. A cooperative effort by
Meharry's Department of Family and Community Health, Fisk University,
and Tennessee State University, it offered an undergraduate program leading to the baccalaureate or a two-year graduate course for the Master of
Science in Public Health degree. Being based in a medical center and
managed by a consortium of public, private, and graduate institutions, the
program had as its goal an increase of blacks, American Indians, and citizens of Hispanic heritage in the designing and management of public and
institutional health services. Some of the teaching methods employed in
the program, including game simulation and psychodrama, reached toward the farther shores of educational experiment and innovation.[36]

The new Meharry's emphasis upon preventive medicine and interdisciplinary study and its pride in a black heritage came together in the

Maternal and Child Health/Family Planning Center. Organized under the graduate division and funded by the Agency for International Development, its staff taught citizens of African nations to be teachers and administrators, researchers, and consultants in nutrition, midwifery, pediatrics, well-child care, family planning, and other subjects. In its early years, center fellows and Meharry faculty members studied in Ghana, Liberia, and Nigeria. In the academic year 1973–74, the center launched a field project in Botswana to train practicing nurses. Another undertaking by the center was made possible with support from the Office of Economic Opportunity. With its grants, the staff gave practitioner training for registered nurses who expected to work in rural communities in the southern United States.[37]

Meharry's own hospital was another site that experienced a shortage of nurses with consequent problems in patient care. Continual reform of the nursing service including salary incentives and provision of opportunities for professional development was one outcome. Another was the revival of nursing education at Meharry. In 1971, nine years after the School of Nursing closed, Meharry began a pilot program for training pediatric nurse practitioners.

Requests were soon being received from nurses seeking advanced instruction in other specialties. In response to this demand the School of Medicine organized in 1972 a Department of Nursing Education and commenced programs to prepare nurse practitioners in adult and family medicine, mental health, midwifery, maternal-child health, and family planning. From the staff of Hubbard Hospital and from all over the nation, classes were assembled. Each participant was already working or qualified as a registered nurse. According to department head Evelyn Kennedy Tomes, Meharry intended to "add to fundamental skills. Then they can go into areas that have heretofore been for physicians only."[38]

As required by the ever-larger expectations of medicine, other members of the health care team extended physicians' and dentists' time to attend more patients. To help meet the demand, the program in medical technology was converted from three years to one; a division of X-ray technology was established in the School of Medicine; and, in dentistry, the dental hygiene curriculum was broadened in scope. The first and last of these were offered in cooperation with Tennessee State University.[39]

The need for improvements in the School of Dentistry had been clear for some time when in 1971 it was placed on probation by the accrediting council of the American Dental Association. A major capital improvements drive was begun immediately, which supported the building of additional classrooms, a fully equipped outpatient clinic, diagnostic facilities, and surgical, orthodontic, and cellular biology laboratories. Fiscal and administrative affairs were reorganized, and Dr. Thomas P. Logan, a physician as well as a dentist, was appointed dean. The most critical need was for more faculty members, and these, too, were found.[40]

The academic year 1969 saw the introduction of a drastically revised curriculum. Under it, clinical experiences were begun in the freshman and sophomore years, while basic sciences were extended into the junior and senior years. The new study plan also placed students on the teams that treated patients at the neighborhood health centers and at Hubbard Hospital. In 1974 a Department of Hospital Dentistry was begun at the latter site. Meharry thus became the first dental school in the nation to have a four-year curriculum for its students that was based in a hospital. The idea for the training of dentists in that setting may be traced at least as far back as 1939, when Dr. Edward L. Turner wrote in the college's *Bulletin*: "I believe this school has a unique opportunity to develop an unusual type of dental teaching where medicine is stressed in teaching and dental aspects of diseases are amply stressed in medicine."

The social aspects of dental health were another part of the reforms. In the words of Dr. William H. Allen, immediate past dean of the school, "The approach of dentistry at Meharry is to take the whole patient and his community into account in preventing, diagnosing, and treating disease."[41] In pursuit of this standard, the dental faculty undertook efforts to improve the quality of teaching in the school and to raise the scores of students on national standard examinations. Each dental department set up instructional objectives, and a review course in educational psychology and teaching methods was made available for all faculty members. The Study Habits Analysis Group, comprising psychologists, faculty members, and young alumni, worked with individual students to help them concentrate their approach to their work.

The goal of the academic changes in the School of Dentistry on the eve of Meharry's centenary was the enhancement of the future practitioner's clinical judgment and his capability for recognizing health problems that required referral to other specialists. The task was without exact boundaries. As Dean Thomas Logan expressed it: "The definition of dentistry is no longer fixed but is changing almost daily to include additional tasks, concepts, duties, and goals. The School of Dentistry must have a system of education that prepares students to meet changes that are occurring or that are likely to occur in the graduate's lifetime."[42]

In the outpatient clinic, Meharry dentists and dental students applied a high degree of technical skill and experience. Fractured jaws, dislodged teeth, and dental caries were treated there. To the clinic, in keeping with a Meharry tradition, students and faculty members each year brought students from the public schools for instruction in the fundamentals of preventive care.

When Dr. Eugenia Mobley succeeded to the chief administrative post of Meharry's School of Dentistry in 1976, she expected to preside over an era when the dentist, like his physician colleague, would practice preventive medicine. Every patient who came to Meharry's dental clinic underwent a battery of examinations, including blood pressure, urinalysis, heart and respiratory rate tests, and a nutritional evaluation. Dr. Mobley, one of only two women deans of a dental school in the United States, explained: "Dentistry used to be seen as a corrective sort of science, since the dentist corrected only those problems that already existed. We now say it's more of a preventive science, preventing the occurrence of disease."[43]   As the centennial year approached, Meharry's School of Dentistry passed several milestones. Full accreditation was restored, Federal assistance delivered it from deficit financing, and passing scores on national standard examinations were won by greater numbers of its advanced students. As was true throughout Meharry, the challenge was to attain specific short-term goals while pursuing a vision of comprehensive health and the highest standards of teaching and research.

The new attention to development matters was reflected in research performed in the School of Dentistry. Growth and development of the human head was a long-term project that assembled more information about the facial skeleton of black people than had ever before been known. Research in mental health and dental care strengthened the school's pioneer course offerings that connected dental practice and the behavioral sciences. The effects of smoking upon dental health, basic research in infant teething, and oral aspects of sickle cell anemia were included in the lively research program that added to the school's academic strengths.

Health conditions among minority and poor people were by no means the exclusive interest of Meharry researchers in this period. To a greater degree and depth than ever before, however, they sought the causes of persistently disproportionate rates of untimely death and illness found among these groups. School of Medicine investigators conducted basic and applied studies in sickle cell anemia, disorders of the eye in the Negro population, and the consequences of racism upon children. They investigated keloids, the disfiguring disease that was, after sickle cell anemia, most commonly associated with black people as a group.

The existence of high levels of DDT in the milk of poor Southern white women was a finding of a major research project conducted in this period. All levels of society were affected by the problem of drug abuse, which Meharry scientists studied through an interdisciplinary approach.

Research in pursuit of ways to reduce the risk in pregnancies among teenage and pre-teen girls addressed another problem found in both black and white communities. Injury and death from accidents among very young children knew no racial lines; thus Meharry's inquiry into the epidemiology of such accidents was widely relevant. Projects entitled "the biochemistry of schizophrenia" and "low blood sugar as it relates to the sudden infant death syndrome" further indicated the range of investigation in the School of Medicine.

Meharry appeared poised to become, early in its second century, a major research institution. Committed to offering comprehensive care in a poor community, it had an unusual opportunity to demonstrate that scientific rigor was not the whole of medicine; yet it could also affirm the importance of basic research, which was sometimes lost in public and press preoccupation with dramatic "breakthroughs."

The first major event in the celebration of Meharry's centenary anticipated an expanding future of scientific work, while also honoring the college's first black president. Harold Dadford West had died in 1974, but the achievements of his life—distinguished research scientist, pioneering Negro educator, and friend of all people—were ideals that Meharry itself proclaimed. Recalling his predecessor's "high human values," President Lloyd Elam accepted from architects the keys to the Harold D. West Basic Sciences Center at dedication ceremonies held on February 26, 1976. In design and use the four-story glass and brick structure enacted several currents in the life of modern Meharry. It invited interdisciplinary exchange, research, and teaching by bringing together all of the college's basic sciences departments—anatomy, biochemistry and nutrition, microbiology, pathology, pharmacology, and physiology. So that related aspects of these subjects could be taught concurrently, laboratories and classrooms were made adaptable to requirements of one field. An atrium, balconies, and bridges spanning the interior expressed the theories of contemporary architecture that shaped space to permit spontaneity and free movement. An observer could stand at any point in the great open central area and see a variety of interrelated activity going forward at the same moment.[44]

The Class of 1976 graduated on May 30. Accelerated programs under the nation's war effort had resulted in two classes in 1944; thus, this was the college's 101st commencement. Under the early summer sun, the procession formed at the West Basic Sciences Center and marched, gowns fluttering and tassels swinging, to the new outdoor amphitheater adjacent to the Community Mental Health Center. Round and full, the notes of Felix Mendelssohn's march echoed against the buildings and the low hills, mixing with the sound of shuffling feet. Dr. James R. Cowan, assistant secretary of defense and member of Meharry's Class of 1944, told the graduates to "keep an eye on the three E's: expectations of medical care; economics of medical care; and ecumenical view of professional roles." Selections by the Meharry Singers spoke of "good news" and "feeling the spirit."

The ninety-three new physicians and twenty-seven new dentists walked across the stage, receiving from President Lloyd Elam the diploma conferred as an outward sign of the skills and understanding they had acquired at Meharry. Standing with them were twenty-six nurse practitioners, twenty master's degree recipients in health care administration and planning; ten new medical technologists; and nine new dental hygienists. Two received a Master of Medical Science degree, and Meharry's first Doctor of Philosophy was awarded his diploma. It was the largest commencement in the history of the college, with more than twice as many graduates as Meharry had presented in classes only a decade earlier. By several indices—race, sex, undergraduate colleges represented—it was also the most diverse.[45]

Continuing education was a major interest and the new Meharry campus the main attraction when the National Medical Association and the National Dental Association chose Nashville as the site of their 1976 conventions. In August, when the surrounding hills appeared blue in the hot and humid air, the two associations of black doctors assembled at convention sites downtown and on the campus.

The highlight of the NDA meeting, attended by 2,000 dentists, dental technologists, and dental hygienists, was the groundbreaking for Meharry's new School of Dentistry. A fund drive for the facility had been a major activity of alumni throughout the nation in the centennial year. On August 4, President Elam, Dean Eugenia Mobley, a trustee, an alumnus, and a student each turned a spadeful of earth. Out of the site on the corner of Eighteenth Avenue, North, and Meharry Boulevard would rise an $8.4 million, five-story building, housing the medical, surgical, and restorative specialties of dentistry. A week after the groundbreaking, the Kresge Foundation announced major gifts in support of the construction.[46]

Increasing the availability and equality of health care for black people was the leading objective of the National Medical Association, president-elect Arthur Coleman told 3,000 of his colleagues who assembled in Nashville. Their guests included the governor of Tennessee, the mayor of Metropolitan Nashville, and the president of the National Association for the Advancement of Colored People. In addition to remarks from these officials and scientific sessions in virtually all disciplines of medicine, the NMA convention heard presentations about malpractice insurance, professional advertising, and the perennial challenge of increasing the number of black students enrolled in medical school.[47]

The opening of the new academic year was the college's true centenary, and Convocation Day, October 4, was designated the official 100th anniversary. The campus community, gathering in the Kresge Learning Resources Center, joined in singing "Happy Birthday, Meharry" and in listening to speeches on the college, past, present, and future.

As the second century began, Dr. Ralph Hines said, still larger numbers of students would be enrolled, and Meharry would achieve wider recognition for the quality and range of its scientific research. Meharry's director of hospital and health services, Florence Gaynor, predicted that the view of health as a positive concept would increasingly influence the care and treatment of patients. "Health care is a continuous process of education and prevention," she continued. "Meharry is committed to providing leadership and social sensitivity along with community and health service. . . . We are aware of the future. As evidenced by our new campus, we have already begun to build for tomorrow."[48]

The new hospital tower was dedicated on November 10. It was the climax and last major event of the centennial year. "These buildings represent a commitment to and for future generations," said Victor Johnson, chairman of the Board of Trustees as he formally opened the facility. The addition of 400 beds multiplied Meharry's capacity to serve the community and the region. A plaque naming the tower for George Russell was unveiled during the ceremony. "What we lacked in money, we made up for in hope," the former General Motors executive told the gathering of celebrants and well-wishers. Having directed the team that raised $55 million for Meharry between 1969 and 1974, Russell admonished that further efforts were required to assure Meharry's long-term financial strength against the ravages of inflation and the cost of giving care to poor people. "I hope Nashville and the nation help Meharry move forward," he said.[49]

Conceived in the pious works of white missionaries and philanthropists, Meharry thus began its second century as an example of black peoples' fortitude. Of all the institutions in the United States, it was the best known and the most admired among nations of the nonwhite Third World.

Every new Meharry graduate—physician and dentist, research scientist, hygienist and technician, planner, and nurse practitioner—was trained to advance the work of health and healing. Yet each one also represented the prospect that a black child or a poor child could aspire to goals that the society had for so long held beyond his reach. After health and life, hope was the greatest gift that Meharrians could give. Having earned the distinction of the college's diploma against the odds, each graduate imparted hope to whomever they met.

In the days after the Civil War, their spiritual and corporeal ancestors wandered toward Nashville in bewildered elation at being set free from slavery. Many of them found their way to the rude benches and the primer and the songbook in the missionary schools. At the commencement in the 100th year of the college and the 200th year of the nation, Meharrians celebrated their persistence and continuing struggle with a joyful noise.

Nashville, from where Meharry's graduates traveled throughout the nation and the world, had been transformed into a major national center for health research and patient care. But the challenge there and everywhere was to deliver from the healers' hands to the suffering man and woman, especially those who were black and poor, the preventive measure, cure, or comfort that medicine had available.

To Meharrians whose callings kept them near their alma mater, the past was as vivid as the present. They could travel extensively in Nashville and its environs, seeing signs on every hand of generations from Meharry who had hallowed these city spaces.

At Greenwood Cemetery winter wind and summer breezes stirred the grass on the graves of the founders, John Braden and George Hubbard. In the libraries and archives, in uncollected accounts and stories, in early rolls and records, the pioneer faculties and students awaited just, enduring memorials.

There was Meharry's first graduate, Dr. James M. Jamison, who had gone west with the declining century; Dr. John Bass, who exhorted his class-mates at the first commencement to "decrease the mortality among our people"; and Dr. Georgia E. L. Patton Washington, the first Meharrian to return to Africa to practice medicine.

Nearby were legacies of Dr. Robert Fulton Boyd, who defied the era of Jim Crow to run for mayor of Nashville. The work of his peers endured as well: the physicians and teachers, Henry T. Noel, William A. Reed, Charles O. Hadley, Thomas Henry Elliott; Drs. James B. Singleton, Donley Tur-pin, and their colleagues of the early dental faculties; Drs. Josie Wells and John Henry Hale, builders of hospitals; and Dr. Charles Victor Roman, historian of Meharry.

There was also Dr. Michael J. Bent, who anticipated Meharry's future direction with his studies of poverty, disease, and their connection; Dr. William Beck, beloved physician of Nashville, who fought against the nemesis of tuberculosis; Dr. Harold West, internationally renowned re-search scientist, humanitarian, and the first black president; and Dr. Mat-thew Walker, who with his contemporaries helped to bring the trans-forming spirit of the civil rights movement to Meharry. For each of these there were thousands of graduates over three generations whose names were preserved only on class rosters, but whose practices saved innumera-ble lives from illnesses that assaulted black Americans out of proportion to their numbers in the nation.

In tribute to all of them, Meharrians sang their anthems in that memo-rial year, when the future seemed as open to development as the past.

Notes

Chapter 1

1. Frances Meharry, *History of the Meharry Family in America* (Lafayette, Ind.: Lafayette Printing Co., 1925), p. 369. There are several versions of this story, differing in details but similar in substance.

2. Henderson H. Donald, *The Negro Freedmen* (New York: H. Schuman, 1952), pp. 4–5.

3. As a result of the war and Reconstruction, the Negro population of Davidson County, Tennessee (of which Nashville was the county seat) rose from 15,999 in 1860 to 25,412 in 1870. *Population of the United States in 1860, Eighth Census, 1860* (Washington, D.C.: Government Printing Office, 1864), "Population of Cities, Towns, &c," table no. 3, p. 467; *Ninth Census of the United States, 1870* (Washington, D.C.: Government Printing Office, 1872), "Statistics of the Population," table no. 2, p. 62.

4. Charles Röbert, *Nashville and Her Trade for 1870* (Nashville: Roberts and Purvis, 1870), p. 47.

5. Nashville *Republican Banner,* December 14, 1865.

6. Paul David Phillips, "A History of the Freedmen's Bureau in Tennessee" (Ph.D. diss., Vanderbilt University, 1964), pp. 71–72 and 179.

7. U.S., *Statutes at Large,* vol. 13, chap. 90; Alrutheus Ambush Taylor, *The Negro in Tennessee, 1865–1880* (Washington, D.C.: Associated Publishers, 1941), p. 13.

8. Stanley J. Folmsbee, Enoch Mitchell, and Robert Corlew, *Tennessee: A Short History* (Knoxville: University of Tennessee Press, 1969), p. 364.

9. Ellen Lillard Carr, "The Struggle of the Freedmen's Bureau to Effect Social Rehabilitation in Nashville and Davidson County" (M.A. thesis, Fisk University, 1967), p. 54; Nashville *Republican Banner,* October 21, 1866.

10. Carr, "Struggle of the Freedmen's Bureau," pp. 29–52.

11. Oliver Otis Howard, *Autobiography,* 2 vols. (New York: Baker and Taylor Co., 1907), 2: 316, 319.

12. Carr, "Struggle of the Freedmen's Bureau," pp. 124– 26 and 130; Henry Lee Swint, *The Northern Teacher in the South, 1862–1870* (Nashville: Vanderbilt University Press, 1941), p. 79.

13. Swint, *The Northern Teacher,* pp. 80– 82.

14. Carr, "Struggle of the Freedmen's Bureau," pp. 123– 24 and 137– 39.

15. Phillips, "Freedmen's Bureau," p. 235.

16. Howard, *Autobiography,* 2: 390– 91.

17. Phillips, "Freedmen's Bureau," p. 239.

18. Caleb Patterson, *The Negro in Tennessee, 1790–1865* (Austin: University of Texas, 1922), pp. 104– 25; J. Beverly Shaw, *The Negro in the History of Methodism* (Nashville: Parthenon Press, 1954), pp. 139– 40; Private Acts, *Acts of the State of Tennessee,* 34th General Assembly, 1865– 66, chap. 115.

19. Special Order No. 134 1/2, Bureau of Refugees, Freedmen, and Abandoned Lands, State of Tennessee, August 30, 1866; W. W. Clayton, *History of Davidson County, Tennessee* (Philadelphia: J. W. Lewis and Co., 1880; reprinted, Nashville: Charles Elder and Son, 1971), pp. 263– 64; Clark Memorial Methodist Church, *A Century of Witness for Christ, 1867–1967* (Nashville: Clark Memorial Methodist Church, 1967), unpaginated; R. Bartley J. Campbelle, Sr., ed., "The History of Clark Memorial Methodist Church," mimeographed (Nashville: the author, n.d.), unpaginated.

20. *The Christian Educator,* 2, no. 1 (October, 1890): 30.

21. The year after the incorporation of Central Tennessee College the references to "general and theological education" and "colored people" were by amendment stricken from the original legislative act. Private Acts, *Acts of the State of Tennessee,* 35th General Assembly, 1867– 68, chap. 17.

22. Emory Stevens Bucke, ed., *The History of American Methodism,* 3 vols. (New York: Abingdon Press, 1964), 2: 362– 64.

23. Clayton, *Davidson County,* p. 263.

24. D. W. Clark, "Education of the Freedmen" in *Reports of the Freedmen's Aid Society of the Methodist Episcopal Church, 1866–1875* (Cincinnati: Western Methodist Book Concern, 1893), preface to the 1868 report [i].

25. Methodist Episcopal Church, Northern Annual Conference Records, vol. 1, Report of the Committee on the Education of Freedmen, October 12, 1866.

26. Grace Harrison, "Hubbard Hospital and Meharry Medical College for Negroes, Nashville, Tennessee" (M.A. thesis, University of Chicago, 1945), pp. 6– 7; Mary E. Braden, *John Braden, A Pioneer in Negro Education* (Morristown, Tenn.: the author, 1935), 30 pages, passim; *Nashville Banner,* June 11, 1900; Central Tennessee College, *Biographical Sketch and Memorial of Reverend John Braden, D.D.* (Nashville: Central Tennessee College, 1900), 9 pages, passim. Clayton, *Davidson County,* p. 264.

27. Clayton, *Davidson County,* p. 264.

28. Ibid.

29. Catalog of Central Tennessee College for 1882– 1883, quoted in Charles Victor Roman, *Meharry Medical College, A History* (Nashville: Sunday School Publishing Board of the National Baptist Convention, 1934), p. 24.

30. Minutes of the Board of Trustees of Central Tennessee College, May 1872, available at the Methodist Board of Higher Education and Ministry, Nashville.

31. *Reports of the Freedmen's Aid Society,* Third Annual Report, p. 8.

32. Alrutheus Ambush Taylor, *The Negro in Tennessee, 1865–1880* (Washington, D.C.: Associated Publishers, 1941), p. 192.

Chapter 2

1. Dr. Jones is quoted in Charles Röbert, *Nashville and Her Trade for 1870* (Nashville: Roberts and Purvis, 1870), p. 467.

2. Henrietta Huxley to Eliza Huxley Scott, letter, September 1888, Huxley Papers, Imperial College of Science and Technology, London.

3. *Second Report of the Board of Health to the Honorable City Council of the City of Nashville for the Year Ending July 4, 1877,* pp. 129–32.

4. Henderson H. Donald, *The Negro Freedman* (New York: H. Schuman, 1952), p. 154.

5. Paul David Phillips, "A History of the Freedmen's Bureau in Tennessee" (Ph.D. diss., Vanderbilt University, 1964), pp. 101–04.

6. Ibid., p. 110.

7. W. W. Clayton, *History of Davidson County, Tennessee* (Philadelphia: J. W. Lewis and Co., 1880; reprinted, Nashville: Charles Elder and Son, 1971), pp. 294–95; *Ordinances of the City of Nashville,* 1875, title 9, chap. 48.

8. Clayton, *Davidson County,* p. 295.

9. Jesse C. Burt, *Nashville, Its Life and Times* (Nashville: Tennessee Book Co., 1959), p. 73; "Reports on the Cholera Epidemic of 1873 in the United States," *House Executive Document,* 43rd Congress, Second Session (1875), pp. 142–46; minutes of the Nashville Board of Health, reprinted in Nashville *Daily American,* August 16, 1876. The unnamed visitor's allusion was to Coleridge's poem, "Cologne" (1828):

In Kohln, a town of monks and bones,
And pavements fang'd with murderous stones
And rags and hags, and hideous wenches;
I counted two and seventy stenches,
All well-defined, and several stinks!
Ye Nymphs that reign o'er sewers and sinks,
The river Rhine, it is well known
Doth wash your city of Cologne;
But tell me, Nymphs, what power divine
Shall henceforth wash the river Rhine?

10. *Second Report of the Board of Health,* p. 23.

11. Nashville *Daily American,* July 20, 1876.

12. Donald, *The Negro Freedman,* pp. 85–92. For an account of a voodoo practitioner of Nashville, "Indian Mary," see Nashville *Daily American,* August 10, 1886.

13. Dr. Hubbard's statement appeared in *Report of the Freedmen's Aid Society for 1888* (Cincinnati: the Society, 1893), p. 45.

14. *Second Report of the Board of Health,* p. 80.

15. Nashville *Colored Tennessean,* March 31, 1866; Miss H. E. Peek, Keeper of the Archives, Cambridge University, to James M. Smith, letter, March 21, 1977; *Nashville Banner,* April 11, 1903.

16. Bureau of the Census, *United States Census Reports,* 1880 (Washington, D.C.: U.S. Government Printing Office, 1883), Mortality and Vital Statistics, vol. 1, table 1, p. 3; table 2, p. 7; table 4, pp. 26–27.

17. Ibid., vol. 1, table 10, p. xxix.

18. Address by the Reverend John Braden at the dedication of the Meharry Medical Department buildings, October 13, 1880. A summary of Braden's remarks is given in the minutes of the Board of Trustees of Central Tennessee College, available at the Methodist Board of Higher Education and Ministry, Nashville.

19. G. W. Hubbard, "Half a Century Among the Freedmen" (undated manuscript, c. 1910); G. W. Hubbard to the Reverend James R. Joy, May 31, 1909. Both these documents are available at the archives, Meharry Medical College Library, Nashville.

20. *Bulletin of Meharry Medical College,* 80th Anniversary Issue 52, no. 2 (April 1956): 11.

21. Hubbard, "Half a Century."

22. *Bulletin of Meharry Medical College* 52, no. 2 (April 1956): 13.

23. Ibid.

24. Frances Meharry, *History of the Meharry Family in America* (Lafayette, Ind.: Lafayette Printing Co., 1925), p. 369.

25. Minutes of the Board of Trustees of Central Tennessee College, 1879, available at the Methodist Board of Higher Education and Ministry, Nashville.

26. *Chicago Tribune,* January 14, 1948.

27. Minutes of the Board of Trustees of Central Tennessee College, 1874, 1875, 1876, 1888, and 1889; James P. Brawley, *Two Centuries of Methodist Concern: Bondage, Freedom, and Education of Black People* (New York: Vantage Press, 1974), pp. 384–85.

28. Minutes of the Board of Trustees of Central Tennessee College, 1877.

29. L. A. Falk and N. A. Quaynor-Malm, "Early Afro-American Medical Education in the United States: The Origins of Meharry Medical College in the Nineteenth Century," *Proceedings of the XXIII Congress of the History of Medicine* (1972), p. 350.

30. Charles Victor Roman, *Meharry Medical College, A History* (Nashville: Sunday School Publishing Board of the National Baptist Convention, 1934), p. 203.

31. Obituary of Dr. Sneed, *Nashville American,* March 18, 1907; Sneed Family Papers, 1796–1856 at the Tennessee State Library and Archives, Nashville. Various authors have erroneously spelled Sneed's name as "Snead."

32. *Catalog of the Meharry Medical Department, Central Tennessee College,* 1887, p. 5; *Catalogue of the Meharry Medical, Dental, and Pharmaceutical Departments, Central Tennessee College,* 1899–1900, p. 4; *Catalogue of the Meharry Medical, Dental, and Pharmaceutical Colleges, Walden University,* 1900–1901, p. 4. A photograph of "Dr. J. Frank McKinley, Graduate of the Medical Department of the University of

Michigan; noted physician" appears in Booker T. Washington, N. B. Wood, and Fannie Barrier Williams, *A New Negro for a New Century* (Chicago: American Publishing House, 1900), p. 167. It has not been verified that Dr. J. F. McKinley of Meharry and Dr. J. Frank McKinley are the same man.

33. *Nashville Tennessean,* December 11, 1910.

34. Clayton, *Davidson County,* p. 267; *Nashville Banner,* January 9, 1899.

35. F. L. Roberts, *Yearbook of the Sixty-second Session of the West Wisconsin Conference of the Methodist Episcopal Church* (Eau Claire: West Wisconsin Conference, 1916), p. 77.

Chapter 3

1. From an address by George W. Hubbard on October 19, 1916, reprinted in *Meharry Annual and Military Review* (Nashville: the College, 1919), p. 12. This yearbook is available at the archives, Meharry Medical College Library.

2. Nashville *Daily American,* February 24, 27, 1880.

3. Kansas State Board of Health, *Third Annual Report* (1887), "Register of Physicians and Accoucheurs," p. 252; *Topeka Capital,* December 31, 1921.

4. *Proceedings of the Commencement of 1878,* available at the archives, Meharry Medical College Library; Nashville *Daily American,* February 23, 1878.

5. *Catalogue of the Meharry Medical Department of Central Tennessee College,* 1887, p. 5. This and other early catalogs subsequently cited are available at the archives, Meharry Medical College Library.

6. Ibid.

7. *Catalog of the Meharry Medical Department of Central Tennessee College,* 1887, p. 5; *Catalogue of the Meharry Medical, Dental, and Pharmaceutical Departments,* 1892–93, p. 2.

8. Nashville *Daily American,* May 15, 1879.

9. *Sixth Annual Announcement of the Meharry Medical Department of Central Tennessee College,* 1881, p. 3.

10. Ibid., p. 4.

11. Sources on the life of Dr. Hadley include *The Nashville Globe,* October 13, 1911, and "Dr. C. O. Hadley," *Bulletin of Meharry Medical College,* Alumni Edition 45, no. 7 (April 1949): 18.

12. *Sixth Annual Announcement,* p. 4.

13. *Catalogue of the Meharry Medical Department of Central Tennessee College,* 1887, p. 2.

14. Charles Victor Roman, *Meharry Medical College, A History* (Nashville: Sunday School Publishing Board of the National Baptist Convention, 1934), p. 90.

15. Sources on the life of Dr. Elliott include *The Nashville Globe,* June 14, 1907, and Harold D. West, "The History of Meharry Medical College" (unpublished manuscript), p. 51. A copy of the West manuscript is available at the archives, Nashville Academy of Medicine.

16. *Catalogue of the Meharry Medical, Dental, and Pharmaceutical Departments,* 1899–1900, pp. 9–11.

17. J. Edward Perry, *Forty Cords of Wood; Memoirs of a Medical Doctor* (Jefferson City, Mo.: Lincoln University, 1947), p. 125.

18. West, "Meharry Medical College," pp. 50–51; *Bulletin of Meharry Medical College,* 80th Anniversary Issue 52, no. 2 (April 1956): 17.

19. *Catalogue of the Meharry Medical, Dental, and Pharmaceutical Departments,* 1899–1900, pp. 7–9.

20. Roman, *Meharry Medical College,* p. 45.

21. *Nashville American,* February 3, 1897.

22. Minutes of the Board of Trustees, Central Tennessee College, 1884, available at the Methodist Board of Higher Education and Ministry, Nashville; *First Annual Announcement of the School of Dentistry, Meharry Medical Department of Central Tennessee College,* 1886–87, p. 2, available at the archives, Meharry Medical College Library; Nashville *Daily American,* October 9, 1886. The subsequent discussion also relies upon an unpublished paper by J. B. Singleton, Jr., "The Meharry Medical College School of Dentistry with Divisions of Dental Hygiene and Dental Technology," mimeographed (Nashville: the School of Dentistry, 1971).

23. D. R. Stubblefield, *In Memoriam, Dr. William Henry Morgan* (Nashville: n.p., 1901?), 30 pages, passim.

24. Minutes of the Board of Trustees of Central Tennessee College, 1884.

25. D. H. Turpin, "The Dental Department" in Roman, *Meharry Medical College,* pp. 158–60; *The Nashville Globe,* March 22, 1907.

26. Grace Harrison, "Hubbard Hospital and Meharry Medical College for Negroes, Nashville, Tennessee" (M.A. thesis, University of Chicago, 1945), pp. 19–21; W. C. Baines, "The Pharmaceutical Department" in Roman, *Meharry Medical College,* p. 160; Nashville *Daily American,* February 23, 1890; John J. Mullowney, "What Future for the Negro Pharmacist?" *Journal of the National Medical Association* 24, no. 3 (November 1932): 27–29.

27. *Proceedings of the Commencement of 1878;* Nashville *Daily American,* May 1, 1884.

28. L. A. Falk and N. A. Quaynor-Malm, "Early Afro-American Medical Education in the United States: The Origins of Meharry Medical College in the Nineteenth Century," *Proceedings of the XXIII Congress of the History of Medicine* (1972), p. 352. Montague Cobb, in his paper on black women physicians, "Our Lady Asclepiads," *Journal of the National Medical Association* 60, no. 2 (March 1968): 136, lists Osceola Queen, Class of 1891, as the first female graduate. The class picture, however, shows that Dr. Queen was a man.

29. *Nashville Banner,* February 8, 1893; March 9, 1893; George W. Hubbard, "Dr. Georgia E. L. Patton Washington," *The Christian Educator* 12, no. 2 (December–January 1900–1901): 5–6.

30. Roman, *Meharry Medical College,* pp. 64, 74, 106–07; *The Nashville Globe,* September 17, 1909; *The Meharry News* 7, no. 2 (April, May, June 1921): 12.

31. *Nashville American,* February 3, 1897.

32. Perry, *Forty Cords of Wood,* p. 126, 129–31.

33. Roman, *Meharry Medical College,* p. 86. Sources on the life of Dr. Perry include W. Montague Cobb, "John Edward Perry, M.D., 1870– ," *Journal of the National Medical Association* 48, no. 4 (July 1956): 292–96.

34. Roman, *Meharry Medical College*, 224 pages, passim. Other sources on the life of Dr. Roman are "Dr. Charles Victor Roman," *Journal of the National Medical Association* 26, no. 4 (November 15, 1934): 172–73; W. Montague Cobb, "Charles Victor Roman," *Journal of the National Medical Association* 45, no. 4 (July 1953): 301–04; J. L. Nichols and W. H. Crogman, *Progress of a Race or, The Remarkable Advancement of the American Negro*, rev. ed. (Naperville, Ill.: J. L. Nichols, 1920), pp. 426–27; and John A. Kenney, *The Negro in Medicine* (Tuskegee, Ala.: Tuskegee Institute Press, 1912), p. 13.

35. *The Christian Record* (Nashville), September 2, 1848.

36. Nashville *Daily American,* December 17, 18, 1882; Falk and Quaynor-Malm, "Early Afro-American Medical Education," p. 351.

37. Nashville *Republican Banner,* August 15, 1875.

38. *Catalogue of the Meharry Medical Department of Central Tennessee College*, 1887, p. 6; Nashville *Daily American,* December 6, 1882.

39. "Our Graduates," *The Christian Educator* 1, no. 4 (July 1890): 163; James T. Haley, comp., *Afro-American Encyclopedia or, the Thoughts, Doings, and Sayings of the Race* (Nashville: Haley and Florida, 1896), pp. 59–62, 226; G. F. Richings, *Evidences of Progress Among Colored People* (Philadelphia: G. S. Ferguson Co., 1903), pp. 266–67; J. W. Gibson and W. H. Crogman, *Progress of a Race or, The Remarkable Advancement of the American Negro*, rev. ed. (Naperville, Ill.: J. L. Nichols, 1902), p. 588; Howard N. Rabinowitz, *Race Relations in the Urban South, 1865–1890* (New York: Oxford University Press, 1978), pp. 92–93.

40. D. W. Culp, ed., *Twentieth Century Negro Literature* (Naperville, Ill.: J. L. Nichols, 1902), pp. 215–20; *The Nashville Globe,* June 17, 1910.

41. *Catalog of the Meharry Medical, Dental, and Pharmaceutical Departments*, Central Tennessee College, 1886–87, p. 5.

42. Minutes of the Board of Trustees of Central Tennessee College, 1883.

43. Nashville *Daily American,* August 1, 1884.

44. *Catalog of the Meharry Medical, Dental, and Pharmaceutical Departments*, Central Tennessee College, 1893–94, p. 6.

45. Perry, *Forty Cords of Wood*, p. 123.

46. William Waller, ed., *Nashville in the 1890s* (Nashville: Vanderbilt University Press, 1970), p. 85; Nashville *Daily American,* September 28, 1893; October 13, 1893; *Nashville Banner,* September 26, 1893.

47. Roman, *Meharry Medical College*, p. 30.

48. Minutes of the Board of Trustees of Central Tennessee College, 1884; Roman, *Meharry Medical College*, p. 39; Nashville *Daily American,* September 14, 1884.

49. Roman, *Meharry Medical College*, pp. 119–20; Cyril A. Crichlow, "The Last of His Generation," *The Brown Book*, pp. 13–18. This latter fragment, about which further bibliographic information is unavailable, may be seen in the George W. Hubbard file at the United Methodist Publishing House, Nashville. See also T. Manuel Smith, "The Pioneering Influence of Dr. George W. Hubbard on Medical Education," *Journal of the National Medical Association* 45, no. 6 (November 1953): 427–29.

Chapter 4

1. James P. Brawley, *Two Centuries of Methodist Concern: Bondage, Freedom, and the Education of Black People* (New York: Vantage Press, 1974), p. 505. Sources on the life of John M. Walden include Charles Victor Roman, *Meharry Medical College, A History* (Nashville: Sunday School Publishing Board of the National Baptist Convention, 1934), pp. 211–17 and Nashville *Daily American,* May 31, 1884.

2. Lucius Salisbury Merriam, *Higher Education in Tennessee* (Washington, D.C.: Government Printing Office, 1893), pp. 271–72; Brawley, *Two Centuries of Methodist Concern,* p. 385.

3. *The Nashville Globe,* March 20, 1908. Some contemporary observers posited a connection between an increase in numbers of black doctors and an improvement in health conditions among black people. For example, the *Globe* for April 5, 1907, reported that the previous decade had witnessed a 600 percent increase in black physicians practicing at Memphis and a proportionate decrease in the weekly mortality rate among black people there.

4. Harold D. West, "The History of Meharry Medical College" (unpublished manuscript), pp. 48–49. A copy of the West manuscript is available at the archives, Nashville Academy of Medicine.

5. Ibid., p. 52; *The Nashville Globe,* February 17, 1908; "Arthur Melvin Townsend, M.D., 1875–1959," *Journal of the National Medical Association* 51, no. 4 (July 1959): 323–24; *The Nashville Globe,* April 24, 1959.

6. Roman, *Meharry Medical College,* p. 92. In 1927 Stewart became one of the first alumni trustees of Fisk University.

7. Herbert M. Morais, *The History of the Negro in Medicine* (New York: Publishers Co., 1967), pp. 66–67.

8. Sources on the life of Dr. Lynk include Myles V. Lynk, *Sixty Years of Medicine; An Autobiography* (Memphis, Tenn.: Twentieth Century Press, 1951), 125 pages; "M. V. Lynk, M.S., M.D., LL.B.," *Journal of the National Medical Association* 33, no. 1 (January 1941): 46–47; and G. James Fleming and Christian E. Burckel, eds., *Who's Who in Colored America* (Yonkers-on-Hudson, N.Y.: Christian E. Burckel and Associates, 1950), p. 348.

9. Morais, *The Negro in Medicine,* pp. 66–70.

10. Roman, *Meharry Medical College,* p. 185.

11. *Nashville American,* August 19, 1903; *Nashville Banner,* August 20, 1903.

12. J. Edward Perry, *Forty Cords of Wood; Memoirs of a Medical Doctor* (Jefferson City, Mo.: Lincoln University, 1947), pp. 390–94; *Nashville Banner,* August 26, 28, 1913.

13. Roman, *Meharry Medical College,* p. 102.

14. Ibid., pp. 61–63.

15. Perry, *Forty Cords of Wood,* p. 123.

16. Roman, *Meharry Medical College,* p. 52. The subsequent discussion of the work of Dr. Daniel Hale Williams at Nashville is indebted to Helen Buckler, *Daniel Hale Williams, Negro Surgeon* (New York: Pitman Co., 1968), pp. 194–201.

17. Williams reported the case in "Stab Wound of the Heart and Pericardium—Suture of the Pericardium—Recovery—Patient Alive Three Years Afterward," *Medical Record* 51, no. 13 (March 27, 1897): 437–39.

18. Roman, *Meharry Medical College,* p. 52.

19. Ibid., pp. 72–73; *Catalogue of Meharry Medical, Dental, and Pharmaceutical Colleges,* 1900–01, p. 11; *The Nashville Globe,* September 4, 1908.

20. See, for example, *The Nashville Globe,* November 15, 1907 and February 14, 1916.

21. *Journal of the National Medical Association* 53, no. 8 (1966): 227; *Nashville Tennessean,* January 7, 1965; William A. Reed, Jr., to James Summerville, interview, January 6, 1977, Nashville.

22. Sources on the life of Dr. McMillan include *The Nashville Globe,* June 19, 1908; Axel C. Hansen, "George W. Hubbard Hospital, 1910–1961," *Journal of the National Medical Association* 54 (1962): 5; and "Julius Augustus McMillan, M.D., 1871–1949," *Journal of the National Medical Association* 48, no. 5 (September 1956): 374.

23. This discussion of the origins of Hubbard Hospital relies upon Roman, *Meharry Medical College,* pp. 71–77 and passim.

24. *The Nashville Globe,* August 27, 1909.

25. Cyril A. Crichlow, "The Last of His Generation," *The Brown Book,* p. 16. This fragment, about which further bibliographic information is unavailable, may be seen in the George W. Hubbard file at the United Methodist Publishing House, Nashville.

26. *The Nashville Globe,* December 16, 1910; *Nashville Banner,* December 17, 1908; January 21, December 31, 1909; March 14, August 15, December 15, 1910; November 29, 1912; *Nashville Tennessean,* July 18, 1937; Grace Harrison, "Hubbard Hospital and Meharry Medical College for Negroes, Nashville, Tennessee" (M.A. thesis, University of Chicago, 1945), pp. 23–25.

27. Hulda M. Lyttle, "The Nurse Training Department," in Roman, *Meharry Medical College,* pp. 160–63; Harrison, "Hubbard Hospital and Meharry Medical College," pp. 25–26. A list of contemporaneous nurse training departments at black hospitals is given in Monroe N. Work, ed., *Negro Year Book, 1918–1919* (Tuskegee, Ala.: Tuskegee Institute, 1919), pp. 424–26.

28. Morais, *The Negro in Medicine,* p. 89.

29. Abraham Flexner, *Medical Education in the United States and Canada, A Report to the Carnegie Foundation for the Advancement of Teaching* (New York: Carnegie Foundation, 1910), 346 pages, passim; Carlton B. Chapman, "The Flexner Report," *Daedalus* 103, no. 1 (Winter 1974): 105–17.

30. Brawley, *Two Centuries of Methodist Concern,* pp. 389–90; Harrison, "Hubbard Hospital and Meharry Medical College," pp. 32–33.

31. Minutes of the Tennessee Annual Conference of the Methodist Episcopal Church, Northern Branch, 1905–1925, pp. 248–49. These manuscript minutes are available in the Manuscripts Section, Tennessee State Library and Archives, Nashville.

32. Roman, *Meharry Medical College,* p. 32; Brawley, *Two Centuries of Methodist Concern,* p. 506.

33. Brawley, *Two Centuries of Methodist Concern,* p. 388.

34. Ibid., pp. 506–07; "Annual Report of the Board of Education for Negroes of the Methodist Episcopal Church for the Year July 1, 1920 to July 1, 1921," *The Christian Educator* [no volume or issue number assigned], (November 1921), pp. 4–5.

35. The life of Dr. Anderson is treated in W. Montague Cobb, "John Wesley Anderson, M.D., 1861–1947," *Journal of the National Medical Association* 45, no. 6 (November 1953): 442–44.

36. Roman, *Meharry Medical College,* pp. 101–08; Brawley, *Two Centuries of Methodist Concern,* p. 389; "Dr. George W. Hubbard Retires," *Journal of the National Medical Association* 13, no. 1 (January–March 1921): 30–31.

Chapter 5

1. John J. Mullowney, *America Gives a Chance* (Tampa, Fla.: Tribune Press, 1940), pp. 90–102, 117.

2. Charles Victor Roman, *Meharry Medical College, A History* (Nashville: Sunday School Publishing Board of the National Baptist Convention, 1934), pp. 125–28, 132–33.

3. *Meharry News* 7, no. 1: 3, quoted in Roman, *Meharry Medical College,* pp. 150–52.

4. Roman, *Meharry Medical College,* p. 133.

5. Ibid., pp. 128–32; "Report . . . Council on Medical Education and Hospitals of the American Medical Association," mimeographed, (Chicago?: American Medical Association, 1931), unpaginated. A copy of this document is available at the archives, Nashville Academy of Medicine.

6. Mullowney, *America,* pp. 116–19.

7. Ibid.; Grace Harrison, "Hubbard Hospital and Meharry Medical College for Negroes, Nashville, Tennessee" (M.A. thesis, University of Chicago, 1945), p. 39; Paul H. Dietrich, "George W. Hubbard Hospital Report for Seven Months Ending April 30, 1922," mimeographed (Nashville: Meharry Medical College, 1922), unpaginated.

8. Minutes of the Faculty, Meharry Medical College, vol. 1 (March 1, 1921–April 12, 1938), various pagings, January 9, 1923. These minutes are available at the archives, Meharry Medical College Library.

9. Harrison, "Hubbard Hospital and Meharry Medical College," pp. 45–48.

10. Roman, *Meharry Medical College,* pp. 128–32; Mullowney, *America,* pp. 119–21; Harold D. West, "The History of Meharry Medical College" (unpublished manuscript), p. 59. A copy of the West manuscript is available at the archives, Nashville Academy of Medicine.

11. Minutes of the Board of Trustees of Meharry Medical College, February 1928, quoted in Mullowney, *America,* pp. 121–22; Harrison, "Meharry Medical College," pp. 49–51.

12. John J. Mullowney, "The New Meharry Medical College Plant, Nashville, Tenn.," *Journal of the National Medical Association* 22, no. 3 (July–September 1930): 146–47.

13. Benjamin Walter, "Ethnicity and Residential Succession: Nashville, 1850–1920," in James F. Blumstein and Benjamin Walter, eds., *Growing Metropolis: Aspects of Development in Nashville* (Nashville: Vanderbilt University Press, 1975), pp. 3–31.

14. *Meharry News,* Catalogue Edition 28, no. 1 (July 1931): 10–15; Axel C. Hansen, "George W. Hubbard Hospital, 1910–1961," *Journal of the National Medi-*

cal Association 54, no. 1 (January 1962): 4–7; Minutes of the Faculty, vol. 1, passim.

15. Herbert M. Morais, *The History of the Negro in Medicine* (New York: Publishers Co., 1967), p. 93; Roman, *Meharry Medical College,* p. 134.

16. These details concerning Dr. Quinland's career rely upon John Edward Perry, *Forty Cords of Wood; Memoirs of a Medical Doctor* (Jefferson City, Mo.: Lincoln University, 1947), p. 409; *Meharry-Hubbard Newsletter* 3, no. 8 (April 15, 1953): 3; Morais, *The Negro in Medicine,* p. 92; Meharry Medical College, *The Centennial Lecture Series, January–December, 1976,* p. 24. Facts about Dr. Bent's life are given in *Bulletin of Meharry Medical College,* 80th Anniversary Issue 52, no. 2 (April 1956): 17; Mullowney, *America,* pp. 149–50.

17. Elbridge Sibley, *Differential Mortality in Tennessee, 1917–1928* (Nashville: Fisk University Press, 1930), 152 pages, passim; Dept. of Social Science, Fisk University, *A Social Study of Negro Families in the Area Selected for the Nashville Negro Federal Housing Project with a Supplementary Study of the Social and Economic Status of the Negro in Nashville* (Nashville: Fisk University, 1934), 109 pages, passim; Stewart Sandy Clark, "A Study of Negro Education in Davidson County, Tennessee" (M.A. thesis, George Peabody College for Teachers, 1919), p. 84.

18. Bureau of Educational Research, Howard University, "The Health Status and Health Education of Negroes in the United States," *Journal of Negro Education* 6, no. 3 (July 1937): 263–349.

19. Michael J. Bent and Ellen F. Greene, *Rural Negro Health: A Report on a Five-Year Experiment in Health Education in Tennessee* (Nashville: Julius Rosenwald Fund, 1937), 85 pages, passim; *Bulletin of Meharry Medical College* 35, no. 2 (October 1938): 31.

Other scholars and public health workers were independently reaching conclusions similar to Bent and Greene's. See, for example, Winfred B. Nathan, "Health Education in Negro Public Schools," *Journal of Negro Education* 6, no. 3 (July 1937): 523–30.

20. James E. McCulloch, ed., *The New Chivalry–Health: Proceedings of the Southern Sociological Congress, Houston, Texas, May 8–11, 1915* (Nashville: Southern Sociological Congress, 1915), p. 396.

21. *The Meharrian* (yearbook), 1945, unpaginated; *Bulletin of Meharry Medical College* 35, no. 2 (October 1938): 27; Mullowney, *America,* pp. 155–58; Minutes of the Faculty, vol. 1, February 1928; *Nashville Banner,* June 6, 1952; William A. Beck, "The Early Diagnosis and Treatment of Pulmonary Tuberculosis," *Journal of the National Medical Association* 45, no. 4 (September 1948): 212–14.

22. Elizabeth C. Tandy, "Infant and Maternal Mortality Among Negroes," *Journal of Negro Education* 6, no. 3 (July 1937): 322–49.

23. E. Perry Crump, "Retrospect: Pediatrics," *The Meharrian,* 1951, unpaginated; Mullowney, *America,* pp. 158–60.

24. Mullowney, *America,* pp. 154–55.

25. E. Y. Williams, "The Incidence of Mental Disease in the Negro," *Journal of Negro Education* 6, no. 3 (July 1937): 391–92; *The Meharrian,* 1946, unpaginated; *Bulletin of Meharry Medical College,* catalog edition for the School of Medicine 50, no. 4 (December 1954): 26, 54; *The Tennessean* (Nashville), July 15, 1976.

26. Thomas A. LaSaine and J. Grace Harrison, "Medical Social Seminars," *Bulletin of Meharry Medical College* 35, nos. 3 and 4 (combined issue for January and April 1939): 21–22; Thomas A. LaSaine, "Teaching the Social Component of Medical Care at Meharry Medical College," *Journal of the National Medical Association* 32, no. 6 (November 1940): 248–51.

27. Harrison, "Hubbard Hospital and Meharry Medical College," p. 38; *The Nashville Globe,* December 9, 1910.

28. Marshall, Texas *News Messenger,* June 27, 1976; Charles Whited, "Faith, Hope, and Cerebral Sweat," *Nashville Tennessean Magazine,* July 23, 1961.

29. James W. Martin, "A Study of the Negro Physician with Particular Reference to Certain Tennessee Counties" (M.A. thesis, George Peabody College for Teachers, 1921), 74 pages, passim.

30. Lester C. Lamon, *Black Tennesseans, 1900–1930* (Knoxville: University of Tennessee Press, 1977), pp. 14–15, 209–13.

31. Walter E. Hogan, "Changing Conceptions of the Aim of Negro Education as Seen in the History of Colored Schools in Nashville, Tennessee" (M.A. thesis, George Peabody College for Teachers, 1917), pp. 93–94.

32. Lamon, *Black Tennesseans,* pp. 288–92.

33. Mullowney, *America,* p. 164.

34. Minutes of the Faculty, vol. 1, passim.

35. Harrison, "Hubbard Hospital and Meharry Medical College," pp. 65, 67–68; West, "Meharry Medical College," pp. 93–94; "Report of the President of Meharry Medical College, 1938–39," *Bulletin of Meharry Medical College* 36, no. 2 (October 1939): 4–5.

36. Harrison, "Hubbard Hospital and Meharry Medical College," pp. 65, 67–68; West, "Meharry Medical College," pp. 93–94; "Annual Report of Meharry Medical College for the Year 1936–37 by John J. Mullowney, President," *Bulletin of Meharry Medical College* 34, no. 2 (October 1937): 5; Minutes of the Faculty, vol. 1, October 13, 1936.

37. Harrison, "Hubbard Hospital and Meharry Medical College," pp. 66–67; "Annual Report of Meharry Medical College for the Year 1936–37 by John J. Mullowney, President," *Bulletin of Meharry Medical College* 34, no. 2 (October 1937): 5; Edward L. Turner, "Selecting Medical Students and Elimination of Misfits," *Journal of the National Medical Association* 36, no. 1 (January 1944): 15–19.

38. *The Nashville Globe,* March 31, 1944; John A. Kenney, "In Memoriam, Dr. John Henry Hale," *Journal of the National Medical Association* 36, no. 4 (July 1944): 130–31.

39. "Annual Report of the President, Meharry Medical College, Nashville, Tennessee, July 1, 1939–June 30, 1940," *Bulletin of Meharry Medical College* 37, no. 2 (October 1940): 3.

40. Ibid.; *Bulletin of Meharry Medical College,* Alumni Edition 41: no. 1C (December 1941): 2; Guerney D. Holloway, "School of Clinical Laboratory Technology," *The Meharrian* (1949), unpaginated.

41. *Bulletin of Meharry Medical College* 36, no. 2 (October 1939), pp. 6, 11; "Annual Report of the President, Meharry Medical College, Nashville, Tennessee, July 1, 1939–June 30, 1940," pp. 3–4.

42. Michael J. Bent, "Research in the School of Medicine," *Bulletin of Meharry Medical College* 36, no. 2 (October 1939): 9–10; "Annual Report of the President, Meharry Medical College, Nashville, Tennessee, July 1, 1939–June 30, 1940," pp. 5–6; *Bulletin of Meharry Medical College,* Alumni Edition 43, no. 5 (February 1947): 4; Committee on Research, *Horizon in Research, Progress Report, The Development of Negro Talent* (Nashville: Meharry Medical College, 1948), unpaginated; Morais, *The Negro in Medicine,* pp. 102–10.

43. "Annual Report, July 1, 1939–June 30, 1940," pp. 1–2; Emma L. White, "Report of the Proposed Grading System at Meharry Medical College, 1939–1940," *Journal of the National Medical Association* 33, no. 1 (January 1941): 42–45.

44. *Meharry News,* catalogue edition 33, no. 1 (July 1936): 41–46.

45. Bent, "Medical Education," p. 8.

46. *Meharry News* 33, no. 2 (October 1936): 6.

47. Data on licensing board failure rates are available in *Journal of the American Medical Association* 134, no. 3 (May 17, 1947): 256–59. These data are assembled in Helen Edith Walker, *The Negro in the Medical Profession* (Charlottesville: University of Virginia, 1949), pp. 36–37. In the spring of 1948, the faculty bulletin from Meharry reported: "For the last two years not a single medical or dental graduate failed a state or national board examination." *Bulletin of Meharry Medical College,* Faculty Edition 44, no. 6 (April 1948): 4.

A detailed description of Meharry admissions policies in the post-Depression period is found in "Meharry Aims for Quality Product," *Bulletin of Meharry Medical College,* Alumni Edition 45, no. 7 (April 1949): 4. For enrollment statistics of the time, see Charles S. Johnson, *Into the Main Stream, A Survey of the Best Practices in Race Relations in the South* (Chapel Hill: University of North Carolina, 1947), p. 244.

48. Paul B. Cornely, "The Economics of Medical Practice and the Negro Physician," *Journal of the National Medical Association* 43, no. 2 (March 1951): 84–92.

49. Gunnar S. Myrdal, *An American Dilemma,* 2 vols. (New York: Harper and Brothers, 1944), 1: 322–25.

50. Dietrich, "George W. Hubbard Hospital Report"; Hulda M. Lyttle, "The School of Nursing, 1921–1938," *Bulletin of Meharry Medical College* 34, no. 3 (January 1938): 21; Hulda M. Lyttle, "A School for Negro Nurses," *American Journal of Nursing* 39, no. 2 (February 1939): 133–38.

51. *The Meharrian,* 1951, unpaginated.

52. *Meharry News,* catalogue edition 33, no. 1 (July 1936): 107–09; Johnson, *Into the Main Stream,* pp. 255–56; *Nashville Tennessean,* October 24, 1947; *Meharry Medical College Faculty Bulletin* 46, no. 2 (April 1950): 14; Mary Lee Brown, "Retrospect: Public Health Nursing," *The Meharrian,* 1951, unpaginated; *Bulletin of Meharry Medical College* 58, no. 8 (August 1962): 2. For an account of the daily work of public health nurses in Nashville, see *Nashville Tennessean,* July 15, 1945.

53. James R. Patterson, comp., *Souvenir History, 1924 Dental Class, Meharry Medical College, 20th Anniversary Reunion at Meharry, Friday, March 17, 1944* (Nashville: the College, 1944), pp. 16–17.

54. John J. Mullowney, "First Formal Instruction in Dentistry in America,"

Journal of the National Medical Association 28, no. 4 (November 1936): 165–68; John J. Mullowney, "The Future of the Negro in Dentistry and What Can Be Done About It," *Journal of the National Medical Association* 30, no. 1 (February 1938): 23–26.

55. Clifton O. Dummett, "A Chronology of Significant Events in the Progress of the Negro in American Dentistry," *Bulletin of the National Dental Association* 16, no. 2 (January 1958): 48–49; Donley H. Turpin, "Report of the School of Dentistry," *Bulletin of Meharry Medical College* 36, no. 2 (October 1939): 11–12; M. Don Clawson, "Changing Patterns in Dental Education at Meharry," *TIC Magazine* [no volume or issue number assigned] (March 1948), 2–7.

56. Donley H. Turpin, "The Progress of the Dental Department," *Bulletin of Meharry Medical College* 35, nos. 3 and 4 (January and April 1939): 15; *Bulletin of Meharry Medical College,* Alumni Edition 48, no. 2 (April 1952): 5; J. B. Singleton, "The Meharry Medical College School of Dentistry," mimeographed (Nashville: Meharry Medical College, 1971), pp. 10–12; "Dentistry at Meharry," *The Meharri-dent* 3, no. 1 (June 1945): 5–6; Edward L. Turner, "The Meharry Medical College School of Dentistry," *TIC Magazine* [no volume or issue number assigned] (September 1950), p. 3; Clarence Utley, "The History of Dental Technology," *The Meharri-dent* 7, no. 1 (January 1950): 5; William H. Allen to James Summerville, interview, April 1, 1977, Nashville, Tennessee; Eugenia L. Mobley, "The Present Status of the Dental Hygienist," *The Meharri-dent* 9, no. 1 (January 1952): 7.

57. Dummett, "Progress of the Negro in American Dentistry," pp. 48–49; Singleton, "Meharry Medical College School of Dentistry," pp. 3–4; Turner, "Meharry Medical College School of Dentistry," pp. 1–3; R. F. Sanford, "A Tribute to Our Late Donley H. Turpin, Dean Emeritus of the School of Dentistry, Meharry Medical College," *The Meharri-dent* 5, no. 3 (June 1948): 2–3; "Dentistry at Meharry," *The Meharri-dent* 2, no. 1 (March 1943): 4; Clifton O. Dummett, "Dentistry at Meharry, Present Day and Future Trends in Dental Education," *The Meharri-dent* 2, no. 3 (September 1943): 4; Clyde Richard Broadus, "Dental Health as a Community Health Problem," *The Meharri-dent* 5, no. 1 (January 1948): 5; James L. Scales, "Dental Public Health Program at Meharry Medical College," *The Meharri-dent* 4, no. 3 (June 1946): 5; Theodore E. Bolden, "A Study of the Oral Health Status of a Selected Number of Students at Meigs, Ford Green, and Pearl Elementary Schools," *The Meharri-dent* 4, no. 6 (June 1947): 4–5; *Nashville Tennessean,* October 17, 1947; *The Nashville Globe,* April 2, 1948; William H. Allen to James Summerville, interview, April 1, 1977, Nashville.

58. "C. O. Dummett Named Dean of Meharry School of Dentistry," *National Negro Health News* 15, no. 4 (October–December 1947): 18.

59. For brief treatments of the life and career of Dr. Allen, see "Faculty Biography," *The Meharri-dent* 6, no. 2 (March 1949): 29–30; 7, no. 1 (January 1950): 3; *Nashville Banner,* June 13, 1969.

60. Morais, *The Negro in Medicine,* pp. 94–95.

61. Minutes of the Faculty, vol. 1, April 13, 1937.

62. Lyttle, "The School of Nursing," pp. 21–22; "Meharry Medical College to Offer Graduate Course," *Bulletin of Meharry Medical College* 34, no. 3 (January

1938): 16–18; W. S. Quinland, "Postgraduate Course in Medicine," *Bulletin of Meharry Medical College* 35, nos. 3 and 4 (January and April 1939): 15–17. See also Paul B. Cornely, "Post Graduate Medical Education and the Negro Physician," *Journal of the National Medical Association* 30, no. 1 (February 1938): 18–22, wherein the author recommends the establishment of short refresher courses at Meharry and Howard.

63. Minutes of the Faculty, vol. 1, passim; *Bulletin of Meharry Medical College,* Alumni Edition 39, no. 4 (April 1943): 9; Harrison, "Hubbard Hospital and Meharry Medical College," pp. 77–78; "Meharry Medical Society," *The Meharrian,* 1943, unpaginated; "Annual Report of the President, Meharry Medical College, Nashville, Tennessee, July 1, 1939–June 30, 1940," p. 2; Harold D. West, "Retrospect: Biochemistry," *The Meharrian,* 1951, unpaginated.

64. Matthew Walker, "Mound Bayou—Meharry's Neighbor," *Journal of the National Medical Association* 65, no. 4 (July 1973): 309–11; Hodding Carter, "He's Doing Something About the Race Problem," *Saturday Evening Post,* 218, no. 34 (February 23, 1946): 31–32; Vernon Lane Wharton, *The Negro in Mississippi, 1865–1890* (Chapel Hill: University of North Carolina Press, 1947), p. 42; J. F. Huddleston as told to Gail Falk, "The Story of Mound Bayou: Negro Pioneers Turned Forests into Farms," *The Southern Courier,* January 7–8, 1967; Kelly Miller Smith to James Summerville, interview, August 21, 1979, Nashville.

65. *Bulletin of Meharry Medical College,* Alumni Edition 48, no. 2 (April 1952): 2–3; "The President Elect," *Journal of the National Medical Association* 45, no. 6 (November 1953): 446.

66. Walker, "Mound Bayou," pp. 309–11.

67. *Bulletin of Meharry Medical College,* Alumni Edition 44, no. 6 (April 1948): 2; Meharry Medical College, *Meharry Medical College, 1876–1941* (Nashville: the College, 1941), unpaginated; "Annual Report of the President, Meharry Medical College, Nashville, Tennessee, July 1, 1938–June 30, 1940," p. 6.

68. "Annual Report of the President, Meharry Medical College, Nashville, Tennessee, July 1, 1939–June 30, 1940," pp. 6–7; "Meharry Medical College Endowment Program, 1940–41," pp. 7–9; *Nashville Tennessean,* April 15, 1944; General Education Board, *Annual Report, 1944* (New York: The Board, 1944), p. 41; "Meharry Gets $4,000,000 Gift for Endowment Fund," *Journal of the National Medical Association* 36, no. 3 (May 1944): 107.

69. General Education Board, *Annual Report, 1944,* p. 41.

70. "Cooperation with Fisk University," *Bulletin of Meharry Medical College* 36, no. 2 (October 1939): 17–18; Harrison, "Hubbard Hospital and Meharry Medical College," pp. 87–88; West, "Meharry Medical College," pp. 112–14.

71. Redding S. Sugg, Jr., and George Hilton Jones, *The Southern Regional Education Board; Ten Years of Regional Cooperation in Higher Education* (Baton Rouge: Louisiana State University Press, 1960), pp. 1–7. In terms of facilities alone, black students had even less chance than whites for advanced studies. See Edward N. Saveth, "Jim Crow and the Regional Plan," *The Survey* 85, no. 9 (September 1949): 477 and "Negro Higher and Professional Education in the United States," *Journal of Negro Education* 17, no. 3 (Summer 1948): 221–426.

72. *Nashville Tennessean,* April 23, 1944; Sugg and Jones, *Southern Regional Education Board,* p. 7.

73. "President's Report to the Board of Trustees of Meharry Medical College, May 22, 1942," p. 19. The governor of Tennessee, James Nance McCord, and his legal adviser, Cecil Sims, a leading member of the Nashville bar, were two of the chief architects of the plan that eventually emerged. Dr. William T. Sanger, president of the Medical College of Virginia, was another figure who played a role in the attempt to convince Meharry to abandon its independent status. Sugg and Jones, *Southern Regional Education Board,* pp. 9, 12–15.

74. A copy of the Southern Regional Education Compact is appended to Sugg and Jones, *Southern Regional Education Board,* pp. 159–62.

75. "President's Report to the Board of Trustees of Meharry Medical College, May 22, 1942," p. 19.

76. *New York Times,* January 19, 1948.

77. Saveth, "Jim Crow and the Regional Plan," pp. 478–79.

78. *Missouri ex rel. Gaines v. Canada,* 305 U.S. 337 (1938). For a discussion of the issues before the Supreme Court in the Gaines case and the significance of the decision, see Richard Kluger, *Simple Justice* (New York: Knopf, 1975), pp. 202–04 and 212–13.

79. *Time* Magazine 60, no. 11 (September 15, 1952): 91–92; *Bulletin of Meharry Medical College,* Alumni Edition 44, no. 2 (August 1947): 3; *Bulletin of Meharry Medical College,* Alumni Edition 44, no. 6 (April 1948): 2–4; Murray C. Brown, "The Regional Plan," *Meharry Medical College Faculty Bulletin* 4, no. 2 (April 1949): 4; Harold D. West, "Regional Education Becomes a Reality," *Bulletin of Meharry Medical College,* Special Issue 47, no. 2 (June 1951): 5–10; *The Nashville Globe,* October 24, 1947; *Nashville Tennessean,* April 29, 1962.

80. Sugg and Jones, *Southern Regional Education Board,* pp. 50–60.

81. "Dr. Turner Dies," *Journal of the National Medical Association* 52, no. 3 (May 1960): 200; Ward Darley, "Edward Lewis Turner, M.D.," *Journal of Medical Education* 35, no. 3 (March 1960): 287.

82. Turner, "The Meharry Medical College School of Dentistry," pp. 2–3; *Bulletin of Meharry Medical College,* Alumni Edition 48, no. 2 (April 1952): 5.

83. This slogan was reproduced on the cover of the *Faculty Bulletin* throughout the years of Dr. Clawson's administration. According to Dr. Turner it was selected by the faculty to be the motto for Meharry shortly after he assumed office.

84. "Annual Report of the President, Meharry Medical College, Nashville, Tennessee, July 1, 1939– June 30, 1940," p. 4; *Nashville Tennessean,* June 8, 1948.

85. "President's Report to the Board of Trustees of Meharry Medical College, May 22, 1942," p. 19; *Nashville Tennessean,* March 19, 1946, July 11, 1949.

86. *Nashville Tennessean,* June 22, 1948.

87. Ibid., July 3, 1947.

88. *Nashville Banner,* November 8, 1947; *Nashville Tennessean,* June 8, 22, 23, 26, 1948.

89. *Nashville Tennessean,* July 11, 1949.

90. The studies of the Committee on the Costs of Medical Care, from which this example is taken, are abstracted in Richard Harrison Shryock, *The Development of Modern Medicine* (New York: Knopf, 1947), pp. 413–20.

91. *Nashville Tennessean,* July 10, 11, 12, 28, 30, August 5, 1949; *Nashville Banner,* July 11, 23, 26, 1949; *The Nashville Globe,* July 22, August 5, 1949; *Pittsburgh Courier,* August 6, 1949; *Bulletin of Meharry Medical College,* Alumni Edition 46, no. 2 (April 1950): 3. The 1949 contract, adopted for the relief of Meharry and for the continued support of General Hospital as a teaching service, was similar to one first proposed by Harvie Branscomb, Chancellor of Vanderbilt University, in 1947. For details of the Branscomb plan, see *Nashville Banner,* November 8, 1947.

Chapter 6

1. Sources on the life and career of Dr. Lambert include *The Meharri-dent* 8, no. 1 (January 1951): 7; *Bulletin of Meharry Medical College,* Alumni Edition 48, no. 2 (April 1952): 2; and *Nashville Banner,* June 30, 1950. The *Meharri-dent* and the *Bulletin* are available at the archives, Meharry Medical College Library.

2. Amos Christie to James Summerville, interview, February 17, 1977, Nashville.

3. *Bulletin of Meharry Medical College,* Catalog Edition 46, no. 4 (December 1950): 45–47.

4. *Bulletin of Meharry Medical College,* Special Issue 47, no. 2 (June 1951): 18–19; *Bulletin of Meharry Medical College* 50, no. 4 (December 1954): 31.

5. Amos Christie to James Summerville, interview; *Meharry-Hubbard Newsletter* 2, no. 12 (June 15, 1952): 2–3. The latter publication is available at the archives, Meharry Medical College Library.

6. Dr. West's research interests are summarized in W. Montague Cobb and Calvin C. Sampson, "Harold Dadford West, Ph.D., LL.D., F.A.I.C.," *Journal of the National Medical Association* 66, no. 5 (September 1974): 448–49.

7. "Retrospect: Biochemistry," *The Meharrian* (1951), unpaginated; *Bulletin of Meharry Medical College,* Alumni Edition 48, no. 2 (April 1952): 2; "Dr. Harold D. West New President of Meharry," *Journal of the National Medical Association* 44, no. 4 (July 1952): 316–17; Cobb and Sampson, "Harold Dadford West," pp. 448–49.

8. *Nashville Banner,* October 18, 21, 1952; Harold Dadford West, "Inaugural Address," *Journal of the National Medical Association* 45, no. 1 (January 1953): 17–20; "Annual Report to the Board of Trustees, Meharry Medical College, 1954–55," p. 5. Dr. West's annual and semiannual reports to the trustees are variously titled. Sometimes dates are included in the title, at other times not. The author has preserved the original title, adding a clarifying note in brackets when necessary to show when the report was made by Dr. West. All of his reports to the trustees cited hereafter are available at the archives, Meharry Medical College Library.

9. *Nashville Banner,* June 24, 1953; "Semi-Annual Report of the President to the Board of Trustees, Meharry Medical College, June, 1953–January, 1954," p. 1.

10. *Nashville Tennessean,* December 15, 1955, June 9, 1956; "Semi-Annual Report of the President to the Board of Trustees, Meharry Medical College, June, 1955–December, 1955," pp. 7–14.

11. Hubbard Hospital *Newsletter* 1, no. 2 (January 26, 1951), unpaginated; *Nashville Tennessean,* July 3, 1947.

12. *Nashville Tennessean,* December 15, 1955; "Annual Report [of the President] to the Board of Trustees, Meharry Medical College, May 25, 1956," pp. 1–2.

13. "Semi-Annual Report of the President to the Board of Trustees, June, 1955–December, 1955," pp. 7–14; *Nashville Banner,* April 23, 1956.

14. *Nashville Banner,* June 24, 1953; *Nashville Tennessean,* January 31, 1956; "Semi-Annual Report of the President to the Board of Trustees, Meharry Medical College, June, 1953–January, 1954," pp. 6–7; "Annual Report of the President to the Board of Trustees, Meharry Medical College, June, 1953–May, 1954," p. 11.

15. "Annual Report [of the President] to the Board of Trustees, Meharry Medical College, May 25, 1956," pp. 13–16; Administrative Committee Minutes, September 11, 1956. The latter are available at the archives, Meharry Medical College Library.

16. Report of the Liaison Committee of the American Medical Association quoted in "[Annual] Report of the President [to the Board of Trustees], June 7, 1963," p. 2; *Nashville Tennessean,* June 23, 1953; *Nashville Banner,* June 24, 1953.

17. "Annual Report of the President to the Board of Trustees, Meharry Medical College, April 10, 1959," pp. 10–11.

18. "[Annual] Report of the President to the Board of Trustees of Meharry Medical College, June 8, 1962," pp. 6–11.

19. M. Elizabeth Carnegie, "Are Negro Schools of Nursing Needed Today?" *Journal of the National Medical Association* 56, no. 3 (May 1964): 233.

20. Committee on Policy Minutes, November 22, 1960. This advisory group to the president of Meharry was formerly called the Administrative Committee. These minutes are available at the archives, Meharry Medical College Library.

21. "Annual Report [of the President] to the Board of Trustees, Meharry Medical College, May 17, 1957," pp. 15–16; Committee on Policy Minutes, December 2, 1958, March 8, July 5, September 13, 1960; *Nashville Tennessean,* August 4, December 1, 1960; *Nashville Banner,* August 4, 1960; "Biography of a Nursing School," *Bulletin of Meharry Medical College* 58, no. 2 (August 1962): 1–6; "Report of the President to the Board of Trustees, Meharry Medical College, November 6, 1964," p. 5.

22. "Report of the President to the Board of Trustees, Meharry Medical College, November 6, 1964," p. 12; Warren Leslie Bennett, "Alumni Relations at Meharry Medical College," *The Meharri-dent* 21, no. 2 (June 1963): 43–45.

23. "Annual Report of the President to the Board of Trustees, 1953–1954," p. 10; "Annual Report [of the President] to the Board of Trustees, Meharry Medical College, May 17, 1957," p. 13.

24. *Nashville Tennessean,* January 8, 1953; "Annual Report of the President to the Board of Trustees, Meharry Medical College, April 10, 1959," n.p.

25. *Nashville Banner,* November 25, 1959; *Nashville Tennessean,* October 24, 1960.

26. "[Annual] Report of the President to the Board of Trustees of Meharry Medical College, June 8, 1962," p. 13.

27. "[Annual] Report of the President, Meharry Medical College, Nashville, Tennessee, June 7, 1963," p. 6; "[Annual] Report of the President to the Board of Trustees of Meharry Medical College, June 8, 1962," pp. 7–8.

28. "President's Report to the Board of Trustees of Meharry Medical College, May 22, 1942," pp. 4–5; "Meharry Biological Research Fund," *Bulletin of Meharry Medical College,* Alumni Edition 44, no. 2 (August 1947): 1–2; "Research," *The Meharrian* (1949), unpaginated; George W. Hillard, "The Cancer Teaching Program at Meharry Medical College, 1949–1950," *Bulletin of Meharry Medical College* 46, no. 2 (April 1950): 11; A. F. MacLeish, "Gold in a Lead Pot," *Bulletin of Meharry Medical College,* Special Issue 47, no. 2 (June 1951): 11–17; *Nashville Tennessean,* February 7, 1960, March 3, 1962, April 16, 1963; *Nashville Banner,* May 1, 1962; *Meharry Medical College Quarterly Digest* 1, no. 4 (October 1963): 4–5. The last publication is available at the archives, Meharry Medical College Library.

29. *Nashville Banner,* February 20, 1958, August 16, 1966; *Nashville Tennessean,* December 9, 1961, February 14, 1965, August 8, 1966; "Cardiovascular Unit Receives Support," *Meharry Medical College Quarterly Digest* 4, no. 4 (July 1966): 4–6.

30. *Nashville Tennessean,* February 28, 1964.

31. Ibid., March 11, 1964.

32. Ibid., July 24, 1966.

33. Ibid., September 23, 1957; *The Meharrian* (1960), p. 155.

34. Meharry Medical College, *The Centennial Lecture Series,* p. 24. These paperbound program notes are available at the archives, Meharry Medical College Library.

35. Ibid., p. 25; "Horace M. Frazier, M.D.," *Meharry Medical College Quarterly Digest* 8, no. 4 (July 1970): 28–29.

36. Birdie L. Rolfe to James Summerville, interview, March 5, 1977, Nashville; *Nashville Tennessean,* July 2, 1952; *Meharry-Hubbard Newsletter* 2, no. 14 (July 15, 1952): 1–2; "Rolfe New Dean of Meharry," *Journal of the National Medical Association* 44, no. 5 (September 1952): 395; *Nashville Banner,* July 1, 1957; "Daniel Thomas Rolfe, B.S., M.D., 1902–1968," *Journal of the National Medical Association* 60, no. 6 (November 1968): 530–31; *Meharry Medical College Quarterly Digest* 7, no. 2 (January 1969): 2–3.

37. The Ewell Neill Dental Society was named for Dr. Ewell P. Neill (1878–1955), professor of prosthetic dentistry.

38. E. Perry Crump and Michael J. Bent, "The New Horizon," *The Meharrian* (1949), unpaginated.

39. Harold D. West to Eugene H. Dibble, Jr., letter, February 8, 1957; Administrative Committee Minutes, November 19, 1957, November 8, 1960; *Nashville Tennessean,* October 13, 1961, January 9, 1966; "Professional News," *Journal of the National Medical Association* 58, no. 2 (March 1966): 141.

40. E. C. Beguesse, "An Incumbent Speaks," *The Meharrian* (1951), unpaginated.

41. *Bulletin of Meharry Medical College,* catalog edition for the School of Medicine 50, no. 4 (December 1954): 46–81; *Bulletin of Meharry Medical College,* catalog edition for the School of Medicine 55, no. 4 (December 1959): 53–88; *Bulletin of Meharry Medical College,* catalog edition for the School of Medicine [no volume or issue number assigned] (June 1965): 51–83.

42. *Bulletin of Meharry Medical College,* catalog edition for the School of Dentistry 53, no. 3 (September 1957): 38–50, 57–59; "[Annual] Report of the President to the Board of Trustees of Meharry Medical College, June 8, 1962," pp. 4–6.

43. "Report of the President to the Board of Trustees, Meharry Medical College," November 6, 1964," p. 2.

44. *Nashville Tennessean,* June 2, 1963.

45. *Nashville Banner,* August 5, 1957.

46. *Time* Magazine 59, no. 2 (January 14, 1952): 71–72.

47. Herbert M. Morais, *The History of the Negro in Medicine* (New York: Publishers Co., 1967), pp. 154–58; Marcus M. Goldstein, "Longevity and Health Status of Whites and Non-Whites in the United States," *Journal of the National Medical Association* 46, no. 2 (March 1954): 83–104.

48. *Nashville Banner,* April 17, 1964; *Nashville Tennessean,* April 18, 1964. An account of an early lawsuit to force the city to permit black physicians to minister to their patients at General Hospital is given in *The Nashville Globe,* December 22, 1944.

49. *Nashville Tennessean,* December 14, 1952, October 4, 1955; *Meharry-Hubbard Newsletter* 2, no. 24 (December 15, 1952): 1; "Annual Report [of the President] to the Board of Trustees, May 20, 1955," p. 9; *Nashville Tennessean,* October 4, 1955; *Nashville Banner,* August 9, 1955; "Nashville Academy of Medicine Admits Three," *Journal of the National Medical Association* 47, no. 4 (July 1955): 264.

50. Morais, *The Negro in Medicine,* p. 157.

51. *Nashville Tennessean,* March 15, 1946, May 30, 1947, June 12, December 15, 1953, June 25, 1954.

52. *Nashville Tennessean,* February 3, May 24, 1953; "Pedodontic Phase of the Child Care Program of Meharry Medical College," *The Meharri-dent* 11, no. 1 (June 1953): 5, 18; William H. Allen to James Summerville, interview, April 1, 1977, Nashville, Tennessee.

53. *Nashville Banner,* November 27, 1956.

54. For a review of the health-related programs under the Economic Opportunity Act, see Lisle C. Carter, Jr., "Health and the War on Poverty," *Journal of the National Medical Association* 58, no. 3 (May 1966): 173–78.

55. William Greenburg, "The First Twenty Years are the Hardest," *Nashville Tennessean Magazine,* September 24, 1967, pp. 18–20.

56. Matthew Walker, "The Affiliation of Taborian Hospital with Meharry Medical College and Development of the O.E.O. Planning Grant," *Meharry Medical College Quarterly Digest* 4, no. 3 (April 1966), unpaginated; Matthew Walker, "Progress Report: The Nashville Community Health Center," *Meharry Medical College Quarterly Digest* 5, no. 1 (October 1966): 14; Ralph H. Hines to James Summerville, interview, April 26, 1977, Nashville, Tennessee.

57. *Nashville Banner,* October 4, 1966.

Chapter 7

1. *Nashville Tennessean,* February 28, 1960.

2. *The Nashville Globe,* December 20, 1946; G. James Fleming and Christian E. Burckel, eds., *WHO'S WHO in Colored America,* 7th ed. (Yonkers-on-Hudson, N.Y.: Christian E. Burckel and Associates, 1950), p. 346; *Nashville Tennessean,* March 25, 1972.

3. For a discussion of *Robert W. Kelley, et al. v. Board of Education of Nashville* (139 F. Supp. 578) see Hugh Davis Graham, *Crisis in Print: Desegregation and the Press in Tennessee* (Nashville: Vanderbilt University Press, 1967), pp. 170–87.

4. John Vahaly, Jr., and Benjamin Walter, "Black Residential Succession in Nashville, 1930 to 1960," in James F. Blumstein and Benjamin Walter, eds., *Growing Metropolis, Aspects of Development in Nashville* (Nashville: Vanderbilt University Press, 1975), pp. 100–07.

5. Graham, *Crisis in Print,* pp. 191–203.

6. G. W. Hubbard, "The Education of Colored Physicians, Dentists, and Pharmacists," *Christian Educator* 2, no. 4 (July 1891): 158.

7. Administrative Committee (a.k.a. Committee on Policy) Minutes, November 18, 1955, December 8, 1955. These minutes are available at the archives, Meharry Medical College Library.

8. "Report of the President to the Executive Committee of the Board of Trustees, March 28, 1959," p. 1; *Nashville Tennessean,* October 3, 1958, July 22, 1965; Committee on Policy Minutes, May 16, 1961; F. Tremaine Billings to James Summerville, interview, April 26, 1977, Nashville, Tennessee; Harold D. West to Eugene H. Dibble, Jr., letters, November 25, December 23, 1958; Eugene H. Dibble, Jr., "Statement at the Annual Meeting of the Board of Trustees, Meharry Medical College, April 10, 1959" (mimeographed: Meharry Medical College, 1959), unpaginated; [Annual] Report of the President to the Board of Trustees, June 12, 1964," p. 3. See also W. Byers Unger, "Preprofessional Courses for Medical Students and Criteria for Admission to Medical School," *Journal of the National Medical Association* 48, no. 3 (May 1956): 165–66 and Ruth M. Raup and Elizabeth A. Williams, "Negro Students in Medical Schools in the United States," *Journal of Medical Education* 39, no. 5 (May 1964): 444–50.

The West-Dibble correspondence is available at the archives, Nashville Academy of Medicine. Reports of President West to the Board of Trustees are available at the archives, Meharry Medical College Library.

9. The oft-quoted WHO definition may be found in National Health Assembly, *America's Health* (New York: Harper and Brothers, 1949), p. 236. For a provocative rejoinder, see Daniel Callahan, "Health and Society: Some Ethical Imperatives," *Daedalus* 106, no. 1 (Winter 1977): 26.

10. Dr. Gregg is quoted in John Edward Hubbard, "Integrating Preventive and Social Medicine in the Medical Curriculum," *New England Journal of Medicine* 251, no. 13 (September 23, 1954): 518.

11. Iago Galdston, *The Meaning of Social Medicine* (Cambridge: Harvard University Press, 1954), p. 19.

12. Leon R. Kass, "Regarding the End of Medicine and the Pursuit of Health," *The Public Interest* 40 [no issue number assigned] (Summer 1975): 11. See also E. Gartly Jaco, "Twentieth Century Attitudes Toward Health and Their Effect on Medicine," *New England Journal of Medicine* 209, no. 1 (July 4, 1963): 21.

13. National Health Assembly, *America's Health*, p. 72. The concepts of universal availability, prevention, coordination, and comprehensiveness of health care were being discussed in American medicine by the early 1930s. See Roger I. Lee and Lewis W. Jones, *The Fundamentals of Good Medical Care* (Chicago: University of Chicago Press, 1933), pp. 6–10, 93–96, 102–09, 296–97.

14. National Health Assembly, *America's Health*, pp. 235–37. A role for the lay public in health planning had been contemplated before World War II. See Association of Teachers of Preventive Medicine, Committee on Medical Care Teaching, *Readings in Medical Care* (Chapel Hill: University of North Carolina Press, 1958), pp. 100–02.

15. John H. Knowles, "The Responsibility of the Individual," *Daedalus* 106, no. 1 (Winter 1977): 57–58; Iago Galdston, *Medicine in Transition* (Chicago: University of Chicago Press, 1965), pp. 66–67.

16. Henry E. Sigerist, "Medical Care for All the People" in Henry Sigerist, *On the Sociology of Medicine,* ed., Milton I. Roemer (New York: MD Publications, 1960), p. 234; Herman Miles Somers and Anne Ramsay Somers, *Doctors, Patients, and Health Insurance* (Washington, D.C.: Brookings Institution, 1961), pp. 134–37, 161; Merlin K. Duval, "The Provider, the Government, and the Consumer," *Daedalus* 106, no. 1 (Winter 1977): 186.

17. Edwin L. Crosby, "The Hospital Administrator," *Modern Hospital* 71, no. 2 (August 1948): 57.

18. Committee on Medical Care Teaching, *Medical Care*, pp. 381–82, 387.

19. Somers and Somers, *Doctors, Patients, and Health Insurance,* p. 78; E. Richard Weinerman and William A. Steiger, "Ambulatory Service in the Teaching Hospital," *Journal of Medical Education* 39, no. 11 (November 1964): 1020–21; Anne Ramsay Somers, "Conflict, Accommodation, and Progress: Some Socio-Economic Observations on Medical Education and the Practicing Profession," *Journal of Medical Education* 38, no. 6 (June 1963): 467; Galdston, *Medicine in Transition,* pp. 62–63.

20. John Knowles, quoted in Michael Crichton, *Five Patients* (New York: Knopf, 1970), p. 209. See also George A. Silver, "The Hospital and Social Medicine," *New England Journal of Medicine* 269, no. 10 (September 5, 1963): 505, 508 and Richard A. Carter, "Role of the University in Providing Personal Preventive Health Services," mimeographed (Nashville: the author, 1975). Dr. Carter's paper is available at the Department of Community and Occupational Health, Meharry Medical College.

21. Eli Ginzberg, *The Limits of Health Reform, The Search for Realism* (New York: Basic Books, 1977), p. 31; George A. Wolf, Jr., "The Financing of Medical Education," *New England Journal of Medicine* 269, no. 3 (July 18, 1963): 133–34.

22. A brief description of the chief Federal undertakings in health since the founding of the first National Institute of Health in 1936 is given in Duval, "Provider, Government, Consumer," p. 186. See also Stewart G. Wolf, Jr., and Ward Darley, eds., "Medical Education and Practice: Relationships and Responsibilities in a Changing Society," *Journal of Medical Education* 40, no. 1 (January 1965), part 2, p. 16.

23. Consultant Group on Medical Education, *Physicians for a Growing America* (Washington, D.C.: U.S. Public Health Service, 1959), pp. 28–35.

24. Committee on Medical Care Teaching, *Medical Care,* p. 222.

25. John M. Cassel, "Potentialities and Limitations of Epidemiology," in Alfred H. Katz and Jean S. Felton, eds., *Health and the Community* (New York: Free Press, 1965), pp. 443–44. Upon becoming Professor of Social Medicine at Cambridge University in 1943, Dr. John A. Ryle said that epidemiology took all disease as its province. Ryle's influential dictum is quoted in Fred B. Rogers, "Extending the Horizons of Preventive Medicine," *Journal of the American Medical Association* 190, no. 9 (November 30, 1964): 837. For a review of curricular changes underway in American medical schools in this period pertinent to the widening concerns of epidemiology, see Walter S. Wiggins, et al., "Medical Education in the United States," *Journal of the American Medical Association.* 178, no. 6 (November 11, 1961): 170–72.

26. W. Montague Cobb and Calvin C. Sampson, "Harold Dadford West, Ph.D., LL.D., F.A.I.C.," *Journal of the National Medical Association* 66, no. 5 (September 1974): 448–49; Henry Moses to James Summerville, interview, March 3, 1977, Nashville, Tennessee.

27. D. T. Rolfe, "The Dean Reports," *Meharry Medical College Quarterly Digest* [no volume or issue number assigned] (January 1963), unpaginated; Theodore E. Bolden, ed., *Research Activities, School of Dentistry, Meharry Medical College* (Nashville: School of Dentistry, 1966), pp. 86–88; Walter S. Wiggins, et al., "Medical Education in the United States," *Journal of the American Medical Association* 178, no. 6 (November 11, 1961): 170–72.

28. "[Annual] Report of the President, Meharry Medical College, Nashville, Tennessee," June 7, 1963, pp. 5–6; William R. Willard, "The Widening Gap Between Two Extreme Groups of Medical Schools," *Journal of the American Medical Association* 185, no. 5 (August 3, 1963): 107; Earl J. McGrath, *The Predominantly Negro Colleges and Universities in Transition* (New York: Teachers College, Columbia University, 1965), p. 76.

29. "[Annual] Report of the President to the Board of Trustees of Meharry Medical College," June 8, 1962, p. 12; Harold D. West to Executive Committee, Board of Trustees (undated memorandum, fall 1963), unpaginated; "Report of the President to the Board of Trustees, Meharry Medical College, Nashville, Tennessee," November 6, 1964, pp. 10, 11.

30. "President's Report to the Executive Committee of the Board of Trustees," December 20, 1957, p. 22; *Nashville Tennessean,* May 20, November 26, 1962.

31. "Psychiatry Notes," *Meharry Medical College Quarterly Digest* 3, no. 3 (April 1965), p. 2; *Nashville Tennessean,* October 31, 1961, January 4, 1964; Ralph H. Hines, "The Emerging Concept of Community Health," *Meharry Medical College*

Quarterly Digest 5, no. 2 (January 1967): 1–2; Ralph H. Hines to James Summerville, interview, April 26, 1977, Nashville, Tennessee; "President's Report to the Executive Committee of the Board of Trustees," December 20, 1957, p. iv.

32. "Report of the President to the Board of Trustees, Meharry Medical College, Nashville, Tennessee," November 6, 1964, pp. 6–8.

33. Warren Leslie Bennett, "Alumni Relations at Meharry Medical College," *The Meharri-dent* 21, no. 2 (June 1963): 43–45; "Annual Report of the Alumni Secretary for the Period Beginning June 7, 1962 and Ending June 9, 1963," *Meharry Medical College Quarterly Digest* 2, no. 2 (January 1964): 8–9. A review of recent trends in black enrollment in medical schools may be found in Edward S. Cooper, "Aspects of Medical Education and Research," *Journal of the National Medical Association* 56, no. 3 (May 1964): 263–66. See also Dietrich C. Reitzes, *Negroes and Medicine* (Cambridge: Harvard University Press, 1958), pp. 3–6 and the "Talent Recruitment Number," *Journal of the National Medical Association* 57, no. 6 (November 1965).

34. Thomas W. Johnson to James Summerville, interview, July 28, 1978, Nashville, Tennessee.

35. Oliver Cope and Jerrold Zacharias, eds., *Medical Education Reconsidered: Report of the Endicott House Summer Study on Medical Education, July, 1965* (Philadelphia: Lippincott, 1966), 95 pages, passim; Oliver Cope, "The Endicott House Conference on Medical Education," in John Knowles, ed., *Views of Medical Education and Medical Care* (Cambridge: Harvard University Press, 1968), pp. 139–76.

36. Maurice C. Clifford, "Meharry Mission," *Meharry Medical College Quarterly Digest* 4, no. 4 (July 1966): 15.

37. Robert Anderson to James Summerville, interview, November 30, 1977, Nashville, Tennessee; Thomas W. Johnson to James Summerville; Ralph H. Hines to James Summerville. Reports on the number of black students in medical schools and the ebb and flow of applicants during this period appeared regularly in the *Journal of the National Medical Association*. A useful summary is Cooper, "Aspects of Medical Education," pp. 263–66.

There was ample precedent for the faculty initiating reforms of educational methods and objectives at Meharry. One of the most influential instances occurred at Case Western Reserve University in the 1950s. For a case study, see Peter V. Lee, "Reorganization of the Medical Curriculum," *Journal of Medical Education* 36, no. 12 (December 1961), part 2: 101–17.

38. *Nashville Tennessean,* December 2, 1965, February 14, May 14, July 26, August 11, 1966; "Grants Given to Tennessee Medical Schools," *Journal of the Tennessee Medical Association* 59, no. 7 (July 1966): 705; Tennessee Mid-South Regional Medical Program, *Continuation Application and Progress Report* (Nashville: the Regional Medical Program, 1968), pp. 4.3–4.4.

39. Robert Anderson to James Summerville; *Nashville Tennessean,* May 26, 1965; *Nashville Banner,* September 30, 1966.

40. *Nashville Tennessean,* November 26, 1962. Dr. West's effort to gain mastery over events through a rigidly organized plan and the centralization of authority is shown in *Standard Procedures Manual for Meharry Medical College,* no. 4, mimeographed (Nashville: the College, 1958?), unpaginated. The manual provided for

"clearing all procedures through one central authority." "Authority" was defined as the "right to act, decide, or command." "In this institution," the document continued, "it emanates from the President." The *Standard Procedures Manual* also noted, foremost in a listing of the college's objectives: "This Institution was created by private capital in the form of gifts and endowment. Its operating organization is obligated to the source of that endowment for its preservation." The *Standard Procedures Manual* is available at the archives, Meharry Medical College Library.

41. Clifford, "Meharry Mission," p. 16.

42. Ralph H. Hines, *The Health Status of Negroes in a Mid-Southern Urban Community*, part 1 (Nashville: Meharry Medical College, 1967), 142 pages, passim; Ralph H. Hines, *The Health Status of Negroes in a Mid-Southern Urban Community*, part 2, Mental Health (Nashville: Meharry Medical College, 1967), 84 pages, passim.

43. Matthew Walker to James Summerville, interview, December 7, 1977, Nashville, Tennessee; Matthew Walker, "Progress Report: The Nashville Community Health Center," *Meharry Medical College Quarterly Digest* 5, no. 1 (October 1966): 14–16; *Nashville Tennessean*, October 21, 1966.

44. The John F. Kennedy Center for Research on Education and Human Development, George Peabody Center for Community Studies, *The Characteristics of the Population and the Social Services for a High Poverty Area in Nashville, Tennessee* (Nashville: the Kennedy Center, 1967), 165 pages, passim. See also Charles V. Mercer and J. R. Newbrough, *The North Nashville Health Study: Research into the Culture of the Deprived* (Nashville: the Kennedy Center, 1967), 98 pages, passim, and Metropolitan Action Commission, "The 1967 Residential Survey of Poverty in the Inner City," mimeographed (Nashville: Council of Community Services, 1968), various pagings.

45. Leslie A. Falk, "Changing Concepts in Comprehensive Health Care. Comprehensive Care in Health Programs," *Journal of the National Medical Association* 64, no. 6 (November 1972): 473; *Nashville Tennessean*, April 6, 1967.

46. "The Meharry North Nashville Neighborhood Health Center," *Journal of the National Medical Association* 59, no. 6 (November 1967): 448.

47. Leslie A. Falk to James Summerville, interviews, December 6, 1977, November 5, 1978, Nashville, Tennessee; Leslie A. Falk to Jude Thomas May, interview, April 9, 1974, Nashville, Tennessee; "Dr. Falk Heads N.H.C.," Meharry Medical College *Intercom* 11, no. 5 (September–October 1967): 8; "Les Falk: Giving Birth to a New Department," *Meharry Medical College Quarterly Digest* 6, no. 3 (April 1968): 10–11.

48. Mrs. Evelyn Graves to James Summerville, interview, October 30, 1978, Nashville, Tennessee.

49. Leslie A. Falk, "Community Participation in the Neighborhood Health Center," *Journal of the National Medical Association* 61, no. 6 (November 1969): 494.

50. *Nashville Tennessean*, September 30, 1969.

51. Meharry Neighborhood Health Center Project, "Facts About the Meharry Neighborhood Health Center," mimeographed (Nashville: the Project, 1968), pp. 9–10.

52. Mrs. Lettie Galloway to James Summerville, interview, October 11, 1978, Nashville, Tennessee; Falk, "Community Participation," pp. 495–96.

53. Falk, "Community Participation," pp. 494–95.

54. Mrs. Evelyn Graves to James Summerville; *Nashville Tennessean,* September 2, 1970; Health Center Project, "The Meharry Neighborhood Health Center," pp. 3, 8–10; Metropolitan Action Commission, "Poverty in the Inner City," Report no. 1 on MAC District V (north Nashville), pp. 8–11.

55. Falk, "Community Participation," p. 495; Mrs. Evelyn Graves to James Summerville; Earnest B. Campbell, "The Matthew Walker Neighborhood Health Center of Meharry Medical College," *Journal of the National Medical Association* 65, no. 4 (July 1973): 298.

56. Mrs. Evelyn Graves to James Summerville.

57. "Meharry Purchases Land for Neighborhood Center," Meharry Medical College *Intercom* 11, no. 6 (November–December 1967): 8; "The 'Center' Becomes a Reality," *Meharry Medical College Quarterly Digest* 7, no. 1 (October 1968): 11; *Nashville Tennessean,* August 14, 1968, June 12, 1969; "Dedication, Matthew Walker Health Center of Meharry Medical College," *Meharry Medical College Quarterly Digest* 8, no. 3 (April 1970): 5–7; "Matthew Walker Health Center: Inspiration for Sunflower County," Meharry Medical College *Intercom* 5, no. 2 (March–June 1970): 8–9; *Nashville Banner,* August 22, 1968.

58. Mrs. Lettie Galloway to James Summerville.

59. Leslie A. Falk, "The Matthew Walker Health Center of Meharry Medical College: OEO-Funded Neighborhood Health Center," *Journal of the Tennessee Medical Association* 63, no. 10 (October 1970): 849; Meharry Medical College, *Ambulatory Services* (Nashville: the College), 16 pages, passim.

60. Mrs. Evelyn Graves to James Summerville.

61. Elizabeth J. Anderson, Leda R. Judd, Jude Thomas May, and Peter K. New, *The Neighborhood Health Center, Its Growth and Problems: An Introduction* (Washington, D.C.: National Association of Neighborhood Health Centers, 1976), pp. 5–6.

62. Kemper Harreld Smith, *The Mission of Tabor* (Mound Bayou, Miss.: Knights and Daughters of Tabor, n.d., 1970?), pp. 6–24; *Washington Post,* June 20, 1974.

63. William R. Willard, "The Development of the Medical School as a Community Resource," *Journal of Public Health* 54, no. 7 (July 1964): 1042–45; Milton Terris, "The Future Growth of Departments of Preventive Medicine," *Archives of Environmental Health* 6, no. 4 (April 1963): 457; Henry J. Bakst, "Summary Report of the Saratoga Springs Conference," *Archives of Environmental Health* 7, no. 5 (November 1963): 509–23.

64. Falk, "Changing Concepts," p. 473.

65. Mrs. Lettie Galloway to James Summerville; Leslie A. Falk, Benjamin Page, and Walter Vesper, "Human Values and Medical Education from the Perspectives of Health Care Delivery," *Journal of Medical Education* 48, no. 2 (February 1973): 155–56; "'Ideal' Approach Developed in Family Practice Residency," Meharry Medical College *Intercom* 4, no. 1 (November 1974): 2.

Chapter 8

1. *Nashville Tennessean,* April 16, 1967; *Newsweek* 69, no. 17 (April 24, 1967): 28; "Tennessee Rebels," *New Republic* 157, no. 11 (September 9, 1967): 9–10; Dr. Edwin Mitchell to Richard Moore, interview, February 18, 1972, Nashville, Tennessee, in Black Oral History Collection, Fisk University Library.

2. *Nashville Tennessean,* May 4, 1971.

3. Eugene J. Lipman and Albert Vorspan, eds., *A Tale of Ten Cities* (New York: Union of American Hebrew Congregations, 1962): 148.

4. The commission's findings are quoted in *Nashville Tennessean,* June 30, 1967. Additional reports on discrimination and black joblessness in Nashville appeared in that newspaper on October 8, 9, and 10, 1967.

5. For a review of the I-40 controversy, see *Nashville Tennessean,* January 10, 1971, and Hubert James Ford, Jr., "Interstate 40 Through North Nashville: A Case Study in Highway Location Decision Making," M.S. thesis, University of Tennessee, 1970, pp. 43–61. Some effects of the expressway on life in north Nashville are recounted in *Nashville Tennessean,* March 1, 1970.

6. *Nashville Tennessean,* February 11, 1969, February 10, 1971.

7. Histories of these institutions are: R. Grann Lloyd, *Tennessee Agricultural and Industrial State University, 1912–1962* (Nashville: Tennessee A & I State University, 1962), 73 pages, and Joe M. Richardson, *A History of Fisk University, 1865–1946* (University, Ala.: University of Alabama Press, 1980), 227 pages.

8. *Nashville Tennessean,* October 12, 1967; "An Alumnus Speaks in Nashville," *Meharry Medical College Quarterly Digest* 6, no. 2 (January 1968): 16–17; Pat Harris, "Dr. Edwin Mitchell: Gentleman from the Ghetto," *Nashville Magazine* 7, no. 3 (March 1969): 23.

9. Dr. Robert Anderson to James Summerville, interview, November 30, 1977, Nashville, Tennessee.

10. Meharry Medical College, *New Developmental Programs: Summary of Proposals* (Nashville: the College, May 1967), 19 pages, passim; Meharry Medical College, *Opening New Doors to Greatness with Meharry Medical College* (Nashville: the College, n.d., 1969?), unpaginated; *Nashville Banner,* June 1, 1970; "$50 Million for Program and Campus Development," *Meharry Medical College Quarterly Digest* 6, no. 4 (July 1968): 1–4; Ralph H. Hines to James Summerville, interview, April 26, 1977, Nashville.

11. *Nashville Banner,* June 16, 1969.

12. *The Tennessean* (Nashville), April 2, 1976.

13. Robert S. Anderson, "Meharry Medical College and the Challenge of Education in the Medical Sciences," *Meharry Medical College Quarterly Digest* 6, no. 2 (January 1968): 10–11; *Nashville Tennessean,* August 10, 1969; "Justification for Development of Graduate Programs at Meharry Medical College," *The Graduate School Manual* (Nashville: Meharry Medical College, 1972), pp. 11–12; Charles W. Johnson, "Meharry's Special Medical and Research Programs," *Journal of the National Medical Association* 65, no. 4 (July 1973): 307–08.

14. Ralph J. Cazort, "An Open Letter to Medical School Alumni," *Meharry Medical College Quarterly Digest* 7, no. 2 (January 1969): 4; Hobart C. Sanders,

"Blueprint for an Active Alumni Association," *Meharry Medical College Quarterly Digest* 6, no. 1 (October 1967): 1; "Enlarged Role of Alumni Association Includes Participation by All Members," *Meharry Today* 3, no. 2 (January 1974): 9.

15. "Minutes of the Annual Meeting of the Meharry Alumni Association," *Meharry Medical College Quarterly Digest* 5, no. 4 (July 1967): 6–8; "Minutes of the Annual Meeting of the Meharry Alumni Association," *Meharry Medical College Quarterly Digest* 6, no. 4 (July 1968): 12–15; Maurice C. Clifford, "Meharry Mission," *Meharry Medical College Quarterly Digest* 4, no. 4 (July 1966): 14–17.

16. For useful discussions of the agenda, achievement, and legacy of the Administrative Committee, see Jacque Srouji, "Meharry: Excellence on a Shoestring," *Nashville Magazine* 6, no. 6 (June 1968): 11–16; *Nashville Tennessean,* November 24, 1967; *Nashville Banner,* November 24, 1967; and "Interim—October '66–June '68," *Meharry Medical College Quarterly Digest* 6, no. 3 (April 1968): 3–5.

17. "Elam New President of Meharry," *Journal of the National Medical Association* 60, no. 2 (March 1968): 150–51; "Dr. Elam Appointed New President," Meharry Medical College *Intercom* 11, no. 6 (November–December 1967), pp. 1, 3; "A Look at the New President," *Meharry Medical College Quarterly Digest* 6, no. 2 (January 1968): 1–4; *Nashville Tennessean,* December 2, 1967; June 10, 1968; Victor S. Johnson to James Summerville, interview, June 22, 1978, Nashville, Tennessee; Lloyd C. Elam, "Meharry Looks Ahead," *Journal of the National Medical Association* 61, no. 1 (January 1969): 40–43. The last-cited article was President Elam's inaugural address.

18. *Nashville Tennessean,* April 29, 1948, October 18, 1966, June 3, 1971; E. Perry Crump, et al., "Participation in a Longitudinal Study of Negro Infants and Children," *Public Health Reports* 75, no. 1 (November 1960): 1085; "C & Y Center Holds Open House May 12," Meharry Medical College *Intercom* 3, no. 2 (March–June 1968: 8; [Annual] Report of the President, Meharry Medical College, June 1969, unpaginated; Dr. E. Perry Crump to James Summerville, interview, December 3, 1978, Nashville.

19. *Nashville Banner,* May 19, 1968, February 10, 1972; *Meharry Medical College: A Report* (Nashville: the College, Summer 1970), unpaginated; "Community Mental Health Center," Meharry Medical College *Intercom* 5, no. 3 (September–October 1970): 14; Henry Tomes, "Meharry's Community Mental Health Center," *Journal of the National Medical Association* 65, no. 4 (July 1973): 300–03; Willie Taylor, "Meharry Mental Health Center: Reaching Out to the Aged," Meharry Medical College *Breakthrough* 4, no. 1 (Winter 1976): 7–10.

20. "Focus: The Patient," *Meharry Medical College Quarterly Digest* 7, no. 3 (April 1969): 8–9; *Nashville Banner,* August 22, 1969; Carl A. Traherne, "Meharry's Comprehensive Health Center," *Journal of the National Medical Association* 65, no. 4 (July 1973): 290–92; *Nashville Tennessean,* April 9, 1971; Meharry Medical College *Intercom* 4, no. 1 (January–February 1969): 10.

21. "All Patient Care Programs are Unified; Changes Will Provide Better Care," *Meharry Today* 4, no. 2 (February–March 1975): 6–7.

22. Lloyd C. Elam, et al., "Health Evaluation Studies Utilizing a Multiphasic Screening Center Operating in Cooperation with a Comprehensive Health Care Program for Persons in an Urban Poverty Area," *Proceedings: Conference Workshop*

on Regional Medical Programs (Washington, D.C.: U.S. Public Health Service, 1968), pp. 1–6; "A Trip Through Multiphasic," *Meharry Medical College Quarterly Digest* 8, no. 5 (October 1970): 14–15; "Evolution of an Electronic Era," *Meharry Medical College Quarterly Digest* 8, no. 1 (October 1969): 6; *Nashville Banner,* October 25, 1969.

23. Center for Health Care Research, *Report of the Center for Health Care Research of Meharry Medical College for July 1, 1969 to June 30, 1971* (Nashville: the Center, 1971), 215 pages, passim; Samuel Wolfe, "The Meharry Medical College Center for Health Care Research," *Journal of the National Medical Association* 65, no. 4 (July 1973): 293–95; *Nashville Tennessean,* December 30, 1970, January 23, 1972; *The Tennessean* (Nashville), November 17, 1974; "Center for Health Care Research Data Shows Massive Unmet Needs," *Meharry Today* 4, no. 2 (February–March 1975): 1, 5; William B. Neser, *Quality Standards of Care in Alternative Health Care Systems* (Nashville: Meharry Medical College, 1975), pp. i–ii.

24. "Robert Wood Johnson Foundation Gives Meharry $5 Million Training Grant," *Meharry Today* 2, no. 1 (November 1972): 1; *The Tennessean* (Nashville), October 13, 1972; *Nashville Banner,* October 13, 1972.

25. "Kresge Center Programs Provide Services," *Meharry Today,* 3, no. 3 (March 1974): 10–12; *Nashville Tennessean,* August 27, 1969; *The Tennessean* (Nashville), April 2, 7, 1973; *Nashville Banner,* April 7, 1973. Besides the gift from the Kresge Foundation, Meharry received $2.9 million from the U.S. Department of Health, Education, and Welfare to build the Learning Resources Center.

26. Meharry Medical College, *Report to the Nation, 1967–1972* (Nashville: Meharry Medical College, 1972), pp. 24–25; *Nashville Tennessean,* October 10, 1971; Ralph H. Hines and John Coffin, "A Meharry Renaissance," *Black Books Bulletin* 3, no. 2 (September 1975): 16–22; Meharry Medical College, *President's Report, 1975–1976, Centennial Edition* (Nashville: Meharry Medical College, 1976), pp. 23, 31.

27. *The Tennessean* (Nashville), September 8, 1972; *Nashville Banner,* September 8, 1972, November 29, 1973; "Construction Starts on 12-Story Hospital Tower," *Meharry Today* 3, no. 2 (January 1974): 1–3; *The George Russell Tower, Meharry Medical College, Tribute and Cornerstone Ceremony, Nashville, Tennessee, November 22, 1974* (Nashville: Meharry Medical College, 1974), unpaginated; "George Russell Honored at Cornerstone Laying Ceremony for New Hospital," *Meharry Today* 4, no. 2 (February–March 1975): 1–2.

28. *The President's Report, Meharry Medical College* (Nashville: the College, 1971), p. 14.

29. "Task Force Report, Nashville General Hospital/Meharry Medical College," mimeographed (Nashville: Mayor's Task Force, September 13, 1976), unpaginated.

30. Ibid.; *Nashville Banner,* August 12, 1976; *The Tennessean* (Nashville), September 12, 1976.

31. "Task Force Report."

32. Ibid.; *The Tennessean* (Nashville), September 12, 14, 1976; *Nashville Banner,* October 13, 1976.

33. *Nashville Tennessean,* September 9, 1969; *Nashville Banner,* July 23, 1976; "The Admissions Process," *Meharry Medical College Quarterly Digest* 8, no. 4 (July 1970): 16–21.

34. Thomas W. Johnson, et al., "Student Life at Meharry," *Journal of the National Medical Association* 65, no. 4 (July 1973): 315–16; *Nashville Tennessean,* May 21, 1970.

35. Ralph J. Cazort, "Meharry's New Approach to Medical Education," *Journal of the National Medical Association* 65, no. 4 (July 1973): 283–85; Meharry Medical College, Self-Study Office, *Introspect: Self-Study News* 1, no. 8 (November 1975): 5–7; *Nashville Tennessean,* December 9, 1967, January 10, 1972; *Meharry Medical College Quarterly Digest* 8, no. 1 (October 1969): 3. For biographical notes on Dr. Cazort see *Nashville Banner,* November 8, 1967 and *Nashville Tennessean,* December 9, 1967.

36. Jean Dorsett Robinson, "Meharry's Health Care Administration and Planning Program," *Journal of the National Medical Association* 65, no. 4 (July 1973): 306; *Nashville Tennessean,* November 11, 1972.

37. James P. Carter, "The Maternal and Child Health/Family Planning, Training and Research Center," *Journal of the National Medical Association* 65, no. 4 (July 1973): 304–05; *Nashville Banner,* July 5, 1971, October 26, 1976; "Maternal and Child Health Center Completed," *Meharry Today* 2, no. 2 (March 1973): 4; "Maternal and Child Health/Family Planning Center," *Meharry Today* 3, no. 2 (January 1974): 12–13; "Maternal and Child Health/Family Planning Center Focuses on Africa," *Meharry Today* [no volume or issue number assigned] (Fall 1976): 14–15.

38. *Nashville Banner,* April 15, 1974.

39. "Meharry Opens New School of X-Ray Technology," Meharry Medical College *Intercom* 3, no. 8 (September–October 1968), unpaginated; *Report to the Nation, Meharry Medical College, 1967–1972,* p. 15; *President's Report, 1975–1976,* p. 71; *Nashville Tennessean,* January 13, 1972.

40. "School of Dentistry: A Turning Point," Meharry Medical College, *Annual Report, 1971–1972: Another Year, Another Step Forward* (Nashville: the College, 1972), unpaginated; *Report to the Nation, Meharry Medical College, 1967–1972,* pp. 12–13.

41. Quoted in J. B. Singleton, "The Meharry Medical College School of Dentistry with Divisions of Dental Hygiene and Dental Technology," mimeographed (Nashville: the School of Dentistry, 1971), p. 7.

42. Thomas P. Logan, "Meharry's New Approach to Dental Education," *Journal of the National Medical Association* 65, no. 4 (July 1973): 286; "Changes in the School of Dentistry Reflect New Approaches in Curriculum and Teaching," *Meharry Today* 3, no. 4 (May 1974): 4–5; *Report to the Nation, Meharry Medical College, 1967–1972,* pp. 12–13; *Nashville Tennessean,* January 12, 1972; *Nashville Banner,* September 22, 1972.

43. *The Tennessean* (Nashville), May 20, 1979.

44. "Ground Breaking Underway for Basic Sciences Building," *Meharry Today* 3, no. 1 (November 1973): 1–2; *The Tennessean* (Nashville), September 30, 1973,

February 24, 1976; *Nashville Banner,* February 27, 1976. The *Journal of the National Medical Association* dedicated its July 1976 issue as "The Harold D. West Basic Sciences Number."

45. "Meharry Holds Centennial Commencement," *Meharry Today* (Special Commencement Issue, 1976), p. 1.

46. *Nashville Banner,* August 2, 3, 1976; *The Tennessean* (Nashville), August 5, 1976; *The New York Times,* August 2, 1976.

47. *The Tennessean* (Nashville), August 8, 1976; *Nashville Banner,* August 11, 1976. Five previous conventions of the National Medical Association had been held in Nashville—those of 1896, 1903, 1913, 1934, and 1953. Of the seventy-five presidents to this time, more than thirty were Meharry graduates.

48. "Convocation Opens 101st Academic Year," *Meharry Today* (Fall 1976; no volume or issue number assigned): 2–5.

49. *The Tennessean* (Nashville), November 11, 1976. In addition to sheaves of newspaper and journal articles from throughout the nation that noted the 100th anniversary, the November 1976 issue (vol. 68, no. 6) of the *Journal of the National Medical Association* was the "Meharry Centennial Number." Among other papers it contained the commencement address by Dr. Cowan and a statement of Meharry's mission, "Why the Black College is Different," by President Lloyd Elam.

Works Cited

Manuscript Collections

London. Imperial College of Science and Technology. Huxley papers.

Nashville. Archives, Meharry Medical College Library. G. W. Hubbard to Reverend James R. Joy, letter, May 31, 1909.

Nashville. Archives, Meharry Medical College Library. G. W. Hubbard, "Half a Century Among the Freedmen." n.d.

Nashville. Archives, Meharry Medical College Library. Administrative Committee Minutes.

Nashville. Archives, Meharry Medical College Library. Committee on Policy Minutes.

Nashville. Archives, Meharry Medical College Library. Minutes of the Faculty, Meharry Medical College.

Nashville. Archives, Meharry Medical College Library. Reports of the President to the Board of Trustees, 1952–1964.

Nashville. Methodist Board of Higher Education and Ministry. Minutes of the Board of Trustees, Central Tennessee College.

Nashville. Tennessee State Library and Archives, Manuscripts Section. Methodist Episcopal Church, Northern Annual Conference Records, vol. 1. Report of the Committee on the Education of Freedmen.

Nashville. Tennessee State Library and Archives, Manuscripts Section. Minutes of the Tennessee Annual Conference of the Methodist Episcopal Church, Northern Branch, 1905–1925.

Nashville. Tennessee State Library and Archives, Manuscripts Section. Sneed Family Papers, 1796–1856.

Newspapers

The Christian Educator (Cincinnati)
Chicago Tribune
Nashville *Colored Tennessean*

Nashville *Daily American*
Nashville Banner
The Nashville Globe
The New York Times
Marshall, Texas *News Messenger*
Nashville *Republican Banner*
Nashville Tennessean [a.k.a. *The Tennessean*]
Topeka Capital
The Washington Post

Public Documents

Bureau of the Census. *Ninth Census of the United States, 1870.* Washington, D.C.: U.S. Government Printing Office, 1872.

———. *Populations of the United States in 1860. Eighth Census, 1860.* Washington, D.C.: Government Printing Office, 1864.

———. *United States Census Reports, 1880.* Washington, D.C.: U.S. Government Printing Office, 1883.

Kansas State Board of Health, *Third Annual Report,* 1887.

Ordinances of the City of Nashville, 1875, title 9, chap. 48.

Private Acts, *Acts of the State of Tennessee.* 34th General Assembly, 1865–66, chap. 115.

———. 35th General Assembly, 1867–68, chap. 17.

"Reports on the Cholera Epidemic of 1873 in the United States." *House Executive Document,* 43rd Congress, Second Session, 1875.

Second Report of the Board of Health to the Honorable City Council of the City of Nashville for the Year Ending July 4, 1877.

United States Statutes at Large, vol. 13, chap. 90.

Theses, Dissertations, and Unpublished Material

American Medical Association. "Report . . . Council on Medical Education and Hospitals of the American Medical Association." Mimeographed: Chicago(?): American Medical Association, 1931.

Campbelle, R. Bartley J., Sr., ed. "The History of Clark Memorial Methodist Church." Mimeographed. Nashville: the Author, n.d.

Carr, Ellen Lillard. "The Struggle of the Freedmen's Bureau to Effect Social Rehabilitation in Nashville and Davidson County." M.A. thesis, Fisk University, 1967.

Carter, Richard A. "Role of the University in Providing Personal Preventive Health Services." Mimeographed. Nashville: the Author, 1975.

Clark, Stewart Sandy. "A Study of Negro Education in Davidson County, Tennessee." M.A. thesis, George Peabody College for Teachers, 1919.

Dibble, Eugene H., Jr., "Statement at the Annual Meeting of the Board of Trustees, Meharry Medical College, April 10, 1959." Mimeographed. Nashville: Meharry Medical College, 1959.

Dietrich, Paul H. "George W. Hubbard Hospital Report for Seven Months Ending April 30, 1922." Mimeographed. Nashville: Meharry Medical College, 1922.

Ford, Hubert James, Jr. "Interstate 40 Through North Nashville: A Case Study in Highway Location Decision Making." M.S. thesis, University of Tennessee, 1970.

Harrison, Grace. "Hubbard Hospital and Meharry Medical College for Negroes, Nashville, Tennessee." M.A. thesis, University of Chicago, 1945.

Hogan, Walter E. "Changing Conceptions of the Aim of Negro Education as Seen in the History of Colored Schools in Nashville, Tennessee." M.A. thesis, George Peabody College for Teachers, 1917.

Martin, James W. "A Study of the Negro Physician with Particular Reference to Certain Tennessee Counties." M.A. thesis, George Peabody College for Teachers, 1921.

Mayor's Task Force. "Task Force Report, Nashville General Hospital/Meharry Medical College." Mimeographed. Nashville: Mayor's Task Force, September 13, 1976.

Meharry Medical College. "Meharry Medical College Endowment Program, 1940–41." Mimeographed. Nashville: the College, 1941.

———. "Standard Procedures Manual for Meharry Medical College." Mimeographed. Nashville: the College, 1958(?).

Meharry Neighborhood Health Center Project. "Facts About the Meharry Neighborhood Health Center." Mimeographed. Nashville: the Project, 1968.

Metropolitan Action Commission. "The 1967 Residential Survey of Poverty in the Inner City." Mimeographed. Nashville: Council of Community Services, 1968.

Phillips, Paul David. "A History of the Freedmen's Bureau in Tennessee." Ph.D. dissertation, Vanderbilt University, 1964.

"President's Report to the Board of Trustees of Meharry Medical College, May 22, 1942." Mimeographed. Nashville: the College, 1942.

Singleton, J. B., Jr. "The Meharry Medical College School of Dentistry with Divisions of Dental Hygiene and Dental Technology." Mimeographed. Nashville: the School of Dentistry, 1971.

West, Harold D. "The History of Meharry Medical College." Mimeographed. Nashville: Meharry Medical College, 1974.

West, Harold D. to Executive Committee, Board of Trustees (undated memorandum, fall 1963).

Interviews and Letters

Allen, William H. to James Summerville, interview, April 1, 1977, Nashville.

Anderson, Robert to James Summerville, interview, November 30, 1977, Nashville.

Billings, F. Tremaine to James Summerville, interview, April 26, 1977, Nashville.

Christie, Amos to James Summerville, interview, February 17, 1977, Nashville.

Crump, E. Perry to James Summerville, interview, December 3, 1978, Nashville.

Falk, Leslie A. to Jude Thomas May, interview, April 9, 1974, Nashville.

Falk, Leslie A. to James Summerville, interviews, December 6, 1977, and November 5, 1978, Nashville.

Galloway, Mrs. Lettie to James Summerville, interview, October 11, 1978, Nashville.

Graves, Mrs. Evelyn to James Summerville, interview, October 30, 1978, Nashville.

Hines, Ralph H. to James Summerville, interview, April 26, 1977, Nashville.

Johnson, Thomas W. to James Summerville, interview, July 28, 1978, Nashville.

Johnson, Victor S. to James Summerville, interview, June 22, 1978, Nashville.

Mitchell, Edwin to Richard Moore, interview, February 18, 1972, Nashville, in Black Oral History Collection, Fisk University Library.

Moses, Henry to James Summerville, interview, March 3, 1977, Nashville.

Peek, Miss H. E. to James M. Smith, letter, March 21, 1977.

Reed, William A., Jr., to James Summerville, interview, January 6, 1977, Nashville.

Rolfe, Mrs. Birdie L. to James Summerville, interview, March 7, 1977, Nashville.

Smith, Kelly Miller to James Summerville, interview, August 21, 1979, Nashville.

Walker, Matthew to James Summerville, interview, December 7, 1977, Nashville.

West, Harold D. to Eugene H. Dibble, Jr., letters, February 8, 1957, November 25, December 23, 1958.

Articles

"The Admissions Process." *Meharry Medical College Quarterly Digest* 8: 4 (July 1970): 16–21.

"All Patient Care Programs are Unified; Changes Will Provide Better Care." *Meharry Today* 4: 2 (February–March 1975): 6–7.

"An Alumnus Speaks in Nashville." *Meharry Medical College Quarterly Digest* 6: 2 (January 1968): 16.

Anderson, Robert S. "Meharry Medical College and the Challenge of Education in the Medical Sciences." *Meharry Medical College Quarterly Digest* 6: 2 (January 1968): 7–12.

"Annual Report of the Alumni Secretary for the Period Beginning June 7, 1962 and Ending June 9, 1963." *Meharry Medical College Quarterly Digest* 2: 2 (January 1964): 8.

"Annual Report of the Board of Education for Negroes of the Methodist Episcopal Church for the Year July 1, 1920 to July 1, 1921." *The Christian Educator,* November 1921, pp. 4–5.

"Annual Report of Meharry Medical College for the Year 1936–37 by John J. Mullowney, President." *Bulletin of Meharry Medical College* 34: 2 (October 1937): 5.

"Annual Report of the President, Meharry Medical College, Nashville, Tennessee, July 1, 1939–June 30, 1940." *Bulletin of Meharry Medical College* 37: 2 (October 1940): 3, 6–23.

"Arthur Melvin Townsend, M.D., 1875–1959." *Journal of the National Medical Association* 51: 4 (1959): 323–24.

Bakst, Henry J. "Summary Report of the Saratoga Springs Conference." *Archives of Environmental Health* 7: 5 (1963): 509–23.

Beck, William A. "The Early Diagnosis and Treatment of Pulmonary Tuberculosis." *Journal of the National Medical Association* 45: 4 (1948): 212–14.

Bennett, Warren Leslie. "Alumni Relations at Meharry Medical College." *The Meharri-dent* 21: 2 (June 1963): 43–45.

Bent, Michael J. "Research in the School of Medicine." *Bulletin of Meharry Medical College* 36: 2 (October 1939): 9–10.

"Biography of a Nursing School." *Bulletin of Meharry Medical College* 58: 2 (August 1962): 1–6.

Bolden, Theodore E. "A Study of the Oral Health Status of a Selected Number of Students at Meigs, Ford Green, and Pearl Elementary Schools." *The Meharri-dent* 4: 6 (June 1947): 7–11.

Broadus, Clyde Richard. "Dental Health as a Community Health Problem." *The Meharri-dent* 5: 1 (January 1948): 5.

Brown, Murray C. "The Regional Plan." *Meharry Medical College Faculty Bulletin* 4: 2 (April 1949): 4.

Bureau of Educational Research, Howard University. "The Health Status and Health Education of Negroes in the United States." *Journal of Negro Education* 6: 3 (1937): 263–349.

"C. O. Dummett Named Dean of Meharry School of Dentistry." *National Negro Health News* 15: 4 (1947): 18.

"C & Y Center Holds Open House May 12." Meharry Medical College *Intercom* 3: 2 (March–June 1968): 8.

Callahan, Daniel. "Health and Society: Some Ethical Imperatives." *Daedalus* 106: 1 (Winter 1977): 23–33.

Campbell, Earnest B. "The Matthew Walker Neighborhood Health Center of Meharry Medical College." *Journal of the National Medical Association* 65: 4 (1973): 296–99.

"Cardiovascular Unit Receives Support." *Meharry Medical College Quarterly Digest* 4: 4 (July 1966): 4–6.

Carnegie, M. Elizabeth. "Are Negro Schools of Nursing Needed Today?" *Journal of the National Medical Association* 56: 3 (1964): 230–36.

Carter, Hodding. "He's Doing Something About the Race Problem." *Saturday Evening Post,* February 23, 1946, p. 31.

Carter, James P. "The Maternal and Child Health/Family Planning, Training and Research Center." *Journal of the National Medical Association* 65: 4 (1973): 304–05.

Carter, Lisle C., Jr. "Health and the War on Poverty." *Journal of the National Medical Association* 58: 3 (1966): 173–78.

Cazort, Ralph J. "Meharry's New Approach to Medical Education." *Journal of the National Medical Association* 65: 4 (1973): 283–85.

———. "An Open Letter to Medical School Alumni." *Meharry Medical College Quarterly Digest* 7: 2 (January 1969): 4.

"The 'Center' Becomes a Reality." *Meharry Medical College Quarterly Digest* 7: 1 (October 1968): 11.

"Center for Health Care Research Shows Massive Unmet Needs." *Meharry Today* 4: 2 (February–March 1975): 1.

"Changes in the School of Dentistry Reflect New Approaches in Curriculum and Teaching." *Meharry Today* 3: 4 (May 1974): 4–5.

Chapman, Carlton B. "The Flexner Report." *Daedalus* 103: 1 (1974): 105–17.

Clawson, M. Don. "Changing Patterns in Dental Education at Meharry." *TIC Magazine* [no volume or issue number assigned] (March 1948): 2–7.

Clifford, Maurice C. "Meharry Mission." *Meharry Medical College Quarterly Digest* 4: 4 (July 1966): 14–17.

Cobb, W. Montague. "John Wesley Anderson, M.D., 1861–1947." *Journal of the National Medical Association* 45: 6 (1953): 442–44.

———. "Our Lady Asclepiads." *Journal of the National Medical Association* 60: 2 (1968): 136.

———, and Sampson, Calvin C. "Harold Dadford West, Ph.D., LL.D., F.A.I.C." *Journal of the National Medical Association* 66: 5 (1974): 448–49.

"Community Mental Health Center." Meharry Medical College *Intercom* 5: 3 (September–October 1970): 14.

"Construction Starts on 12-Story Hospital Tower." *Meharry Today* 3: 2 (January 1974): 1–3.

"Convocation Opens 101st Academic Year." *Meharry Today* [no volume or issue number assigned] (Fall 1976): 2–5.

Cooper, Edward S. "Aspects of Medical Education and Research." *Journal of the National Medical Association* 56: 3 (1964): 263–66.

"Cooperation with Fisk University." *Bulletin of Meharry Medical College* 36: 2 (October 1939): 17–18.

Cornely, Paul B. "The Economics of Medical Practice and the Negro Physician." *Journal of the National Medical Association* 43: 2 (1951): 84–92.

———. "Post Graduate Medical Education and the Negro Physician." *Journal of the National Medical Association* 30: 1 (1958): 18–22.

Crosby, Edwin L. "The Hospital Administrator." *Modern Hospital* 71: 2 (1948): 56–58.

Crump, E. Perry, et al. "Participation in a Longitudinal Study of Negro Infants and Children." *Public Health Reports* 75: 1 (1960): 1085.

"Daniel Thomas Rolfe, B.S., M.D., 1902–1968." *Journal of the National Medical Association* 60: 6 (1968): 530–31.

Darley, Ward. "Edward Lewis Turner, M.D." *Journal of the National Medical Association* 35: 3 (1960): 287.

"Dedication, Matthew Walker Health Center of Meharry Medical College." *Meharry Medical College Quarterly Digest* 8: 3 (April 1970): 5–7.

"Dentistry at Meharry." *The Meharri-dent* 2: 1 (March 1943): 4.

"Dentistry at Meharry." *The Meharri-dent* 3: 1 (June 1945): 5–6.

"Dr. C. O. Hadley." *Bulletin of Meharry Medical College* 45: 7 (1949): 18.

"Dr. Charles Victor Roman." *Journal of the National Medical Association* 26: 4 (1934): 172–73.

"Dr. Elam Appointed New President." Meharry Medical College *Intercom* 11: 6 (November–December 1967): 1.

"Dr. Falk Heads N. H. C." Meharry Medical College *Intercom* 11: 5 (September–October 1967): 8.

"Dr. George W. Hubbard Retires." *Journal of the National Medical Association* 13: 1 (1921): 30–31.

"Dr. Harold D. West New President of Meharry." *Journal of the National Medical Association* 44: 4 (1952): 316.

"Dr. Turner Dies." *Journal of the National Medical Association* 52: 3 (1960): 200.

"Dr. William A. Reed, Sr." *Journal of the National Medical Association* 58: 3 (1966): 227.

Dummett, Clifton O. "A Chronology of Significant Events in the Progress of the Negro in American Dentistry." *Bulletin of the National Dental Association* 16: 2 (1958): 48.

———. "Dentistry at Meharry, Present Day and Future Trends in Dental Education." *The Meharri-dent* 2: 3 (September 1943): 4.

Duval, Merlin K. "The Provider, the Government, and the Consumer." *Daedalus* 106: 1 (Winter 1977): 185–92.

Elam, Lloyd C. "Meharry Looks Ahead." *Journal of the National Medical Association* 61: 1 (1969): 40–43.

"Elam New President of Meharry." *Journal of the National Medical Association* 60: 2 (1968): 150–51.

"Enlarged Role of Alumni Association Includes Participation by All Members." *Meharry Today* 3: 2 (January 1974): 9.

"Evolution of an Electronic Era." *Meharry Medical College Quarterly Digest* 8: 1 (October 1969): 6.

Falk, Leslie A. "Changing Concepts in Comprehensive Health Care. Comprehensive Care in Health Programs." *Journal of the National Medical Association* 64: 6 (1972): 471–75.

———. "Community Participation in the Neighborhood Health Center." *Journal of the National Medical Association* 61: 6 (1969): 493–97.

———. "The Matthew Walker Health Center of Meharry Medical College: O.E.O.-Funded Neighborhood Health Center." *Journal of the Tennessee Medical Association* 63: 10 (1970): 849.

———; Page, Benjamin; and Vesper, Walter. "Human Values and Medical Education from the Perspectives of Health Care Delivery." *Journal of Medical Education* 48: 2 (1973): 152–57.

———, and Quaynor-Malm, N.A. "Early Afro-American Medical Education in the United States: The Origins of Meharry Medical College in the Nineteenth Century." *Proceedings of the XXIII Congress of the History of Medicine* (1972), pp. 346–56.

"$50 Million for Program and Campus Development." *Meharry Medical College Quarterly Digest* 6: 4 (July 1968): 1–4.

"Focus: The Patient." *Meharry Medical College Quarterly Digest* 7: 3 (1969): 8.

"George Russell Honored at Cornerstone Laying Ceremony for New Hospital." *Meharry Today* 4: 2 (February–March 1975): 1–2.

"Go for the Honkies." *Newsweek*, April 24, 1967, p. 28.

Goldstein, Marcus M. "Longevity and Health Status of Whites and Non-Whites in the United States." *Journal of the National Medical Association* 46: 2 (1954): 83–104.

"Grants Given to Tennessee Medical Schools." *Journal of the Tennessee Medical Association* 59: 7 (1966): 705.

Greenburg, William. "The First Twenty Years are the Hardest." *Nashville Tennessean Magazine*, September 24, 1967, pp. 18–20.

"Ground Breaking Underway for Basic Sciences Building." *Meharry Today* 3: 1 (November 1973): 1.

Hansen, Axel C. "George W. Hubbard Hospital, 1910–1961." *Journal of the National Medical Association* 54: 1 (1962): 1–12.

"Harold D. West Basic Sciences Number." *Journal of the National Medical Association* 68: 4 (July 1976).

Harris, Pat. "Dr. Edwin Mitchell: Gentleman from the Ghetto." *Nashville Magazine* 7: 3 (1969): 23.

Hillard, George W. "The Cancer Teaching Program at Meharry Medical College, 1949–1950." *Bulletin of Meharry Medical College* 46: 2 (April 1950): 11.

Hines, Ralph H. "The Emerging Concept of Community Health." *Meharry Medical College Quarterly Digest* 5: 2 (January 1967): 1–5.

———, and Coffin, John. "A Meharry Renaissance." *Black Books Bulletin* 3: 2 (1975): 16–22.

"Horace M. Frazier, M.D." *Meharry Medical College Quarterly Digest* 8: 4 (July 1970): 28–29.

Hubbard, G. W. "The Education of Colored Physicians, Dentists, and Pharmacists." *The Christian Educator* 2: 4 (July 1891): 155–62.

Hubbard, John Edward. "Integrating Preventive and Social Medicine in the Medical Curriculum." *New England Journal of Medicine* 251: 13 (1954): 513–19.

Huddleston, J. F., as told to Gail Falk. "The Story of Mound Bayou: Negro Pioneers Turned Forests into Farms." *The Southern Courier,* January 7–8, 1967.

"'Ideal' Approach Developed in Family Practice Residency." Meharry Medical College *Intercom* 4: 1 (1974): 2.

"Interim—October '66–June '68." *Meharry Medical College Quarterly Digest* 6: 3 (April 1968): 3–5.

Jaco, E. Gartly. "Twentieth Century Attitudes Toward Health and Their Effect on Medicine." *New England Journal of Medicine* 269: 1 (1963): 18–22.

Johnson, Charles W. "Meharry's Special Medical and Research Programs." *Journal of the National Medical Association* 65: 4 (1973): 307.

Johnson, Thomas W., et al. "Student Life at Meharry." *Journal of the National Medical Association* 65: 4 (1973): 315–16.

"Julius Augustus McMillan, M.D., 1871–1949." *Journal of the National Medical Association* 48: 5 (1956): 374.

Kass, Leon R. "Regarding the End of Medicine and the Pursuit of Health." *The Public Interest* 40 (Summer 1975): 11–42.

Kenney, John A. "In Memoriam, Dr. John Henry Hale." *Journal of the National Medical Association* 36: 4 (1944): 130–31.

Knowles, John H. "The Responsibility of the Individual." *Daedalus* 106: 1 (Winter 1977): 57–80.

"Kresge Center Programs Provide Services." *Meharry Today* 3: 3 (1974): 10–12.

LaSaine, Thomas A. "Teaching the Social Component of Medical Care at Meharry Medical College." *Journal of the National Medical Association* 32: 6.

———, and Harrison, J. Grace. "Medical Social Seminars." *Bulletin of Meharry Medical College* 35: 3 and 4 (1939): 21–22.

Lee, Peter V. "Reorganization of the Medical Curriculum." *Journal of Medical Education* 36: 12 (1961), part 2: 101–17.

"Les Falk: Giving Birth to a New Department." *Meharry Medical College Quarterly Digest* 6: 3 (April 1968): 10–11.

Logan, Thomas P. "Meharry's New Approach to Dental Education." *Journal of the National Medical Association* 65: 4 (1973): 286–87.

"A Look at the New President." *Meharry Medical College Quarterly Digest* 6: 2 (January 1968): 1–4.

Lyttle, Hulda M. "A School for Negro Nurses." *American Journal of Nursing* 39: 2 (1939): 133–38.

———. "The School of Nursing, 1921–1938." *Bulletin of Meharry Medical College* 34: 3 (1938): 20–22.

MacLeish, A. F. "Gold in a Lead Pot." *Bulletin of Meharry Medical College,* Special Issue 47: 2 (June 1951): 11–17.

"Maternal and Child Health Center Completed." *Meharry Today* 2: 2 (March 1973): 4.

"Maternal and Child Health/Family Planning Center." *Meharry Today* 3: 2 (January 1974): 12–13.

"Maternal and Child Health/Family Planning Center Focuses on Africa." *Meharry Today* [no volume or issue number assigned] (Fall 1976): 14–15.

"Matthew Walker Health Center: Inspiration for Sunflower County." Meharry Medical College *Intercom* 5: 2 (March–June 1970): 8–9.

"Medical Licensure Statistics for 1946." *Journal of the American Medical Association* 134: 3 (1947): 255–90.

"Meharry Aims for Quality Product." *Bulletin of Meharry Medical College,* Alumni Edition 45: 7 (April 1949): 4.

"Meharry Biological Research Fund." *Bulletin of Meharry Medical College,* Alumni Edition 44: 2 (August 1947): 1–2.

"Meharry Centennial Number." *Journal of the National Medical Association* 68: 6 (1976).

"Meharry Gets $4,000,000 Gift for Endowment Fund." *Journal of the National Medical Association* 36: 3 (1944): 102.

"Meharry Holds Centennial Commencement." *Meharry Today,* Special Commencement Issue [no volume or issue number assigned] (1976): 1.

"Meharry Medical College to Offer Graduate Course." *Bulletin of Meharry Medical College* 34: 3 (January 1938): 16–18.

"The Meharry North Nashville Neighborhood Health Center." *Journal of the National Medical Association* 59: 6 (1967): 448.

"Meharry Opens New School of X-Ray Technology." Meharry Medical College *Intercom* 3: 8 (September–October 1968): unpaginated.

"Meharry Purchases Land for Neighborhood Center." Meharry Medical College *Intercom* 11: 6 (November–December 1967): 8.

"Minutes of the Annual Meeting of the Meharry Alumni Association." *Meharry Medical College Quarterly Digest* 5: 4 (July 1967): 6–8.

"Minutes of the Annual Meeting of the Meharry Alumni Association." *Meharry Medical College Quarterly Digest* 6: 4 (July 1968): 12–15.

Mobley, Eugenia L. "The Present Status of the Dental Hygienist." *The Meharridant* 9: 1 (January 1952): 7.

Mullowney, John J. "First Formal Instruction in Dentistry in America." *Journal of the National Medical Association* 28: 4 (1936): 165–68.

———. "The Future of the Negro in Dentistry and What Can Be Done About It." *Journal of the National Medical Association* 30: 1 (1938): 23– 26.

———. "The New Meharry Medical College Plant, Nashville, Tenn." *Journal of the National Medical Association* 22: 3 (1930): 146– 47.

———. "What Future for the Negro Pharmacist?" *Journal of the National Medical Association* 24: 3 (1932): 27– 29.

"M. V. Lynk, M.S., M.D., LL.B." *Journal of the National Medical Association* 33: 1 (1941): 46– 47.

"Nashville Academy of Medicine Admits Three." *Journal of the National Medical Association* 47: 4 (1955): 264.

Nathan, Winfred B. "Health Education in Public Schools." *Journal of Negro Education* 6: 3 (1937): 523– 30.

"Negro Higher and Professional Education in the United States." *Journal of Negro Education* 17: 3 (1948): 221– 426.

"Negro in Florida." *Time* Magazine, January 14, 1952, pp. 71– 72.

Pedodontic Phase of the Child Care Program at Meharry Medical College." *The Meharri-dent* 11: 1 (June 1953): 5.

"The President-Elect" [Dr. Matthew Walker]. *Journal of the National Medical Association* 45: 6 (1953): 446.

"Professional News." *Journal of the National Medical Association* 58: 2 (1966): 141.

"Psychiatry Notes." *Meharry Medical College Quarterly Digest* 3: 3 (April 1965): 2.

Quinland, W. S. "Postgraduate Course in Medicine." *Bulletin of Meharry Medical College* 35: 3 and 4 (January and April 1939): 15– 17.

Raup, Ruth M.; and Williams, Elizabeth A. "Negro Students in Medical Schools in the United States." *Journal of Medical Education* 39: 5 (1964): 444– 50.

"Report of the President of Meharry Medical College, 1938– 39." *Bulletin of Meharry Medical College* 36: 2 (October 1939): 4– 21.

"Robert Wood Johnson Foundation Gives Meharry $5 Million Training Grant." *Meharry Today* 2: 1 (November 1972): 1.

Robinson, Jean Dorsett. "Meharry's Health Care Administration and Planning Program." *Journal of the National Medical Association* 65: 4 (1973): 306.

Rogers, Fred B. "Extending the Horizons of Preventive Medicine." *Journal of the American Medical Association* 190: 9 (1964): 837– 39.

Rolfe, D. T. "The Dean Reports." *Meharry Medical College Quarterly Digest* [no volume or issue number assigned] (January 1963): unpaginated.

"Rolfe New Dean of Meharry." *Journal of the National Medical Association* 44: 5 (1952): 395.

Sanders, Robert C. "Blueprint for an Active Alumni Association." *Meharry Medical College Quarterly Digest* 6: 1 (October 1967): 1.

Sanford, R. F. "A Tribute to Our Late Donley H. Turpin, Dean Emeritus of the School of Dentistry, Meharry Medical College." *The Meharri-dent* 5: 3 (June 1948): 2– 3.

Saveth, Edward N. "Jim Crow and the Regional Plan." *The Survey* 85: 9 (1949): 477.

Scales, James L. "Dental Public Health Program at Meharry Medical College." *The Meharri-dent* 4: 3 (June 1946): 5.

Silver, George A. "The Hospital and Social Medicine." *New England Journal of Medicine* 269: 10 (1963): 504– 08.

Smith, T. Manuel. "The Pioneering Influence of Dr. George W. Hubbard on Medical Education." *Journal of the National Medical Association* 45: 6 (1953): 427–29.

Somers, Anne Ramsay. "Conflict, Accommodation, and Progress: Some Socio-Economic Observations on Medical Education and the Practicing Profession." *Journal of Medical Education* 38: 6 (1963): 466–78.

Srouji, Jacque. "Meharry: Excellence on a Shoestring." *Nashville Magazine* 6: 6 (1968): 11–16.

"Talent Recruitment Number." *Journal of the National Medical Association* 57: 6 (1965).

Tandy, Elizabeth C. "Infant and Maternal Mortality Among Negroes." *Journal of Negro Education* 6: 3 (1937): 322–49.

Taylor, Willie. "Meharry Mental Health Center: Reaching Out to the Aged." Meharry Medical College *Breakthrough* 4: 1 (Winter 1976): 7–10.

"Tennessee Rebels." *New Republic,* September 9, 1967, pp. 9–10.

Terris, Milton. "The Future Growth of Departments of Preventive Medicine." *Archives of Environmental Health* 6: 4 (1963): 456–57.

Tomes, Henry. "Meharry's Community Mental Health Center." *Journal of the National Medical Association* 65: 4 (1973): 300–03.

Traherne, Carl A. "Meharry's Comprehensive Health Center." *Journal of the National Medical Association* 65: 4 (1973): 290–92.

"A Trip Through Multiphasic." *Meharry Medical College Quarterly Digest* 8: 5 (October 1970): 14–15.

Turner, Edward L. "The Meharry Medical College School of Dentistry." *TIC Magazine* [no volume or issue number assigned] (September 1950): 1–3.

———. "Selecting Medical Students and Elimination of Misfits." *Journal of the National Medical Association* 36: 1 (1944): 15–19.

Turpin, Donley H. "The Progress of the Dental Department." *Bulletin of Meharry Medical College* 35: 3 and 4 (1939): 13–15.

———. "Report of the School of Dentistry." *Bulletin of Meharry Medical College* 36: 2 (1939): 11–12.

Unger, W. Byers. "Preprofessional Courses for Medical Students and Criteria for Admission to Medical School." *Journal of the National Medical Association* 48: 3 (1956): 165–66.

Utley, Clarence. "The History of Dental Technology." *The Meharri-dent* 7: 1 (January 1950): 5.

Walker, Matthew. "The Affiliation of Taborian Hospital with Meharry Medical College and Development of the O.E.O. Planning Grant." *Meharry Medical College Quarterly Digest* 4: 3 (April 1966): unpaginated.

———. "Mound Bayou—Meharry's Neighbor." *Journal of the National Medical Association* 65: 4 (1973): 309–12.

———. "Progress Report: The Nashville Community Health Center." *Meharry Medical College Quarterly Digest* 5: 1 (October 1966): 14–16.

Weinerman, E. Richard, and Steiger, William A. "Ambulatory Service in the Teaching Hospital." *Journal of Medical Education* 39: 11 (1964): 1020–29.

West, Harold D. "Inaugural Address." *Journal of the National Medical Association* 45: 1 (1953): 17–20.

———. "Regional Education Becomes a Reality." *Bulletin of Meharry Medical College.* Special Issue 47: 2 (June 1951): 5–10.

White, Emma L. "Report of the Proposed Grading System at Meharry Medical College, 1939–1940." *Journal of the National Medical Association* 33: 1 (1941): 42–45.

Wiggins, Walter S., et al. "Medical Education in the United States." *Journal of the American Medical Association* 178: 6 (1961): 579–652.

Willard, William R. "The Development of the Medical School as a Community Resource." *Journal of Public Health* 54: 7 (1964): 1042–45.

———. "The Widening Gap Between Two Extreme Groups of Medical Schools." *Journal of the American Medical Association* 185: 5 (1963): 367–70.

Williams, Daniel Hale. "Stab Wound of the Heart and Pericardium—Suture of the Pericardium—Recovery—Patient Alive Three Years Afterward." *Medical Record* 51: 13 (1897): 437–39.

Williams, E. Y. "The Incidence of Mental Disease in the Negro." *Journal of Negro Education* 6: 3 (1937): 377–92.

Wolf, George A., Jr. "The Financing of Medical Education." *New England Journal of Medicine* 269: 3 (1963): 132–37.

Wolf, Stewart G., Jr., and Darley, Ward, eds. "Medical Education and Practice: Relationships and Responsibilities in a Changing Society." *Journal of Medical Education* 40: 1 (1965) part 2: 16.

Wolfe, Samuel. "The Meharry Medical College Center for Health Care Research." *Journal of the National Medical Association* 65: 4 (1973): 293–95.

Books and Pamphlets

Anderson, Elizabeth J.; Judd, Leda R.; May, Jude Thomas; and New, Peter K. *The Neighborhood Health Center, Its Growth and Problems: An Introduction.* Washington, D.C.: National Association of Neighborhood Health Centers, 1976.

Association of Teachers of Preventive Medicine. Committee on Medical Care Teaching. *Readings in Medical Care.* Chapel Hill: University of North Carolina Press, 1958.

Baines, W. C. "The Pharmaceutical Department." In Charles Victor Roman, *Meharry Medical College, A History.* Nashville: Sunday School Publishing Board of the National Baptist Convention, 1934.

Beguesse, E. C. "An Incumbent Speaks." In *The Meharrian* (yearbook) 1951: unpaginated.

Bent, Michael J., and Greene, Ellen F. *Rural Negro Health: A Report on a Five Year Experiment in Health Education in Tennessee.* Nashville: Julius Rosenwald Fund, 1937.

Bolden, Theodore E., ed. *Research Activities, School of Dentistry, Meharry Medical College.* Nashville: School of Dentistry, 1966.

Braden, Mary E. *John Braden, A Pioneer in Negro Education.* Morristown, Tenn.: the author, 1935.

Brawley, James P. *Two Centuries of Methodist Concern: Bondage, Freedom, and Education of Black People.* New York: Vantage Press, 1974.

Brown, Mary Lee. "Retrospect: Public Health Nursing." In *The Meharrian* (yearbook) 1951: unpaginated.

Bucke, Emory Stevens, ed. *The History of American Methodism.* New York: Abingdon Press, 1964.

Buckler, Helen. *Daniel Hale Williams, Negro Surgeon.* New York: Pitman Co., 1968.

Burt, Jesse C. *Nashville, Its Life and Times.* Nashville: Tennessee Book Co., 1959.

Cassel, John M. "Potentialities and Limitations of Epidemiology." In Alfred H. Katz and Jean S. Felton, eds., *Health and the Community.* New York: Free Press, 1965.

Center for Health Care Research. *Report of the Center for Health Care Research of Meharry Medical College for July 1, 1969 to June 30, 1971.* Nashville: the Center, 1971.

Central Tennessee College. *Biographical Sketch and Memorial of Reverend John Braden, D.D.* Nashville: Central Tennessee College, 1900.

Clark Memorial Methodist Church. *A Century of Witness for Christ, 1867–1967.* Nashville: the Church, 1967.

Clayton, W. Woodford. *History of Davidson County, Tennessee.* Philadelphia: J. W. Lewis and Co., 1880; reprinted, Nashville: Charles Elder and Son, 1971.

Committee on Research. *Horizon in Research, Progress Report, The Development of Negro Talent, 1947–48.* Nashville: Meharry Medical College, 1948.

Consultant Group on Medical Education. *Physicians for a Growing America.* Washington, D.C.: U.S. Public Health Service, 1959.

Cope, Oliver. "The Endicott House Conference on Medical Education." In John Knowles, ed., *Views of Medical Education and Medical Care.* Cambridge: Harvard University Press, 1968.

———, and Zacharias, Jerrold, eds. *Medical Education Reconsidered: Report of the Endicott House Summer Study on Medical Education, July 1965.* Philadelphia: Lippincott, 1966.

Crichlow, Cyril A. "The Last of His Generation." In *The Brown Book.* [Fragment in the George W. Hubbard file, United Methodist Publishing House Library, Nashville. No other information available.]

Crichton, Michael. *Five Patients.* New York: Knopf, 1970.

Crump, E. Perry. "Retrospect: Pediatrics." In *The Meharrian* (yearbook) 1951: unpaginated.

———, and Bent, Michael J. "The New Horizon." In *The Meharrian* (yearbook) 1949: unpaginated.

Culp, D. W., ed. *Twentieth Century Negro Literature.* Naperville, Ill.: J. L. Nichols, 1902.

Department of Social Science, Fisk University. *A Social Study of Negro Families in the Area Selected for the Nashville Negro Federal Housing Project with a Supplementary Study of the Social and Economic Status of the Negro in Nashville.* Nashville: Fisk University Press, 1934.

Donald, Henderson H. *The Negro Freedman.* New York: H. Schuman, 1952.

Elam, Lloyd C., et al. "Health Evaluation Studies Utilizing a Multiphasic Screening Center Operating in Cooperation with a Comprehensive Health Care Program for Persons in an Urban Poverty Area." In *Proceedings: Conference Workshop on Regional Medical Programs.* Washington, D.C.: U.S. Public Health Service, 1968.

"Faculty Biography" [William H. Allen]. *The Meharri-dent* 6: 2 (March 1949): 29–30.

Fleming, G. James, and Burckel, Christian E., eds. *Who's Who in Colored America.* Yonkers-on-Hudson, N.Y.: Christian E. Burckel and Associates, 1950.

Flexner, Abraham. *Medical Education in the United States and Canada, A Report to the Carnegie Foundation for the Advancement of Teaching.* New York: Carnegie Foundation, 1910.

Folmsbee, Stanley J.; Mitchell, Enoch; and Corlew, Robert. *Tennessee: A Short History.* Knoxville: University of Tennessee Press, 1969.

Freedmen's Aid Society. *Reports of the Freedmen's Aid Society of the Methodist Episcopal Church, 1866–1875.* Cincinnati: Western Methodist Book Concern, 1893.

———. *Report of the Freedmen's Aid Society for 1888.* Cincinnati: the Society, 1893.

Galdston, Iago. *The Meaning of Social Medicine.* Cambridge: Harvard University Press, 1954.

———. *Medicine in Transition.* Chicago: University of Chicago Press, 1965.

General Education Board. *Annual Report, 1944.* New York: the Board, 1944.

Gibson, J. W., and Crogman, W. H. *Progress of a Race or, The Remarkable Achievement of the American Negro.* Rev. ed. Naperville, Ill.: J. L. Nichols, 1902.

Ginzberg, Eli. *The Limits of Health Reform, The Search for Realism.* New York: Basic Books, 1977.

Graham, Hugh Davis. *Crisis in Print: Desegregation and the Press in Tennessee.* Nashville: Vanderbilt University Press, 1967.

Haley, James T., comp. *Afro-American Encyclopedia or, the Thoughts, Doings, and Sayings of the Race.* Nashville: Haley and Florida, 1896.

Hines, Ralph H. *The Health Status of Negroes in a Mid-Southern Urban Community.* Two parts. Nashville: Meharry Medical College, 1967.

Holloway, Guerney D. "School of Clinical Laboratory Technology." In *The Meharrian* (yearbook) 1949: unpaginated.

Howard, Oliver Otis. *Autobiography.* 2 vols. New York: Baker and Taylor Co., 1907.

John F. Kennedy Center for Research on Education and Human Development, George Peabody Center for Community Studies. *The Characteristics of the Population and the Social Services for a High Poverty Area in Nashville, Tennessee.* Nashville: the Kennedy Center, 1967.

Johnson, Charles S. *Into the Main Stream, A Survey of the Best Practices in Race Relations in the South.* Chapel Hill: University of North Carolina Press, 1947.

"Justification for Development of Graduate Programs at Meharry Medical College." In *The Graduate School Manual.* Nashville: Meharry Medical College, 1972.

Kenney, John A. *The Negro in Medicine.* Tuskegee, Ala.: Tuskegee Institute Press, 1912.

Lamon, Lester C. *Black Tennesseans, 1900–1930.* Knoxville: University of Tennessee Press, 1977.

Lee, Roger I., and Jones, Lewis W. *The Fundamentals of Good Medical Care.* Chicago: University of Chicago Press, 1933.

Lipman, Eugene J., and Vorspan, Albert, eds. *A Tale of Ten Cities.* New York: Union of American Hebrew Congregations, 1962.

Lloyd, R. Grann. *Tennessee Agricultural and Industrial State University, 1912–1962.* Nashville: Tennessee A & I State University, 1962.

Lynk, Miles V. *Sixty Years of Medicine; An Autobiography.* Memphis, Tenn.: Twentieth Century Press, 1951.

Lyttle, Hulda M. "The Nurse Training Department." In Charles Victor Roman, *Meharry Medical College, A History.* Nashville: Sunday School Publishing Board of the National Baptist Convention, 1934.

McCulloch, James E., ed. *The New Chivalry—Health: Proceedings of the Southern Sociological Congress, Houston, Texas, May 8–11, 1915.* Nashville: Southern Sociological Congress, 1915.

McGrath, Earl J. *The Predominantly Negro Colleges and Universities in Transition.* New York: Teachers College, Columbia University, 1965.

Meharry, Frances. *History of the Meharry Family.* Lafayette, Ind.: Lafayette Printing Co., 1925.

The Meharrian (yearbook) 1945, 1951, 1960.

Meharry Medical College. *Ambulatory Services.* Nashville: the College, 1970(?).

————. *The George Russell Tower, Meharry Medical College, Tribute and Cornerstone Ceremony. Nashville, Tennessee, November 22, 1974.* Nashville: the College, 1974.

————. *The President's Report, Meharry Medical College.* Nashville: the College, 1971.

————. *President's Report, 1975–1976, Centennial Edition.* Nashville: the College, 1976.

————. *Meharry Medical College: A Report.* Nashville: the College, 1970.

————. [Annual] *Report of the President, Meharry Medical College, June, 1969.* Nashville: the College, 1969.

————. *Report to the Nation, 1967–1972.* Nashville: the College, 1972.

————. *The Centennial Lecture Series, January–December, 1976.* Nashville: the College, 1976.

————. *Meharry Annual and Military Review.* Nashville: the College, 1919.

————. *Meharry Medical College, 1876–1941.* Nashville: the College, 1941.

————. *New Developmental Programs: Summary of Proposals.* Nashville: the College, May 1967.

————. *Opening New Doors to Greatness with Meharry Medical College.* Nashville: the College, 1969(?).

Meharry Medical Department, Central Tennessee College. *Proceedings* [of the Commencement of 1878]. Nashville: the Department, 1878.

"Meharry Medical Society." In *The Meharrian* (yearbook) 1943: unpaginated.

Mercer, Charles V., and Newbrough, J. R. *The North Nashville Health Study: Research into the Culture of the Deprived.* Nashville: the Kennedy Center, 1967.

Merriam, Lucius Salisbury. *Higher Education in Tennessee.* Washington, D.C.: Government Printing Office, 1893.

Morais, Herbert M. *The History of the Negro in Medicine.* New York: Publishers Co., 1967.

Mullowney, John J. *America Gives a Chance.* Tampa, Fla.: The Tribune Press, 1940.

Myrdal, Gunnar S. *An American Dilemma.* 2 vols. New York: Harper and Brothers, 1944.

National Health Assembly. *America's Health*. New York: Harper and Brothers, 1949.

Neser, William B. *Quality Standards of Care in Alternative Health Care Systems*. Nashville: Meharry Medical College, 1975.

Nichols, J. L., and Crogman, W. H. *Progress of a Race or, The Remarkable Achievement of the American Negro*. Rev. ed. Naperville, Ill.: J. L. Nichols, 1920.

Patterson, Caleb. *The Negro in Tennessee, 1790–1865*. Austin: University of Texas Press, 1922.

Patterson, James R., comp. *Souvenir History, 1924 Dental Class, Meharry Medical College, 20th Anniversary Reunion at Meharry, Friday, March 17, 1944*. Nashville: the College, 1944.

Perry, J. Edward. *Forty Cords of Wood; Memoirs of a Medical Doctor*. Jefferson City, Mo.: Lincoln University, 1947.

Rabinowitz, Howard N. *Race Relations in the Urban South, 1865–1890*. New York: Oxford University Press, 1978.

Reitzes, Dietrich C. *Negroes and Medicine*. Cambridge: Harvard University Press, 1958.

"Research." In *The Meharrian* (yearbook) 1949: unpaginated.

"Retrospect: Biochemistry." In *The Meharrian* (yearbook) 1951: unpaginated.

Richardson, Joe M. *A History of Fisk University, 1865–1946*. University, Ala.: University of Alabama Press, 1980.

Richings, G. F. *Evidences of Progress Among Colored People*. Philadelphia: G. S. Ferguson Co., 1903.

Röbert, Charles. *Nashville and Her Trade for 1870*. Nashville: Roberts and Purvis, 1870.

Roberts, F. L. *Yearbook of the Sixty-second Session of the West Wisconsin Conference of the Methodist Episcopal Church*. Eau Claire: the Conference, 1916.

Roman, Charles Victor. *Meharry Medical College, A History*. Nashville: Sunday School Publishing Board of the National Baptist Convention, 1934.

"School of Dentistry: A Turning Point." In Meharry Medical College, *Annual Report, 1971–1972: Another Year, Another Step Forward*. Nashville: the College, 1972.

Shaw, J. Beverly. *The Negro in the History of Methodism*. Nashville: Parthenon Press, 1954.

Shryock, Richard Harrison. *The Development of Modern Medicine*. New York: Knopf, 1947.

Sibley, Elbridge. *Differential Mortality in Tennessee, 1917–1928*. Nashville: Fisk University Press, 1930.

Sigerist, Henry E. "Medical Care for All the People." In Henry Sigerist, *On the Sociology of Medicine*. Edited by Milton I. Roemer. New York: MD Publications, 1960.

Smith, Kemper Harreld. *The Mission of Tabor*. Mound Bayou, Miss.: Knights and Daughters of Tabor, 1963.

Somers, Herman Miles, and Somers, Anne Ramsay. *Doctors, Patients, and Health Insurance*. Washington, D.C.: Brookings Institution, 1961.

Stubblefield, D. R. *In Memoriam, Dr. William H. Morgan.* Nashville: n.p., 1901(?).

Sugg, Redding S., Jr., and Jones, George Hilton. *The Southern Regional Education Board: Ten Years of Regional Cooperation in Higher Education.* Baton Rouge: Louisiana State University Press, 1960.

Swint, Henry Lee. *The Northern Teacher in the South, 1862–1870.* Nashville: Vanderbilt University Press, 1941.

Taylor, Alrutheus Ambush. *The Negro in Tennessee, 1865–1880.* Washington, D.C.: Associated Publishers, 1941.

Tennessee Mid-South Regional Medical Program. *Continuation Application and Progress Report.* Nashville: Regional Medical Program, 1968.

Turpin, D. H. "The Dental Department." In Charles Victor Roman, *Meharry Medical College, A History.* Nashville: Sunday School Publishing Board of the National Baptist Convention, 1934.

Vahaly, John, Jr., and Walter, Benjamin. "Black Residential Succession in Nashville, 1930 to 1960." In James F. Blumstein and Benjamin Walter, eds., *Growing Metropolis, Aspects of Development in Nashville.* Nashville: Vanderbilt University Press, 1975.

Walker, Helen Edith. *The Negro in the Medical Profession.* Charlottesville: University of Virginia, 1949.

Waller, William, ed. *Nashville in the 1890s.* Nashville: Vanderbilt University Press, 1970.

Walter, Benjamin. "Ethnicity and Residential Succession: Nashville, 1850–1920." In James F. Blumstein and Benjamin Walter, eds., *Growing Metropolis, Aspects of Development in Nashville.* Nashville: Vanderbilt University Press, 1975.

Washington, Booker T.; Wood, N. B.; and Williams, Fannie Barrier. *A New Negro for a New Century.* Chicago: American Publishing House, 1900.

Wharton, Vernon Lane. *The Negro in Mississippi, 1865–1890.* Chapel Hill: University of North Carolina Press, 1947.

Work, Monroe N., ed. *Negro Year Book, 1918–1919.* Tuskegee, Ala.: Tuskegee Institute, 1919.

Miscellaneous College Publications

Bulletin of Meharry Medical College 35: 2 (October 1938): 31.

———, Alumni Edition 41: 1C (December 1941): 2.

———, Alumni Edition 39: 4 (April 1943): 9.

———, Alumni Edition 43: 5 (February 1947): 4.

———, Alumni Edition 44: 2 (August 1947): 3.

———, Alumni Edition 44: 6 (April 1948): 2, 4.

———, Catalog Edition 46: 4 (December 1950): 45.

———, Special Issue 47: 2 (June 1951): 18.

———, Alumni Edition 48: 2 (April 1952): 2, 3, 5.

———, Catalog Edition for the School of Medicine 50: 4 (December 1954): 26, 31, 46–81.

———, Catalog Edition for the School of Dentistry 53: 3 (September 1957): 38–50, 57–59.

————, Catalog Edition for the School of Medicine 55: 4 (December 1959): 53–88.

————. Catalog Edition for the School of Medicine [no volume or issue number assigned] (June 1965): 51–83.

————, 80th Anniversary Issue 52: 2 (April 1956): 11, 17.

Catalog of the Meharry Medical, Dental, and Pharmaceutical Departments, 1886–87, p. 5.

Catalog of the Meharry Medical Department, Central Tennessee College, 1887, pp. 2, 5, 6.

Catalogue of the Meharry Medical, Dental, and Pharmaceutical Departments, 1892–93, p. 2.

Catalog of the Meharry Medical, Dental, and Pharmaceutical Departments, 1893–94, p. 6.

Catalogue of the Meharry Medical, Dental, and Pharmaceutical Departments, Central Tennessee College, 1899–1900, pp. 4, 7–11.

Catalogue of the Meharry Medical, Dental, and Pharmaceutical Colleges, Walden University, 1900–1901, pp. 4, 11.

First Annual Announcement of the School of Dentistry, Meharry Medical Department of Central Tennessee College, 1886–87, p. 2.

Hubbard Hospital *Newsletter* I: 2 (January 26, 1951): unpaginated.

The Meharri-dent 7: 1 (January 1950): 3.

————. 8: 1 (January 1951): 7.

Meharry-Hubbard Newsletter 2: 12 (June 15, 1952): 2.

————. 2: 14 (July 15, 1952): 1.

————. 2: 24 (December 15, 1952): 1.

————. 3: 8 (April 15, 1953): 3.

Meharry Medical College Faculty Bulletin 46: 2 (April 1950): 14.

Meharry Medical College, Self-Study Office. *Introspect: Self-Study News* 1: 8 (November 1975): 5.

Meharry Medical College Quarterly Digest 1: 4 (October 1963): 4.

———— 7: 2 (January 1969): 2.

———— 8: 1 (October 1969): 3.

Meharry News, Catalogue Edition 28: 1 (July 1931): 10–15.

————, Catalogue Edition 33: 1 (July 1936): 41–46, 107–09.

———— 33: 2 (October 1936): 6.

Sixth Annual Announcement of the Meharry Medical Department, Central Tennessee College, 1881, p. 3.

Index